LIVINGSTONE

n 1994.

0-091-X C3047

e your order by contacting your local medical bookseller or in the United States
Livingstone Fulfillment Centre, 5 S 250 Frontenac Road, Naperville, IL 60563-
08) 416-3939; Fax: (708) 983-5576.
Longman Group UK Ltd., PO Box 88, Harlow, Essex, UK CM19 5SR;
-623925; Fax: +44-279-453450.

ngapore by Longman Singapore Publishers (Pte) Limited

Communications Japan, Churchill Livingstone Japan K.K. 1994
e: K.I.T. Bldg., 2-8-16 Yutenji, Meguro-ku, Tokyo 153, Japan
e: 7F., Manabe-Doshomachi Bldg., 1-4-6 Doshomachi, Chuo-ku, Osaka 541, Japan

RECENT ADVANCES IN

Endothelial C
Dysfunction i

Edited by

George L. King MD
Associate Professor
Department of Medicine
Brigham and Women's Hospital
and Harvard Medical School
Boston, USA

Yukio Shigeta MD PhD
Professor
Third Department of Medicine
Shiga University of Medical Science
Shiga, Japan

CHURCHILL LIVING
OSAKA TOKYO EDINBURGH LO
MELBOURNE MILAN AND N

CHURCHIL

Published by

English edit

ISBN 4-893

You can pla
to Churchil
1711; Tel:
For ROW
Tel: +44-2

Printed in

Contents

SECTION 1: METABOLISM AND EFFECTS OF HYPERGLYCAEMIA

1. Glucose metabolism in endothelial cells 3
   A. Kashiwagi, Y. Shigeta

2. Prostaglandin metabolism in endothelial cells 17
   F. Umeda, M. Kunisaki, T. Hashimoto, H. Nawata

3. Abnormal antithrombogenic function on endothelial cells in diabetes mellitus 33
   K. Oida, H. Maeda, T. Nakai

SECTION 2: NEW APPROACH OF PATHOGENESIS OF DIABETIC VASCULAR COMPLICATIONS

4. Protein kinase C activation in the pathogenesis of diabetic vascular complications 57
   T. Inoguchi, F. Umeda, H. Nawata, G. L. King

5. Regulation of gene expression in vascular cells by glucose and its relationship to diabetic vascular complications 73
   Y. Nishio, G. L. King

6. Specific gene transfection and expression in cultured human endothelial cell 89
   Y. Mitsui, N. Ishida, M. Kondo, M. Matsui

SECTION 3: DYSREGULATION OF VASOMOTOR TONE

7. Endothelium-dependent and -independent vasodilator action of insulin: implications for the role of insulin in vasomotor tone regulation 105
   Y. Ouchi, S.-Z. Han, H. Orimo

8. Endothelium-derived nitric oxide and atherosclerosis 117
K. Hirata, S. Kawashima, M. Yokoyama

9. Endothelial dysfunction in diabetes: role of endothelium-derived relaxing factor 133
T. Taminato, S. Sen, H. Kato, G. Sarwar

SECTION 4: ACCELERATED ATHEROGENESIS

10. A possible mechanism for vascular endothelial cell injury elicited by activated leucocytes: a significant involvement of adhesion molecules, CD11/CD18 and ICAM-1 145
H. Fujita, I. Morita, S. Murota

11. Interaction between endothelial cells and smooth muscle cells through platelet-derived growth factor: direct effects and phenotypic modulation 159
N. Morisaki Y. Saito

12. Regulation of proteoglycans in endothelial cells: implication for atherogenesis and thrombogenesis 173
M. Nishinaga, M. Kobayashi, K. Shimada

13. Modulation of endothelial cell function by glycated proteins 189
H. Takeda, E. Yamaguchi, T. Nishikawa, S. Kobori, M. Shichiri

SECTION 5: ACCELERATED PERMEABILITY AND ANGIOGENESIS

14. Abnormal endothelial cell permeability in diabetes 201
O. Tokunaga, J. L. Fan, T. Yamada

15. Angiogenesis in diabetes 215
H. Ito

16. Transforming growth factor-β: interaction of endothelial cells and pericytes/smooth muscle cells 231
Y. Sato

17. Inhibition of vascular endothelial cell proliferation by the protein kinase C pathway: a possible mechanism underlying the pathogenesis of diabetic vascular complications 245
T. Sasaguri, C. Kosaka

18. Role of insulin-like growth factor-I in proliferative diabetic retinopathy: a modulator of free radical-derived oxidant generation 265
M. B. Grant, E. A. Ellis, S. Caballero

Foreward

The 1st Meeting on Studies of Diabetes Mellitus and Endothelial Cell Dysfunction was held in Japan in 1990, and since then meetings have been held annually. The four organizing committee members alternate in the supervision and chairing of the meetings. The organizing committee members are:

•Tsugihiko Nakai, Associate Professor, Third Department of Internal Medicine, Fukui Medical School, Fukui, Japan

•Hideki Ito, Head of the Endocrinology Section, Tokyo Metropolitan Geriatric Hospital, Tokyo, Japan

•Fumio Umeda, Associate Professor, Third Department of Internal Medicine, Faculty of Medicine, Kyushu University, Fukuoka, Japan

•Atsunori Kashiwagi, Assistant Professor, Third Department of Medicine, Shiga University of Medical Science, Shiga, Japan

The purpose of these meetings is to clarify endothelial cell dysfunction in diabetes using cell biological and molecular biological investigations from front-line investigators in Japan. We also aim at presenting studies on the mechanisms of vascular dysfunction in diabetes and the development of effective diagnostic and therapeutic methods for these abnormalities. The present publication summarizes the significant presentations from the last four annual meetings supplemented where necessary with any other significant recent advances. We deeply appreciate the contributions from the 24 institutes involved in these meetings and from selected experts from overseas.

Acknowledgement

The organizing committee would like to thank Otsuka Pharmaceutical Co., Ltd. for providing an educational grant for the publication of 'Recent Advances in Endothelial Cell Dysfunction in Diabetes'.

Preface

Vascular complications are the major cause of mortality and morbidity in diabetic patients, involving large arteries as well as microvessels. The pathologies are quite diverse, depending on the vascular tissues involved. In general, some of the vascular pathologies are unique to diabetes, such as loss of pericytes in the retina and nodular mesangial enlargement in the renal glomeruli. On the other hand, many of the pathologies are quite similar to those found in other vascular diseases involving the nondiabetic population, such as in the large vessels where the pathology is very similar to atherosclerosis. Furthermore, not all diabetic patients will have all the vascular diseases, both in type or severity.

These findings have provided us with the clue that vascular pathologies in diabetic patients are probably the result of a combination of metabolic and genetic factors. Some of these causal factors are unique to diabetes, such as hyperglycaemia and abnormal insulin levels, as well as factors which may be in common with other diseases, such as hyperlipidaemia. Central to the pathology of vascular disease is the endothelial cells, which line the blood vessels and provide a host of functions that enable the body to survive. They involve the distribution of nutrients, anticoagulation, regulation of blood flow and providing communication between organs. Not surprisingly in diabetes, abnormalities have been found in all these properties. However, it is surprising that detailed studies of abnormality caused by diabetes and its metabolic changes in vascular endothelial cell metabolism and function have been a relatively recent phenomenon.

Over the last few years a great deal of new knowledge has been gathered on this subject and much of it is summarized in this book. The areas covered in the various chapters are critical to the functions of endothelial cells, such as in the metabolism of prostaglandins, which has been a hot topic with regard to abnormalities in diabetes, as well as the metabolism of glucose by vascular cells. This aspect has gained a great deal of importance recently due to the results of the Diabetes Control and Complications Trial, which documented that glucose control can prevent vascular complications, therefore identifying hyperglycaemia as being a primary pathogenic factor for vascular complications. Abnormalities in anticoagulation have also been described in diabetes. Therefore, this area is also described. Another important function of endothelial cells is in the area of haemodynamics, where numerous abnormalities have been found. This area will also be described in relation to exciting findings on the role of nitric oxide. With regard to interaction between various vascular cells and leucocytes, information on this rapidly advancing area is not well known with regard to diabetes, but needs to be further studied. Lastly is the area of growth factors, which are involved in the repair and growth of the various vascular cells. This is a very important topic due to the fact that, in diabetes, abnormality of endothelial cell proliferation is easily found in diabetic proliferative retinopathy and is involved in the inhibition of vascular cells, such as pericytes and arterial endothelial cells. There are several chapters on the various growth factors possibly involved in diabetic complications. This monograph therefore brings together a series of topics which highlight the rapid advances not only in vascular cell biology but also in the understanding of pathogenesis of diabetic vascular complications.

Boston, USA
Shiga, Japan
1994

G. L. K.
Y. S.

Contributors

Sergio Caballero MD
Division of Endocrinology and Metabolism, Department of Medicine, University of Florida, Gainesville, USA

E. Ann Ellis MD
Division of Endocrinology and Metabolism, Department of Medicine, University of Florida, Gainesville, USA

Jiang Lin Fan MD PhD
Department of Pathology, Saga Medical School, Saga, Japan

Hiroshi Fujita MD PhD
Department of Physiological Chemistry, Graduate School, Tokyo Medical and Dental University, Tokyo, Japan

Maria B. Grant MD
Division of Endocrinology and Metabolism, Department of Medicine, University of Florida, Gainesville, USA

Shu-zhong Han MD PhD
Department of Geriatrics, Faculty of Medicine, University of Tokyo, Tokyo, Japan

Toshihiko Hashimoto MD PhD
Third Department of Internal Medicine, Faculty of Medicine, Kyushu University, Fukuoka, Kyushu, Japan

Ken-ichi Hirata MD
First Department of Internal Medicine, Kobe University School of Medicine, Kobe, Japan

Toyoshi Inoguchi MD PhD
Saiseikai Fukuoka General Hospital, Fukuoka, Japan

Norio Ishida PhD
National Institute of Bioscience & Human Technology, Tsukuba, Ibaraki, Japan

Hideki Ito MD
Endocrinology Section, Tokyo Metropolitan Geriatric Hospital, Tokyo, Japan

Atsunori Kashiwagi MD PhD
Third Department of Medicine, Shiga University of Medical Science, Shiga, Japan

Hiroko Kato MD
The Second Division, Department of Medicine, Hamamatsu University of Medicine, Hamamatsu, Japan

Seinosuke Kawashima MD
First Department of Internal Medicine, Kobe University School of Medicine, Kobe, Japan

George L. King MD
Research Division, Joslin Diabetes Center, Department of Medicine, Brigham and Women's Hospital, Harvard Medical School, Boston, USA

Masashi Kobayashi MD
Department of Hematology, Jichi Medical School, Kawachigun, Tochigi, Japan

Shozo Kobori MD
Department of Metabolic Medicine, Kumamoto University School of Medicine, Kumamoto, Japan

Masaaki Kondo
National Institute of Bioscience & Human Technology, Tsukuba, Ibaraki, Japan

Chiya Kosaka MD
National Cardiovascular Center Research Institute, Osaka, Japan

Makoto Kunisaki MD PhD
Third Department of Internal Medicine, Faculty of Medicine, Kyushu University, Fukuoka, Japan

Hajime Maeda MD PhD
Third Department of Internal Medicine, Fukui Medical School, Fukui, Japan

Miwa Matsui
National Institute of Bioscience & Human Technology, Tsukuba, Ibaraki, Japan

Youji Mitsui PhD
National Institute of Bioscience & Human Technology, Tsukuba, Ibaraki, Japan

Nobuhiro Morisaki MD PhD
Second Department of Internal Medicine, School of Medicine, Chiba University, Chiba, Japan

Ikuo Morita PhD
Department of Physiological Chemistry, Graduate School, Tokyo Medical and Dental University, Tokyo, Japan

Sei-itsu Murota MD PhD
Department of Physiological Chemistry, Graduate School, Tokyo Medical and Dental University, Tokyo, Japan

Tsuguhiko Nakai MD PhD
Third Department of Internal Medicine, Fukui Medical School, Fukui, Japan

Hajime Nawata MD PhD
Third Department of Internal Medicine, Faculty of Medicine, Kyushu University, Fukuoka, Japan

Takeshi Nishikawa MD
Department of Metabolic Medicine, Kumamoto University School of Medicine, Kumamoto, Japan

Mansanori Nishinaga MD
Department of Cardiology, Jichi Medical School, Kawachigun, Tochigi, Japan

Yoshihiko Nishio MD
Research Division, Joslin Diabetes Center, Department of Medicine, Brigham and Women's Hospital, Harvard Medical School, Boston, USA

Koji Oida MD PhD
Third Department of Internal Medicine, Fukui Medical School, Fukui, Japan

Hajime Orimo MD PhD
Department of Geriatrics, Faculty of Medicine, University of Tokyo, Tokyo, Japan

Yasuyoshi Ouchi MD PhD
Department of Geriatrics, Faculty of Medicine, University of Tokyo, Tokyo, Japan

Yasushi Saito MD PhD
Second Department of Internal Medicine, School of Medicine, Chiba University, Chiba, Japan

Gram Sarwar MD
The Second Division, Department of Medicine, Hamamatsu University of Medicine, Hamamatsu, Japan

Toshiyuki Sasaguri MD
National Cardiovascular Center Research Institute, Osaka, Japan

Yasufumi Sato MD PhD
First Department of Internal Medicine, Oita Medical University, Oita, Japan

Seikou Sen MD
The Second Division, Department of Medicinc, Hamamatsu University of Medicine, Hamamatsu, Japan

Motoaki Shichiri MD
Department of Metabolic Medicine, Kumamoto University School of Medicine, Kumamoto, Japan

Yukio Shigeta MD PhD
Third Department of Medicine, Shiga University of Medical Science, Shiga, Japan

Kazuyuki Shimada MD
Department of Cardiology, Jichi Medical School, Kawachigun, Tochigi, Japan

Haruo Takeda MD
Department of Metabolic Medicine, Kumamoto University School of Medicine, Kumamoto, Japan

Tomohiko Taminato MD
The Second Division, Department of Medicine, Hamamatsu University of Medicine, Hamamatsu, Japan

Osamu Tokunaga MD PhD
Department of Pathology, Saga Medical School, Saga, Japan

Fumio Umeda MD PhD
Third Department of Internal Medicine, Faculty of Medicine, Kyushu University, Fukuoka, Japan

Takahiro Yamada MD PhD
Department of Pathology, Saga Medical School, Saga, Japan

Eiji Yamaguchi MD
Department of Metabolic Medicine, Kumamoto University School of Medicine, Kumamoto, Japan

Mitsuhiro Yokoyama MD
First Department of Internal Medicine, Kobe University School of Medicine, Kobe, Japan

SECTION 1

Metabolism and Effects of Hyperglycaemia

1

Glucose metabolism in endothelial cells

A. Kashiwagi, Y. Shigeta

INTRODUCTION

Specific abnormalities of glucose metabolism in endothelial cells may exist in diabetes which are causally related to the pathogenesis of micro- and macrovascular complications (Baynes 1991; Brownlee 1992; Gabbay 1973; Schwartz et al 1992; The Diabetes Control and Complication Trial Research Group 1993). Hyperglycaemia may be a major risk factor for microvascular complications (Engerman et al 1977; The Diabetes Control and Complication Trial Research Group 1993), while hyperinsulinaemia together with hyperglycaemia is thought to be one of the major risk factors for atherosclerosis in diabetes (Kannel & McGee 1979; Pyorala 1979; Schwartz et al 1992; Stout 1991). Studies on the effects of high glucose and/or insulin levels on endothelial cell metabolism may therefore be crucial for understanding the pathogenesis of diabetic vascular complications. However, detailed metabolic characterisation of micro- and macrovascular endothelial cells has not yet been fully achieved (King et al 1983). This article overviews those data which are available concerning a number of aspects of glucose metabolism in cells isolated from various micro- and macrovascular endothelial tissues: 1) characterisation of the glucose transporter; 2) stimulation of glucose metabolism by insulin and other cytokines; 3) activation of the polyol pathway and its metabolic consequences; and 4) oxidative stress and glucose metabolism.

CHARACTERISTICS OF THE GLUCOSE TRANSPORTER IN ENDOTHELIAL CELLS

Recent cloning and sequencing studies of glucose transporters suggest several different isoforms for carrier-mediated diffusion of glucose across the cell membrane (Bell et al 1990). Currently used nomenclature identifies the individual transporters according to the chronology of their discovery as GLUT-1 through to GLUT-5. GLUT-1 (glucose transporter isoform 1) is ubiquitously expressed and has been described as the erythrocyte form; GLUT-2 is specifically expressed in liver and pancreatic β cells, and has been termed the hepatic form; and GLUT-3 is found in brain and foetal skeletal muscle (Kayano et al 1988; Mueckler et al 1985; Oka et al 1988; Thorens et al 1988). GLUT-4 is selectively expressed in muscle and fat tissues (Birnbaum 1989; Charron et al 1989; Fukumoto et al 1989; James et al 1989) and is highly responsive to acute insulin exposure via redistribution of the transporters from intracellular vesicles to the plasma membrane (Cushman & Wardzala 1980; Suzuki & Kono 1980). GLUT-5 is considered to be a fructose transporter (Bell et al 1990) and Na^+/glucose cotransporter. It is specifically located in intestinal and renal tubular epithelial cells where it functions as an active glucose transporter (Hediger et al 1987).

The GLUT-1 transporter also appears to be insulin responsive in muscle and adipocytes, but to a much lesser extent than the GLUT-4 isoform (Zorzano et al 1989). GLUT-1 is the principal glucose transporter in both rat brain capillary and bovine aortic endothelial cells when assessed using immunogold electron microscopy (Farrell & Pardridge 1991) and Northern blot analysis, whereas GLUT-2, -3, -4 and -5 mRNA cannot be detected by Northern blot analysis in bovine aortic endothelial cells (Kaiser et al 1993). The GLUT-1 mRNA level in bovine aortic endothelial cells is unaffected by insulin in the medium, and the hexose transport system in bovine aortic endothelial cells also shows little or no adaptation to changes in ambient glucose levels (Kaiser et al 1993). The GLUT-4 transporter can be detected in endothelial cells surrounding skeletal muscle (Vilaro et al 1989) and glomerulus (Brosius et al 1993). It would therefore be interesting to know whether GLUT-4 protein is expressed in retinal and glomerular capillary endothelial cells. GLUT-4 transporter can be translocated from intracellular vesicles to plasma membrane through an activation mechanism mediated by insulin (Cushman et al 1980; Suzuki et al 1980).

With regard to the effect of glucose levels on the glucose transport system, glucose transport activity has been measured in cells exposed long-term to low and high glucose concentrations. Takakura et al (1991) have shown that 3-*O*-[^{3}H]-methyl-D-glucose ([^{3}H]-3MG) uptake in cultured bovine brain microvessel endothelial cells can occur via a carrier-mediated diffusion mechanism which is affected by ambient glucose conditions. Preincubation with high concentrations of glucose for 30 min accelerates [^{3}H]-3MG uptake by bovine brain microvessel endothelial cells by a counter-transport mechanism. In contrast, a decrease in the glucose concentration of the medium for 7 days can induce stimulation of glucose transport (increase in V_{max}) as well as increased levels of GLUT-1 determined by ELISA (Takakura et al 1991). The increase in [^{3}H]-3MG uptake is not observed until after 12 h of glucose starvation, and this response is dependent on protein synthesis. On the other hand, long-term high glucose conditions in the media did not induce any significant down-regulation of the glucose transport rate in bovine brain microvessel endothelial cells at all (Takakura et al 1991).

Brain capillary endothelium is particularly enriched with a glucose transporter, similar to that of human erythrocytes, which allows the selective, stereospecific and saturable transport of large amounts of glucose from blood to brain (Crone 1965; Oldendorf 1971). The brain capillary endothelial cells constitute the blood-brain barrier (Crone 1965; Oldendorf 1971). In rats subjected to long-term hyperglycaemia, the maximum glucose transport capacity of the blood-brain barrier was decreased by 27% (Gjedde & Crone 1981). When the plasma glucose concentration was returned to normal values, the glucose transport rate into brain still remained 20% below normal. This result suggests that repressive changes of the glucose transport mechanism occur in brain endothelial cells in response to increased plasma glucose levels. GLUT-1 is the principal glucose transporter at the blood-brain barrier. It has been shown that immunoreactive GLUT-1 protein is not symmetrically distributed on the plasma membrane of the blood-brain barrier with a 4-fold greater abundance on the abluminal membrane compared with thc luminal membrane, while 40% of the transporter protein is conserved in cytoplasmic space (Farrell & Pardridge 1991). These data indicate that free glucose in endothelial cells is efficiently transported into brain tissues before further metabolism in endothelial cells and that glucose transporter stored in the intracellular vesicular fraction can be rapidly translocated from the cytoplasmic space to the plasma membrane under certain conditions.

[^{3}H]-3MG uptake into cultured endothelial cells of retinal microvessels is also regulated by a facilitative-diffusion type of glucose transport system. GLUT-1 has been identified at a high density in retinal microvessels endothelial cells and it constitutes the principal glucose transporter of the blood-retinal barrier (Harik et al 1990). However, the glucose transport rate in retinal microvessel endothelial cells is not rate-limiting for glucose metabolism, since the endothelial cells contain free sugar when exposed to an extracellular sugar concentrations in the physiological range. This may be significant for transendothelial transfer of glucose from blood to retina and also provide the basis for capillary dysfunction in diabetes mellitus (Betz et al 1983).

The hexose transport system of bovine aortic endothelial cells also shows little or no adaptation to high ambient glucose concentration and Northern blot analysis has also demonstrated that GLUT-1 mRNA levels in bovine aortic endothelial cells are unaffected by the glucose concentration in the medium (Kaiser et al 1993).

DO INSULIN AND OTHER CYTOKINES STIMULATE GLUCOSE METABOLISM IN ENDOTHELIAL CELLS?

It has been reported that a differential insulin stimulation of glucose metabolism may exist between endothelial cells obtained from micro- and macrovasculature. Kaiser et al (1993) have reported that insulin at a concentration of 10 μg/l stimulated [^{14}C]-glucose incorporation into glycogen in calf retinal endothelial cells. Similarly, Allen and Gerritsen (1986) reported that insulin stimulated both 2-deoxy-D-glucose uptake and 3-*O*-methylglucose transport in a dose-dependent manner in cultured bovine retinal endothelial cells (Allen & Gerritsen 1986). The maximum effect was observed at an insulin concentration of 1 μg/l (170 pmol/l). In contrast, insulin did not stimulate glucose uptake in either bovine brain microvessel endothelial cells (Takakura et al 1991) or calf aortic endothelial cells (King et al 1983).

Hypoxia can induce increased GLUT-1 mRNA expression in both bovine aortic and human umbilical vein endothelial cells (Loike et al 1992). The up-regulation of glucose transport activity in endothelial cells exposed to hypoxia requires several hours and a similar up-regulatation of glucose transporter mRNA expression is also found in cells treated with inhibitors of oxidative phosphorylation (Loike et al 1992). We have recently found that H_2O_2 stimulated a 2-fold increase in 2-deoxyglucose uptake by human umbilical vein endothelial cells (Kashiwagi, unpublished data). In bovine aortic endothelial cells, both vascular permeable factor (VPF) and TNF-α stimulated a 3-fold increase in the hexose transport rate and, in combination, these cytokines induced an additive stimulation of the glucose transport rate (Pekala et al 1990). These cytokines caused a specific increase in the amount of message for the GLUT-1/erythrocyte form of transporter, without any changes in mRNA expression for GLUT-2, GLUT-3 and GLUT-4. What is the meaning of these cytokine effects on the stimulation of GLUT-1 mRNA expression in bovine aortic endothelial cells? VPF stimulates endothelial cell growth and angiogenesis, and vascular permeability, while TNF-α inhibits the effect of VPF on endothelial cells. However, both cytokines can act together in tissue factor induction and change the nature of endothelial cells from nonthrombogenic to thrombogenic (Nawroth et al 1988). Stimulation of the glucose transport rate via the induction of GLUT-1 mRNA may therefore be associated with these changes in endothelial cell function.

ACTIVATION OF THE POLYOL PATHWAY AND ITS METABOLIC CONSEQUENCES

Isolated microvessels (primarily capillaries) from bovine retina and cerebral cortex, as well as cultured porcine and canine retinal endothelial cells contain aldose reductase activity (Kennedy et al 1983). High glucose concentration can induce an 8-fold increase in sorbitol accumulation in cultured canine retinal capillary endothelial cells (Kennedy et al 1983). A similar but less remarkable sorbitol accumulation has been reported in human umbilical vein (Hawthorne et al 1989; Lorenzi et al 1987), rat cerebral microvascular (Sussman et al 1988), bovine aortic (Yorek &

Dunlap 1989) and bovine retinal capillary (Lee et al 1989) endothelial cells exposed to high glucose conditions. Hawthorne et al (1989) found that the accumulation reached a maximum level by 24 hours (3-fold higher than the basal level) and was maintained at that level over a period of 14 days.

Is this sorbitol accumulation associated with any other metabolic pathways? Previous studies have found divergent results concerning the association of intracellular sorbitol accumulation with intracellular myo-inositol depletion. Myo-inositol is a substrate for the production of phosphoinositides and their breakdown products, inositol phosphate and diacylglycerol, of which the latter is an activator of protein kinase C (Simmons et al 1986; Winegrad 1987). Therefore, depletion of intracellular myo-inositol levels may cause reduced activation of protein kinase C and Na^+,K^+-ATPase. The effect of long-term exposure to high glucose concentration on myo-inositol depletion depends on the origin of endothelial cells (Hawthorne et al 1989; Lee et al 1989; Sussman et al 1988; Yorek & Dunlap 1989). Bovine aortic endothelial cells showed a 50% decrease in both myo-inositol uptake and its intracellular content (Yorek & Dunlap 1989), but human umbilical vein (Hawthorne et al 1989), retinal capillary (Lee et al 1989) and rat cerebral microvessel (Sussman et al 1988) endothelial cells showed no such decrease. Using bovine retinal capillary endothelial cells, Lee et al (1989) found that high glucose concentration induced a 100% increase in intracellular sorbitol but without any change in the myo-inositol concentration. The activation of protein kinase C may be associated with a decrease in ouabain-inhibitable Na^+,K^+-ATPase activity. However, sorbinil, an inhibitor of aldose reductase, did not significantly affect protein kinase C activity in these cells (Lee et al 1989). It might therefore be speculated that activation of the polyol pathway in endothelial cells exposed to high glucose concentration contributes little to endothelial cell dysfunction in diabetes. The biological significance of activation of the polyol pathway as a shunt pathway of glucose metabolism and osmotic regulator in endothelial cells awaits future studies.

OXIDATIVE STRESS AND GLUCOSE METABOLISM IN ENDOTHELIAL CELLS

Endothelial cells are very sensitive to oxidative stress when overproduced in intra- and extracellular space (Harlan et al 1984; Henning & Chow 1988; Sacks et al 1978; Schraufstatter et al 1988), and this may be one of the earliest events leading to vascular dysfunction in diabetes. Various oxygen radicals are overproduced in the diabetic state by the process of nonenzymatic glycation as well as from other pathophysiological processes associated with diabetes (Brown et al 1988; Mullarkey et al 1990; Weiss et al 1981; Zweier et al 1988). For a better understanding of the mechanisms involved in the increased oxidative stress in diabetic vascular tissues, it is necessary to know the effects of hyperglycaemia on radical scavenger function in endothelial cells.

H_2O_2 is a potentially harmful molecule produced by superoxide dismutase and many other oxidase reactions, whereas catalase and the glutathione redox cycle are the primary means of its enzymatic degradation (Freeman & Crapo 1982). Oxygen radical production and degradation in endothelial cells are summarised in figure 1.1. In a recent study we showed that high glucose concentration impaired glutathione-dependent H_2O_2 degradation by 50% in human umbilical vein endothelial cells without any changes in catalase activity (Kashiwagi et al 1994). Furthermore, this effect depended on D-glucose concentrations in the medium and is specific for D-glucose metabolism, since high raffinose and high L-glucose concentrations had no effect on H_2O_2 degradation.

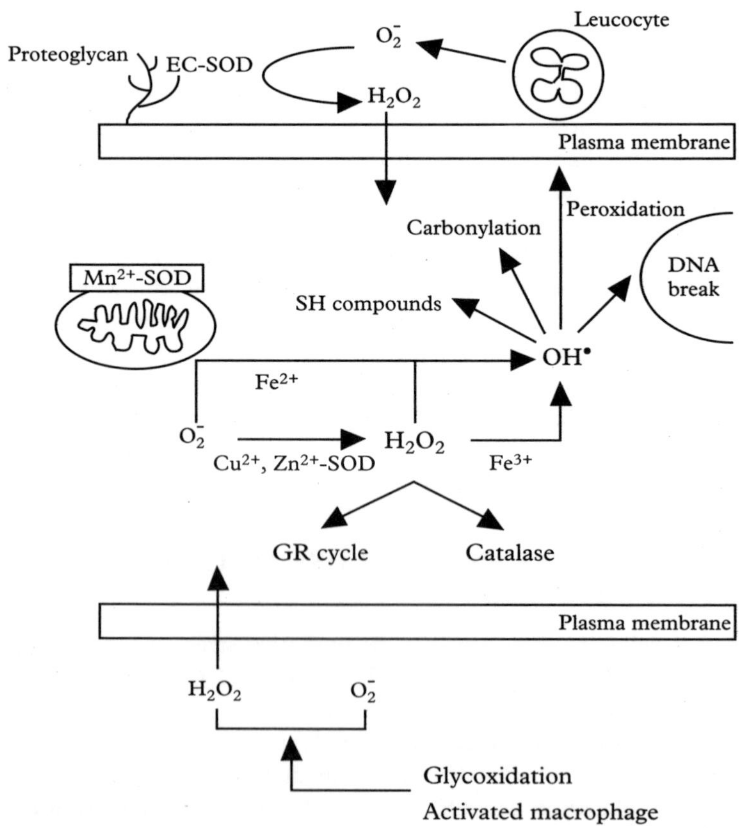

Fig. 1.1 Oxygen radical production and degradation in endothelial cells. *Abbreviations:* EC = endothelial cell; GR = glutathione reductase; SOD = superoxide dismutase.

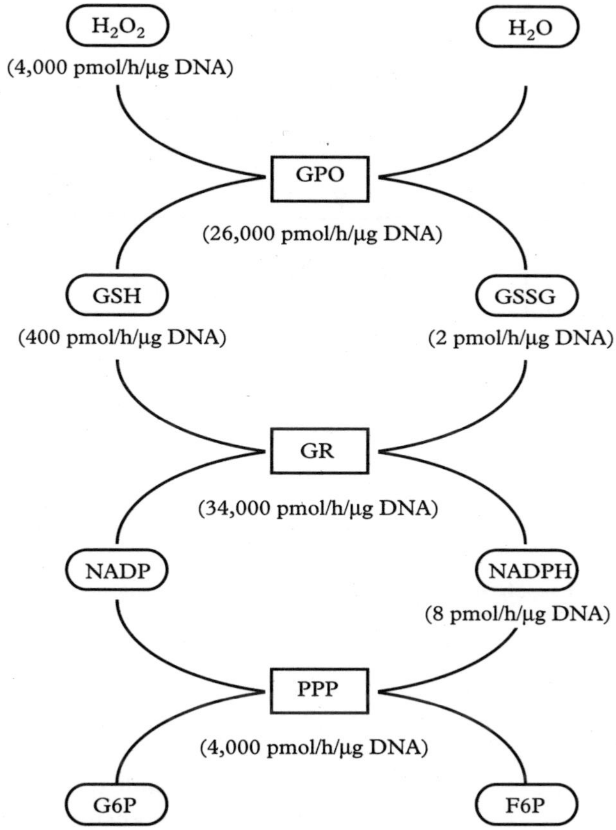

Fig. 1.2 Glutathione redox cycle activity in endothelial cells. *Abbreviations:* F6P = fructose-6-phosphate; G6P = glucose-6-phosphate; GPO = glutathione peroxidase; GR = glutathione reductase; GSH = reduced glutathione; GSSG = oxidized glutathione; PPP = pentose phosphate pathway.

The presence of H_2O_2 in endothelial cells causes rapid activation of the pentose phosphate pathway as well as the glutathione redox cycle (Schraufstatter et al 1985). This resulted in: increased levels of intracellular glutathione; decreased intracellular concentrations of reduced glutathione, ATP, NAD and NADH; a fast rise of intracellular free calcium; impairment of the cytoskeletal system; and finally reduced glycolytic activity (Hyslop et al 1988; Kashiwagi et al 1994; Schraufstatter et al 1985, 1988). Glutathione redox cycle activity is regulated by many factors (Fig. 1.2). NADPH supply would appear to be the major rate-

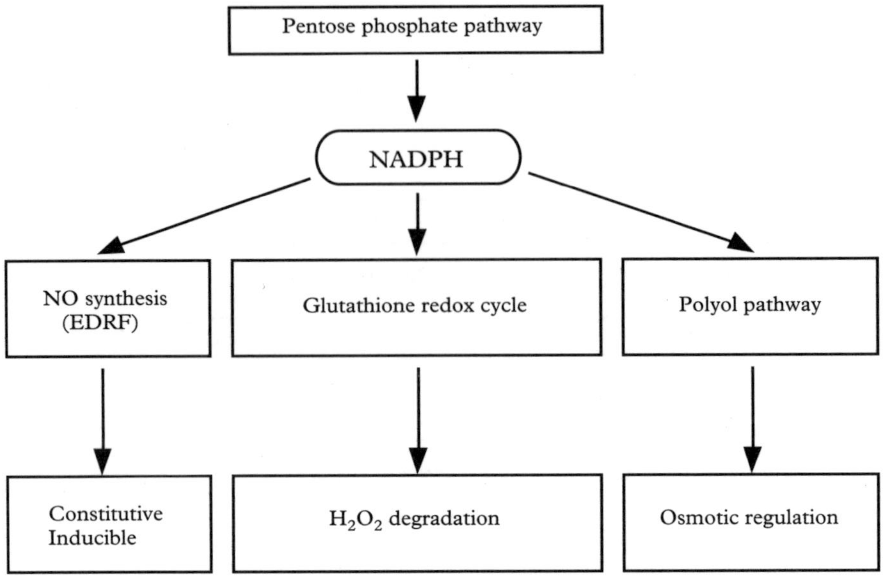

Fig. 1.3 NADPH supply and endothelial cell function. *Abbreviation:* EDRF = endothelial-derived relaxing factor.

limiting step (Kashiwagi et al 1994, Kashiwagi et al 1992). Glycolysis is specifically inactivated by H_2O_2 at the glyceraldehyde-3-phosphate dehydrogenase step by three mechanisms: 1) direct inhibition of the enzyme; 2) a decrease in NAD content; and 3) a shift to low cytosolic pH (Schraufstatter et al 1985). This inhibition may ensure metabolism of glucose 6-phosphate via the pentose phosphate pathway.

We have recently shown that the decrease in H_2O_2 degradation induced by high glucose concentrations in endothelial cells may be closely associated with reduced NADPH supply to the glutathione redox cycle because of impaired activation of the pentose phosphate pathway (Kashiwagi et al 1992). Cultured endothelial cells exposed to high ambient glucose concentrations showed significant increases in both glucose-6-phosphate and fructose-6-phosphate concentrations, a much lesser increase in fructose-1,6-diphosphate, and no change in lactate release into the medium and [6-^{14}C]-glucose oxidation via the tricarboxylic acid cycle. The rate-limiting step in the glycolytic pathway is therefore upstream of glyceraldehyde-3-phosphate dehydrogenase, probably mediated by the response of phosphofructokinase to high glucose conditions. However, lactate release into the medium was less inhibited by H_2O_2 in high glucose compared with normal glucose conditions. Therefore, glucose-6-phosphate flux into the pentose phosphate pathway is remarkable in high glucose versus normal glucose conditions. These results may be coincident with reduced activation of the pentose phosphate pathway in response to high glucose levels.

Excessive active oxygen stress to endothelial cells results in the reduction of intracellular NADPH concentration and the H_2O_2-induced decrease in NADPH is more accentuated in high glucose conditions. As shown in figure 1.3, continuous activation of the polyol pathway (Hawthorne et al 1989; Kennedy et al 1983; Lee et al 1989; Sussman et al 1988; Yorek & Dunlap 1989) and NO synthesis (Moncada et al 1991) further utilise NADPH in endothelial cells exposed to high glucose conditions, which may also accentuate NADPH depletion and then further impair H_2O_2 degradation via the glutathione redox cycle. General glucose metabolism in endothelial cells exposed to high glucose condition is depicted in figure 1.4. However, it should be recalled that the characteristics of glucose metabolism may be differently regulated in micro- and macrovascular endothelial cells.

Other mechanisms of radical scavenger dysfunction have been postulated as being implicated in the aetiology of diabetes. Superoxide dismutase is inactivated by nonenzymatic glycation (Arai et al 1987a, 1987b). Inhibited oxidation mechanisms and reduced content of antioxidant substances (vitamin E and ascorbate) have also been reported in diabetic tissues (Kaplan et al 1982; Yue et al 1989). These results indicate that, in addition to increased oxygen radical production, reduced degradation of other harmful molecules in hyperglycaemic conditions may deteriorate endothelial cell function, which may be one of early events in the course of diabetic vascular dysfunction. Although the clinical relevance of these abnormalities in endothelial cells exposed to high glucose concentrations with respect to the true pathogenesis of diabetic complications awaits future studies, evidence of excessive oxidative stress in diabetes, including increased levels of lipid peroxidation (Jain 1989; Jongkind et al 1989; Sato et al 1979) and autoxidation products (Bucala et al 1993; Wolff & Dean 1987; Makita et al 1992) *in vivo*, suggests that these should be normalised during the treatment of diabetes.

CONCLUSION

It has been proven that GLUT-1 is the principal glucose transporter in endothelial cells originating from both micro- and macrovascular endothelia. The glucose transport rate in macrovascular endothelial cells is not regulated by either insulin or ambient glucose concentrations, while it is significantly regulated in microvascular endothelial cells by both insulin and glucose concentrations. Therefore, insulin deficiency and hyperglycaemia in diabetes may profoundly impair microvascular endothelial cell function. Furthermore, many vasoactive cytokines activate

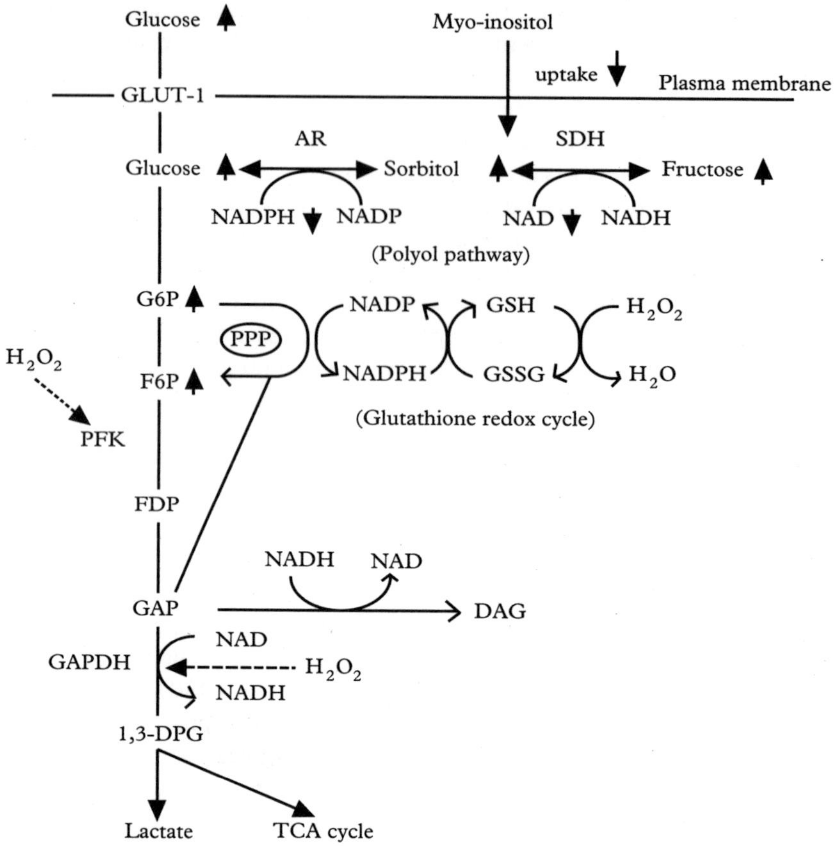

Fig. 1.4 Glucose metabolism in endothelial cells under high glucose conditions. *Abbreviations:* AR = aldose reductase; DAG = diacylglycerol; 1,3-DPG = 1,3-diphosphoglycerate; FDP = fructose diphosphate; F6P = fructose-6-phosphate; GAP = glyceraldehyde phosphate; GAPDH = glyceraldehyde-3-phosphate dehydrogenase; GLUT-1 = glucose transporter isoform 1; G6P = glucose-6-phosphate; GSH = reduced glutathione; GSSH = oxidized glutathione; PFK = phosphofructokinase; SDH = sorbitol dehydrogenase; TCA = tricarboxylic acid.

gene expression of the glucose transporter and may therefore affect its biological activity. Activation of the polyol pathway by high ambient glucose conditions can be found in all micro- and macrovascular endothelial cells, but it is unclear whether the decrease in myo-inositol concentration induced by high glucose conditions has any relation to endothelial cell dysfunction in diabetes. Oxidative stress induces activation of the pentose phosphate pathway, which provides an important oxygen radical scavenger system via the continuous supply of NADPH to the glutathione redox cycle. This radical scavenger function in endothelial cells is significantly impaired by high glucose culture conditions and may therefore be in part associated with the enhancement of oxidative stress-induced vascular dysfunction in diabetes.

REFERENCES

Allen L A, Gerritsen M E 1986 Regulation of hexose transport in cultured bovine retinal microvessel endothelium by insulin. Exp Eye Res 43: 679-686

Arai K, Iizuka S, Tada Y et al 1987a Increase in glycosylated form of erythrocyte Cu,Zn-superoxide dismutase in diabetes and close association of nonenzymatic glycosylation with the enzyme activity. Biochim Biophys Acta 924: 292-296

Arai K, Maguchi S, Fujii S 1987b Glycation and inactivation of human Cu,Zn-superoxide dismutase. J Biol Chem 262: 16969-16972

Baynes J W 1991 Role of oxidative stress in development of complications in diabetes. Diabetes 40: 405-412

Bell G I, Kayano T, Buse J B et al 1990 Molecular biology of mammalian glucose transporters. Diabetes Care 13: 198-208

Betz A L, Bownan P D, Goldstein G W 1983 Hexose transport in microvascular endothelial cells cultured from bovine retina. Exp Eye Res 36: 269-277

Birnbaum M J 1989 Identification of a novel gene encoding an insulin-responsive glucose transporter protein. Cell 57: 305-315

Brosius III F C, Briggs J P, Marcus R G et al 1992 Insulin-responsive glucose transporter expression in renal microvessels and glomeruli. Kidney Int 42: 1086-1092

Brown M L, Jakubowski J A, Leventis L L et al 1988 Elevated glucose alters eicosanoid release from porcine aortic endothelial cells. J Clin Invest 82: 2136-2141

Brownlee M 1992 Glycation products and the pathogenesis of diabetic complications. Diabetes Care 15: 1835-1843

Bucala R, Makita Z, Koschinsky T et al 1993 Lipid advanced glycosylation: pathway for lipid oxidation *in vivo*. Proc Natl Acad Sci USA 90: 6434-6438

Charron M J, Brosius F C, Alper S L et al 1989 A glucose transport protein expressed predominantly in insulin-responsive tissues. Proc Natl Acad Sci USA 86: 2535-2539

Crone C 1965 Facilitated transporter of glucose from blood into brain tissue. J Physiol 181:103-113

Cushman S W, Wardzala L J 1980 Potential mechanism of insulin action on glucose transport in the isolated rat adipose cell. Apparent translocation of intracellular transport systems to the plasma membrane. J Biol Chem 255: 4758-4762

Engerman R, Bloodworth Jr J M, Nelson S 1977 Relationship of microvascular disease in diabetes to metabolic control. Diabetes 26: 760-769

Farrell C L, Pardridge W M 1991 Blood-brain barrier glucose transporter is asymmetrically distributed on brain capillary endothelial laminal and abluminal membranes: an electron microscopic immunogold study. Proc Natl Acad Sci USA 88: 5779-5783

Freeman B A, Crapo J D 1982 Biology of disease: free radicals and tissue injury. Lab Invest 47: 412-426

Fukumoto H, Kayano T, Buse J B et al 1989 Cloning and characterization of the major insulin-responsive glucose transporter expressed in human skeletal muscle and other insulin-responsive tissues. J Biol Chem 264: 7776-7779

Gabbay K H 1973 The sorbitol pathway and the complications of diabetes. N Engl J Med 288: 831-836

Gjedde A, Crone C 1981 Blood-brain glucose transfer: repression in chronic hyperglycemia. Science 214: 456-457

Harik S I, Kalaria R N, Whitney P M et al 1990 Glucose transporters are abundant in cells with "occluding" junctions at the blood-eye barriers. Proc Natl Acad Sci USA 87: 4261-4264

Harlan J M, Levine J D, Callahan K S et al 1984 Glutathione redox cycle protects cultured endothelial cells against lysis by extracellularly generated hydrogen peroxide. J Clin Invest 73: 706-713

Hawthorne G C, Bartlett K, Hetherington C S et al 1989 The effect of high glucose on polyol pathway activity and myoinositol metabolism in cultured human endothelial cells. Diabetologia 32: 163-166

Hediger M A, Coady M J, Ikeda T S et al 1987 Expression cloning and cDNA sequencing of the Na^+/glucose cotransporter. Nature 330: 379-381

Henning B, Chow C K 1988 Lipid peroxidation and endothelial cell injury: implications in atherosclerosis. Free Radical Biol Med 4: 99-106

Hyslop P A, Hinshaw D B, Halsey Jr W A 1988 Mechanism of oxidant- mediated cell injury: the glycolytic and mitochondrial pathways of ADP phosphorylation are major intracellular targets inactivated by hydrogen peroxide. J Biol Chem 263: 1665-1675

Jain S K 1989 Hyperglycemia can cause membrane lipid peroxidation and osmotic fragility in human red blood cells. J Biol Chem 264: 21340-21345

James D E, Strube M, Mueckler M 1989 Molecular cloning and characterization of an insulin-regulatable glucose transporter. Nature 338: 83-87

Jongkind J F, Verkerk A, Baggen R G A 1989 Glutathione metabolism of human vascular endothelial cells under peroxidative stress. Free Radical Biol Med 7: 507-512

Kaiser N, Sasson S, Feener E P et al 1993 Differential regulation of glucose transport and transporters by glucose in vascular endothelial and smooth muscle cells. Diabetes 42: 80-89

Kannel W B, McGee D L 1979 Diabetes and glucose tolerance as risk factors for cardiovascular disease: the Framingham study. Diabetes Care 2: 120-126

Kaplan C W, Pritchard Jr K A, Arnold J H et al 1982 Restoration of the prostacyclin/thromboxane A_2 balance in the diabetic rat: influence of vitamin E. Diabetes 31: 947-951

Kashiwagi A, Asahina T, Ikebuchi M et al 1994 Abnormal glutathione metabolism and increased cytotoxicity caused by H_2O_2 in human umbilical vein endothelial cells cultured in high glucose medium. Diabetologia 37:264-269

Kashiwagi A, Asahina T, Nishio Y et al 1992 An insufficient hexose monophosphate shunt activity as a cause of abnormal radical scavenging function in endothelial cells cultured in high glucose media. Diabetes 41: 18A

Kayano T, Fukumoto H, Eddy R L et al 1988 Evidence for a family of human glucose transporter-like proteins. J Biol Chem 263:15245-15248

Kennedy A, Frank R N, Verma S D 1983 Aldose reductase activity in retinal and cerebral microvessels and cultured vascular cells. Invest Ophthalm Vis Sci 24: 1250-1258

King G L, Buzney S M, Kahn C R et al 1983 Differential responsiveness to insulin of endothelial and support cells from micro- and macrovessels. J Clin Invest 71: 974-979

Lee T S, MacGreger L C, Fluharty S J et al 1989 Differential regulation of protein kinase C and (Na,K)-adenosine triphosphatase activities by elevated glucose levels in retinal capillary endothelial cells. J Clin Invest 83:90-94

Loike J D, Brett C J, Ogawa S et al 1992 Hypoxia induces glucose transporter expression in endothelial cells. Am J Physiol 263: C326-333

Lorenzi M, Toledo S, Boss G R et al 1987 The polyol pathway and glucose 6-phosphate in human endothelial cells cultured in high glucose concentrations. Diabetologia 30: 222-227

Makita Z, Radoff S, Rayfield E J et al 1992 Immunochemical detection of advanced glycosylation end products *in vivo*. J Biol Chem 267: 5133-5138

Moncada S, Palmer R M J, Higgs E A 1991 Nitric oxide: physiology, pathophysiology, and pharmacology. Pharmacol Rev 43: 109-142

Mueckler M, Caruso C, Baldwin S A et al 1985 Sequence and structure of a human glucose transporter. Science 229: 941-945

Mullarkey C J, Edelstein D, Brownlee M 1990 Free radical generation by early glycation products: a mechanism for accelerated atherosclerosis in diabetes. Biochim Biophys Res Comm 173: 932-939

Nawroth P, Handley D, Matsueda G et al 1988 Tumor necrosis factor/cachectin-induced intravascular fibrin formation in METH fibrosarcomas. J Exp Med 168: 637-647

Oka Y, Asano T, Shibasaki Y et al 1988 Studies with antipeptide antibody suggest the presence of at least two types of glucose transporter in rat brain and adipocyte. J Biol Chem 263: 13432-13439

Oldendorf W H 1971 Brain uptake of radiolabeled amino acids, amines and hexoses after arterial injection. Am J Physiol 221: 1629-1639

Pekala P, Marlow M, Heuvelman D et al 1990 Regulation of hexose transport in aortic endothelial cells by vascular permeability factor and tumor necrosis factor-alpha , but not by insulin. J Biol Chem 265: 18051-18054

Pyorala K 1979 Relationship of glucose tolerance and plasma insulin to the incidence of coronary heart disease. Diabetes Care 2: 131-141

Sacks T, Moldow C F, Craddock P R et al 1978 Oxygen radicals mediate endothelial cell damage by complement-stimulated granulocytes: an *in vitro* model of immune vascular damage. J Clin Invest 61: 1161-1167

Sato Y, Hotta N, Sakamoto N et al 1979 Lipid peroxide level in plasma of diabetic patients. Biochem Med 21: 104-107

Schraufstatter I U, Hinshaw D B, Hyslop P A et al 1985 Glutathione cycle activity and pyridine nucleotide levels in oxidant-induced injury of cells. J Clin Invest 76: 1131-1139

Schraufstatter I U, Hyslop P A, Jackson C G 1988 Oxidant-induced DNA damage of target cells. J Clin Invest 82: 1040-1050

Schwartz C J, Kelley J L, Valente A J et al 1992 Pathogenesis of the atherosclerotic lesion. Implications for diabetes mellitus. Diabetes Care 15: 1156-1167

Simmons D A, Kern E F O, Wingrad A I et al 1986 Basal phosphatidylinositol turnover controls aortic Na^+/K^+ ATPase activity. J Clin Invest 77: 503-513

Stout R W 1991 Insulin as a mitogenic factor: role in the pathogenesis of cardiovascular disease. Am J Med 90: 62-65S

Sussman I, Carson M P, Schults V et al 1988 Chronic exposure to high glucose decreases myo-inositol in cultured cerebral microvascular pericytes but not in endothelium. Diabetologia 31: 771-775

Suzuki K, Kono T 1980 Evidence that insulin causes translocation of glucose transport activity to the plasma membrane from an intracellular storage site. Proc Natl Acad Sci USA 77: 2542-2545

Takakura Y, Kuentzel S L, Raub T J et al 1991 Hexose uptake in primary cultures of bovine brain microvessel endothelial cells. I. Basic characteristics and effects of D-glucose and insulin. Biochim Biophys Acta 1070: 1-10

The Diabetes Control and Complication Trial Research Group 1993 The effect of intensive treatment of diabetes on the development and progression of long-term complications in insulin-dependent diabetes mellitus N Engl J Med 329: 977-986

Thorens B, Sarkar H K, Kaback H R et al 1988 Cloning and functional expression in bacteria of a novel glucose transporter present in liver, intestine, kidney, and β pancreatic islet cells. Cell 55: 281-290

Vilaro S, Palacin M, Pilch P F et al 1989 Expression of an insulin-regulatable glucose carrier in muscle and fat endothelial cells. Nature 342: 798-800

Weiss S J, Young J, LoBuglio A F et al 1981 Role of hydrogen peroxide in neutrophil-mediated destruction of cultured endothelial cells. J Clin Invest 68: 714-721

Winegrad A I 1987 Does a common mechanism induce the diverse complications of diabetes? Diabetes 36: 396-406

Wolff S P, Dean R T 1987 Glucose autoxidation and protein modification. Biochem J 245: 243-250

Yorek M A, Dunlap J A 1989 The effect of elevated glucose levels on myoinositol metabolism in cultured bovine aortic endothelial cells. Metabolism 38: 16-22

Yue D K, McLennan S, Fisher E et al 1989 Ascorbic acid metabolism and the polyol pathway in diabetes. Diabetes 38: 257-261

Zorzano A, Wilkinson W K, Kotlian N et al 1989 Insulin-regulated glucose uptake in rat adipocytes is mediated by two transporter isoforms present in at least two vesicle populations. J Biol Chem 264: 12358-12363

Zweier J L, Kuppusamy P, Lutty J A 1988 Measurement of endothelial cell free radical generation: evidence for a central mechanism of free radical injury in postischemic tissues. Proc Natl Acad Sci USA 85: 4046-4050

2

Prostaglandin metabolism in endothelial cells

F. Umeda, M. Kunisaki, T. Hashimoto, H. Nawata

INTRODUCTION

There are many notable common complications in patients with diabetes mellitus which result from biochemical, physiological and morphological changes, such as those in vascular resistance, arterial pressure, blood flow regulation, vascular permeability, vascular cell growth and metabolic pathways like glucose utilization. Based on many pathogenic studies, prostaglandins in the vascular wall are known to have potent bioactivity, playing an important role in the maintenance of vascular homeostasis, whose abnormality may cause thrombus formation and atherosclerosis. In view of the close relationship between abnormal prostaglandin metabolism and diabetic vascular changes, numerous studies have been carried out on the effect of diabetes mellitus on prostaglandin metabolism in various vessels.

In the vascular wall, prostacyclin (PGI_2) produced mainly by endothelial cells acts both as a potent vasodilator and as an inhibitor of platelet adhesion and aggregation (Moncada et al 1976; Moncada & Vane 1978). On the other hand, thromboxane A_2 (TXA_2) released from activated platelets is a potent vasoconstrictor and also a stimulator of platelet aggregation. Homeostasis of the vasculature is therefore maintained by the balance of these vasoactive prostaglandins (Moncada 1982). The imbalance of PGI_2 and TXA_2 production may cause microangiopathy and atherosclerosis in patients with diabetes mellitus. As the abnormality of TXA_2 production by platelets in diabetes mellitus will be described elsewhere in this book, abnormalities in prostaglandin metabolism of vascular endothelial cells relative to the pathogenesis of diabetic vascular complications are specifically discussed in this article.

PGI_2 METABOLISM IN VASCULAR ENDOTHELIAL CELLS

Arachidonic acid, a precursor of prostaglandins, is the most common fatty acid in cellular phospholipids. Release of arachidonic acid from membrane phospholipids in endothelial cells is mediated mainly by the activation of phospholipase A_2 and partially by the activation of diacylglycerol lipase after agonist stimulation (Bicknell & Vallee 1989; Brock & Capasso 1988;

Jaffe et al 1987; Kaya et al 1989; Lo & Fan 1987). Phospholipase A_2 is regulated by many factors, such as intracellular Ca^{2+} or cAMP concentration (Brotherton & Hoak 1982), GTP binding protein (Bicknell & Vallee 1989) and lipocortin (Rothhut et al 1983). Inhibition of prostaglandin synthesis by glucocorticoid is mediated by the stimulation of lipocortin production, which inhibits phospholipase A_2 (De Caterina & Weksler 1986). However, recent studies have demonstrated that glucocorticoid acts through inhibition of cyclooxygenase expression. More recently, Clark et al (1987) found phospholipase A_2-activating protein (PLAP), which specifically stimulates phospholipase A_2 and whose synthesis is enhanced by tumour necrosis factor-α (Clark et al 1988). PLAP has been cloned (Clark et al 1991) and is expressed as a 2.5-kb mRNA in vascular endothelial and smooth muscle cells.

Once released from the membrane phospholipids, arachidonic acid is metabolised by two different enzymes, i.e. cyclooxygenase and lipoxygenase. Prostaglandins could be found in any organ, but certain tissues, such as seminal vesicle, kidney and lung, have a greater capacity for prostaglandin synthesis (Christ & van Dorp 1972). In addition to the classic prostaglandins, such as prostaglandin (PG) E_2, D_2 and $F_{2\alpha}$, more biologically potent prostaglandins, such as prostaglandin endoperoxides (PGG_2 and PGH_2), TXA_2 and PGI_2, have been recently discovered. PGI_2, a major prostaglandin metabolite of the cyclooxygenase pathway in vascular endothelial cells, was found by Moncada et al (1976). Vascular endothelial cells also produce PGE_2, PGD_2, $PGF_{2\alpha}$ and TXA_2, the amounts of which are, however, relatively small (Gerritsen 1987; Ingerman-Wojenski et al 1981).

Synthesis of PGI_2 is regulated by several enzymes, such as phospholipase A_2, cyclooxygenase and PGI_2 synthetase. Since cyclooxygenase is rapidly inactivated in endothelial cells and steady-state enzyme activity is kept at a low level (Wu et al 1988), it is known to act as a rate-limiting enzyme in endothelial cells. On the other hand, PGI_2 synthetase does not act as a rate-limiting enzyme since it has high activity in endothelial cells. PGI_2 is synthesized from PGH_2 by PGI_2 synthetase in the microsomes of vascular endothelial cells. PGI_2 synthetase, which has a broad pH optimum, catalyses the rapid conversion of saturating concentrations of PGH_2 to PGI_2 at 37°C (Salmon et al 1978). Vascular endothelial cells treated with a specific cyclooxygenase inhibitor, indomethacin, can produce PGI_2-like antiaggregating activity when incubated with activated platelets (Bunting et al 1976; Bunting et al 1977; Gryglewski et al 1976). This result indicates that PGI_2 is synthesized not only from its own endogenous precursor, but also from prostaglandin endoperoxides released from platelets (Moncada & Vane 1978). PGI_2 is chemically unstable with a half life of 2-3 min (Dusting et al 1977) and metabolized nonenzymatically to 6-keto-prostaglandin $F_{1\alpha}$ (6-keto-$PGF_{1\alpha}$). However, PGI_2 is more stable in plasma and in blood (Gimeno et al 1980) because it is bound to serum albumin (Blasko et al

1980; Orchard & Robinson 1981; Pifer et al 1981; Wynalda & Fitzpatrick 1980). Moreover, recent reports have demonstrated that circulating PGI_2 is stabilized by apolipoprotein A1 (Apo-A1), a major component of high-density lipoprotein (HDL) in plasma (Yui et al 1988). The antiatherogenic action of HDL or Apo A-1 may work in part through PGI_2 stabilization.

PGI_2 is released from endothelial cells when stimulated by various factors, such as hormones, chemical mediators, cytokines, growth factors, and shear stress (Baenziger et al 1980; Coughlin et al 1980; Kawakami et al 1986; Rossi et al 1985; Weksler et al 1978). Rapid production of PGI_2 depends on the activation of phospholipase A_2, but prolonged production by cytokines and growth factors depends on the increased production of cyclooxygenase (Bicknell & Valle 1989).

PGI_2 PRODUCTION IN DIABETES MELLITUS

Many studies have demonstrated that platelet aggregation and TXA_2 production increase in diabetic patients as well as in animal models of diabetes. Furthermore, altered PGI_2 metabolism has been described in vascular endothelial cells and vascular wall. Johnson et al (1979) and Silberbauer et al (1979) demonstrated that PGI_2 production by vessels

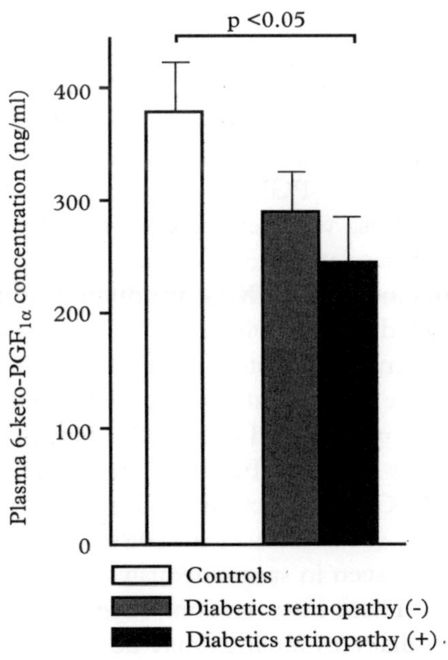

Fig. 2.1 Plasma 6-keto-$PGF_{1\alpha}$ concentrations in diabetic patients with and without retinopathy compared with healthy control subjects. Values are given as means ± SEM. (Reproduced with permission from Watanabe et al 1985)

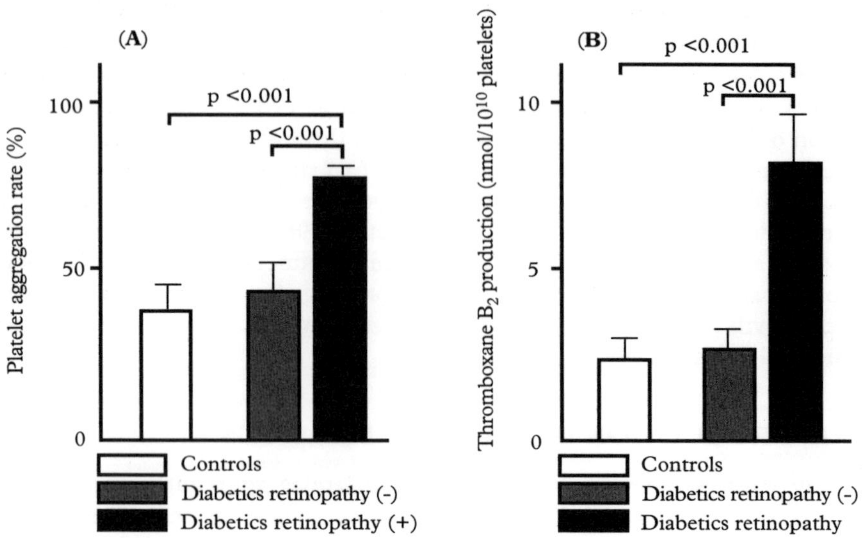

Fig. 2.2 Collagen-induced platelet aggregation rate (**A**) and platelet thromboxane B_2 production during aggregation (**B**) in diabetic patients with and without retinopathy compared with healthy control subjects. Values are given as means ± SEM. (Reproduced with permission from Watanabe et al 1985)

obtained from diabetic patients is reduced compared with controls. The plasma concentration of 6-keto-$PGF_{1\alpha}$, a stable metabolite of PGI_2, is significantly lower in diabetic patients with proliferative retinopathy than in control subjects (Dollery et al 1979). Watanabe et al (1985) have also confirmed that plasma 6-keto-$PGF_{1\alpha}$ concentrations are reduced in diabetic patients, especially in those with retinopathy (Fig. 2.1). They also reported that collagen-induced platelet aggregation rate and platelet thromboxane B_2 (TXB_2), a stable metabolite of TXA_2, production during aggregation are significantly higher in diabetics with retinopathy than in control subjects (Fig. 2.2). Platelets from streptozotocin (STZ)-induced diabetic rats release more TXA_2 than those from controls, whereas their blood vessels show reduced PGI_2 production (Gerrard et al 1980; Harrison et al 1978; Jeremy et al 1985; Watanabe et al 1985). Furthermore, long-term insulin treatment restores the reduced PGI_2 production by aorta and renal cortex in STZ-induced diabetic rats (Harrison et al 1980). Similarly reduced PGI_2 production by vessels is seen in spontaneously diabetic Wistar rats (Subbiah & Deitemeyer 1980). These investigations suggest that reduced production of PGI_2 by vessels in diabetes mellitus may be caused by an abnormality in vascular endothelial cells.

The effects of high glucose levels on PGI_2 production by vascular wall and cultured vascular endothelial cells are controversial. Valentovic and

Lubawy (1985) reported that high concentrations of glucose adversely alter PGI_2 production by incubated normal rat aortic ring. Aanderud et al (1985) demonstrated that high concentrations of glucose do not affect PGI_2 synthesis in cultured human umbilical endothelial cells, but that incubation with serum obtained from patients with type 1 diabetes significantly reduces PGI_2 production. Paton et al (1982) showed that PGI_2 production stimulated by thrombin is significantly reduced in human umbilical endothelial cells cultured with serum obtained from diabetics. These findings have lead to speculation that diabetic sera may have an inhibitory effect on PGI_2 production by cultured vascular endothelial cells irrespective of glucose and insulin levels. However, Jeremy et al (1983) demonstrated that glucose has a stimulatory effect on PGI_2 production by rat aortic ring between concentrations of 10 and 30 mmol/l, but a progressive decrease in stimulation occurs at higher concentrations. Additionally, Ono et al (1988) reported that high concentrations of glucose have an inhibitory effect on PGI_2 production by cultured bovine aortic endothelial cells (Fig. 2.3). These contradictory findings may arise from

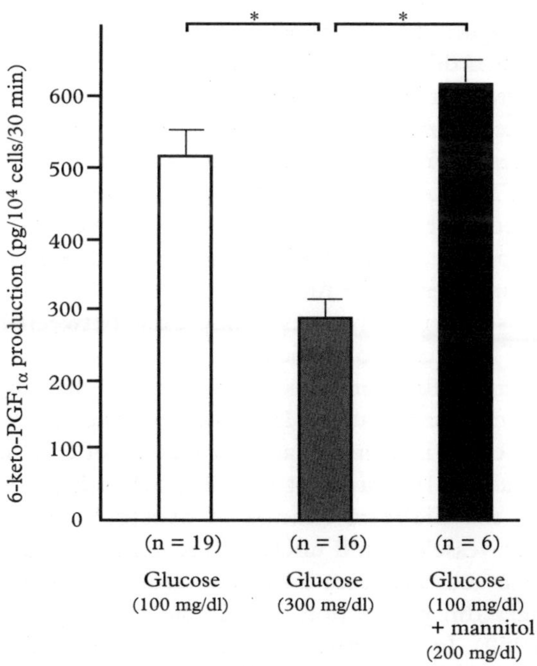

Fig. 2.3 Comparison of 6-keto-$PGF_{1\alpha}$ production by cultured bovine aortic endothelial cells containing two different concentrations of glucose, or glucose plus mannitol. Production of 6-keto-$PGF_{1\alpha}$ was stimulated by the addition of plasma-derived serum 10% for 30 min at 37°C. Values are given as means ± SEM. *Statistical significance:* * $p < 0.01$. (Reproduced with permission from Ono et al 1988)

differences in culture conditions or in the species from which the endothelium was derived.

Aanderud et al (1985) found that insulin does not affect PGI_2 production in cultured endothelial cells. In contrast, Jeremy (1983) showed that insulin has an inhibitory effect on PGI_2 production. However, these authors also showed that combination of insulin with a high concentration of glucose (10 mmol/l) stimulates PGI_2 production in rat aortic ring. From these findings, it seems that altered vascular endothelial cell function and/or alteration in some plasma product, perhaps associated with the hyperglycaemia of diabetes mellitus, may reduce PGI_2 production by vascular wall. The circulating abnormality may include the possibility that some plasma product which stimulates PGI_2 production is decreased in diabetes mellitus. This will be discussed in the next section.

All the above-mentioned abnormalities in prostaglandin metabolism were observed in large vessels or endothelial cells from large vessels. Abnormalities in prostaglandin metabolism in microvessels have also been studied. Homogenates of cremaster muscle from STZ-induced diabetic rats produce more PGE_2 and PGI_2 than the corresponding muscle from normal animals (Myers et al 1985). However, there was no difference in basal or melittin-stimulated production of PGE_2 and PGI_2 by cerebral microvessels comparing STZ-induced diabetic and normal rats (Wey et al 1986). A decreased dilatory response of cerebral arterioles to acetylcholine or ADP is reported for STZ-induced diabetic rats (Mayhan 1989; Mayhan et al 1991). These authors suggest that the decreased response to these agonists may result from the enhanced production of vasoconstrictive products, e.g. TXA_2 or PGH_2, since treatment with indomethacin or the TXA_2/PGH_2 receptor antagonist (SQ 29548) restores the response to normal. It is apparent from these findings that microvessels are somewhat different from large vessels. A fundamental difference in the abnormalities of vascular prostaglandin synthesis may exist between large and small vessels in the STZ-induced diabetic rats .

Altered prostaglandin metabolism has been extensively investigated in the glomerular microcirculation. Increased production of PGE_2, $PGF_{1\alpha}$, and PGI_2 is observed in glomerular microvessels of STZ-induced diabetic rats (Chang et al 1991; Craven et al 1987; Schambelan et al 1985). The mechanism of the diabetic change in prostaglandin metabolism by glomerular microvessels is still unclear, but might be explained in part by aldose reductase activity, since an aldose reductase inhibitor can restore altered prostaglandin production in diabetic animals (Chang et al 1991; Craven et al 1989). In contrast, enhanced TXA_2 production has also been suggested as playing an important role in the pathogenesis of nephropathy in STZ-induced diabetic animals (Craven 1992; Craven & DeRubertis 1990; DeRubertis & Craven 1992; Hora et al 1990). All of these authors have demonstrated that a thromboxane synthetase inhibitor attenuates renal damage in diabetic animals. Finally, decreased PGI_2 production has also been suggested as playing a part in the pathogenesis of diabetic retinopathy (Robertson et al 1990).

PGI_2 PRODUCTION AND ATHEROSCLEROSIS

Patients with diabetes mellitus have an increased susceptibility to atherosclerosis (Colwell et al 1981; Crall & Roberts 1978). Sinzinger et al (1979) have demonstrated that PGI_2 production by atherosclerotic arterial tissue is significantly lower than that by normal arterial tissue. High accumulation of lipid peroxides, which are potent and selective inhibitors of PGI_2 synthetase (Bunting et al 1976), occurs in advanced atherosclerotic lesions (Glavind et al 1952). The exact mechanism of the reduced PGI_2 synthesis in atherosclerosis is still unknown. It should be noted, however, that the reduced PGI_2 production in cultured aortic smooth muscle cells obtained from aged rats is related to decreased PGI_2 synthetase activity (Chang et al 1980).

Many epidemiological studies have revealed that increased levels of low-density lipoprotein (LDL) and decreased levels of HDL are risk factors for ischaemic heart disease. The effects of LDL and HDL on PGI_2 production by vascular wall have been examined by several investigators. Nordoy et al (1978) showed that LDL reduces the inhibitory action of vascular endothelial cells for platelet aggregation, which is partially restored by HDL. Beitz and Forster (1980) also reported that LDL inhibits, whereas HDL stimulates PGI_2 synthesis. Additionally, they showed that there is a linear correlation between PGI_2 synthesis and HDL (positive) or LDL (negative) concentration. They speculated that the effect of HDL on PGI_2 synthesis is due to stimulation of PGI_2 synthetase by HDL. Furthermore, Gryglewski and Szczeklik (1981) have confirmed the inhibitory effect of LDL on PGI_2 production. Analysis of lipoproteins taken from a group of hyperlipidaemic patients revealed that the LDL fraction, but not the HDL fraction, contains lipid peroxides at a concentration several times higher than those in the total serum. It is therefore possible that the lipid peroxide associated with LDL inhibits PGI_2 synthesis.

However, conflicting observations have been reported. Fleischer et al (1982) found that incubation of HDL with porcine aortic endothelial cells for 24 h stimulates PGI_2 production in a dose- and time-dependent fashion. On the other hand, no significant changes in PGI_2 production were observed when endothelial cells were incubated with LDL. The mechanism by which HDL stimulates PGI_2 production by vascular endothelial cells may be complex. Much greater stimulation of PGI_2 production is found by incubation with rat HDL, whose arachidonic acid contents are greater than those of human HDL, whereas similar stimulation of PGI_2 production is observed by the delipidated apoprotein of both human and rat HDL. HDL may therefore stimulate PGI_2 synthesis by providing the cell with arachidonic acid. A recent report by Galle et al (1990) shows that LDL stimulates PGI_2 production by cultured endothelial cells. Ishii et al (1989) also demonstrated that LDL stimulates PGI_2 production by cultured bovine aortic endothelial cells in a dose-dependent manner and that glycation of LDL reduces the stimulatory effect of native LDL on PGI_2 production. Since endothelial cells can bind LDL and utilise its phospholipids and cholesteryl esters containing arachidonic acid (Fielding et al 1979; van Hinsbergh et al 1983), LDL stimulation of PGI_2 production by endothelial cells is in part due to providing arachidonic acid within cells.

There is also evidence of a relation between vitamin E and PGI_2 synthesis in vascular endothelial cells. Vitamin E is known to have antiatherogenic effect because of its antioxidant properties as well as its inhibitory properties against platelet aggregation. Vascular vitamin E content has been considered to be decreased in diabetics. PGI_2 synthesis by the vascular wall is reduced in vitamin E-deficient animals (Chan & Leith 1981; Karpen et al 1981; Okuma et al 1980; Sugimoto et al 1980). Moreover, it has been reported that vitamin E stimulates the production of PGI_2 by cultured endothelial cells (Boogaerts et al 1984; Huang et al 1988; Kunisaki et al 1989; Tran & Chan 1990; Umeda et al 1990). These findings suggest that the reduced PGI_2 production by vascular wall in diabetic patients may be in part due to vitamin E deficiency in tissues. Reduced PGI_2 production in both STZ-induced diabetic and vitamin E-deficient rats is restored by vitamin E supplementation (Karpen et al 1981; Karpen et al 1982). Kunisaki et al (1992) demonstrated that PGI_2 production by bovine vascular endothelial cells cultured with high concentration of glucose is reduced after stimulation by histamine and the Ca^{2+} ionophore, A23187, and that the application of vitamin E restores PGI_2 production. These results led to speculation that the antiatherogenic effect of vitamin E may be mediated in part through stimulation of PGI_2 production by vascular wall, in addition to the prevention of lipid peroxide accumulation and platelet aggregation.

Recently, Kunisaki et al (1993) have reported that cultured bovine aortic endothelial cells have specific binding sites for D-α–tocopherol and that incubation of cells with high glucose medium reduces this specific binding. Since an aldose reductase inhibitor has no effect on this reduction of D-tocopherol binding by high glucose medium (Kunisaki et al 1993), glycation of protein and oxidative damage of cells may be a possible mechanism of reduced binding.

PGI_2-STIMULATORY ACTIVITY IN PLASMA

MacIntyre et al (1978) were the first to report that human plasma contained stimulatory activity for PGI_2 production by cultured aortic endothelial cells. Later, Ritter et al (1983) showed that PGI_2 production is stimulated by a serum factor formed during coagulation, which is antagonized by heparin. Inoguchi et al (1989) also demonstrated the PGI_2-stimulatory activity of human plasma with cultured bovine aortic endothelial cells. This stimulatory activity in plasma may play a major role in the regulation of PGI_2 production by the vascular wall. Decreased PGI_2-stimulatory activity may reduce PGI_2 production and cause vascular lesions.

Inoguchi et al (1989) found that plasma PGI_2-stimulatory activity is reduced in diabetic patients as well as in diabetic animals. Figure 2.4 shows 6-keto-$PGF_{1\alpha}$ production by cultured bovine aortic endothelial cells stimulated by plasma-derived serum (PDS) from diabetic patients and STZ-induced diabetic rats. PDS 2-10% prepared from both diabetic patients and rats show reduced stimulatory activity on 6-keto-$PGF_{1\alpha}$ production. Moreover, stimulation of PGI_2 production by serum is decreased in diabetic patients without microangiopathy, indicating that the abnormality in serum PGI_2-stimulatory activity precedes diabetic angiopathy (Inoguchi et al 1989). PDS from elderly subjects with atherosclerosis has less PGI_2-stimulatory activity than that from young subjects (Umeda et al 1989). However, it is still unknown whether the reduced PGI_2-stimulatory activity might be a result or a cause of atherosclerosis in elderly.

Platelets have stimulatory activity on PGI_2 production by endothelial cells (Inoguchi et al 1991; Seid et al 1983). Inoguchi et al (1991) demonstrated that the nature of this stimulatory activity in platelet extract is different from that of plasma because combined application of plasma and platelet extracts results in a 2-fold increase in PGI_2 production

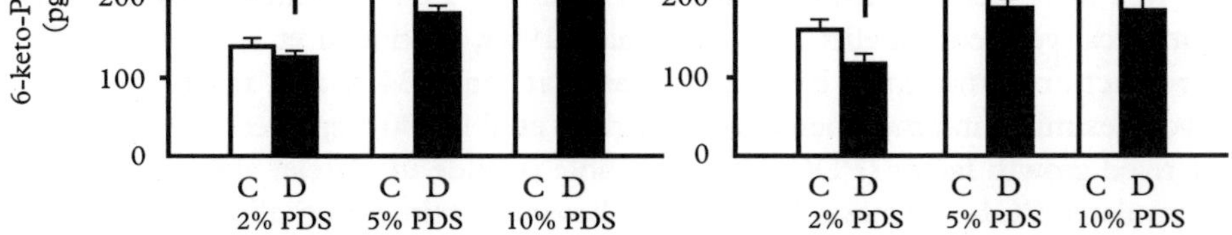

Fig. 2.4 Comparison of 6-keto-$PGF_{1\alpha}$ production by cultured aortic endothelial cells by the addition of plasma-derived serum (PDS) at final concentrations of 2%, 5% and 10% from diabetic patients (D) and controls (C). Rat: streptozotocin-induced diabetic rats (n = 12) and controls (n = 11). Human: noninsulin-dependent diabetes mellitus patients (n = 11) and controls (n = 10). Each experiment was performed in duplicate. Values are given as means ± SEM. *Statistical significance:* * $p < 0.05$, ** $p < 0.01$, *** $p < 0.001$. (Reproduced with permission from Inoguchi et al 1989)

compared with stimulation by plasma alone. Furthermore, they found that platelet extract from patients with noninsulin-dependent diabetes mellitus stimulates PGI_2 production to a greater extent than that from age-matched healthy controls. This might be a compensatory effect for reduced stimulation of PGI_2 production by serum in diabetic patients.

CHARACTERIZATION OF PGI_2-STIMULATORY ACTIVITY IN PLASMA

PGI_2-stimulatory activity (PSA) in PDS was characterized by Inoguchi et al (1989). It is stable at 56°C for 30 min and partially stable at 100°C for 5 min, nondialyzable, resistant to freezing, not extracted by diethyl ether, precipitable with trichloroacetic acid and has no affinity to Con A-Sepharose. Sephadex G50 gel chromatography shows two peaks of PSA, one at 29 kDa and the other at about 17 kDa. Two peaks of PSA are obtained on heparin agarose affinity chromatography, one of which is markedly reduced in PDS from diabetic patients while the other peak is not different between PDS from diabetic patients and control subjects (Fig. 2.5). This reduced PSA in the former peak may be the main factor for reduced PSA in diabetic patients. The latter peak may be responsible for antithrombin III, since PSA of this peak is completely inhibited by antisera against antithrombin III. Yamauchi et al (1989) showed that antithrombin III stimulates PGI_2 production by cultured endothelial cells at physiological concentrations, and that this is inhibited by heparin in a dose-dependent manner.

Many stimulants of PGI_2 production by vascular endothelial cells have been identified. Interleukin-1 induces PGI_2 synthesis in endothelial and smooth muscle cells (Rossi et al 1985). They also found that interleukin-2 and interferons do not stimulate PGI_2 production by these cells. Tumour necrosis factor-α has been reported to stimulate PGI_2 production by vascular endothelial cells, which may play a role in producing decreased blood pressure or shock (Kawakami et al 1986). Transforming growth factor-alpha (TGF-α) as well as epidermal growth factor also stimulate PGI_2 production by human umbilical vein endothelial cells (Ristimaki 1988; Ristimaki et al 1989). PGI_2 production stimulated by TGF-α lasts at least 24 h and is blocked by cycloheximide and indomethacin. Coughlin et al (1980) reported that platelet-derived growth factor (PDGF), a releasable peptide in platelet alpha granules, stimulates PGI_2 synthesis by cultured bovine aortic endothelial cells, aortic smooth muscle and adrenal capillary endothelium. The concentrations of PDGF required to stimulate PGI_2 production are below the levels reported in normal human serum. They postulated that the effect of PDGF on PGI_2 production may be an *in vivo* negative feedback mechanism controlling platelet aggregation. None of these substances, however, seems to correspond to the PGI_2-stimulatory activity in human plasma.

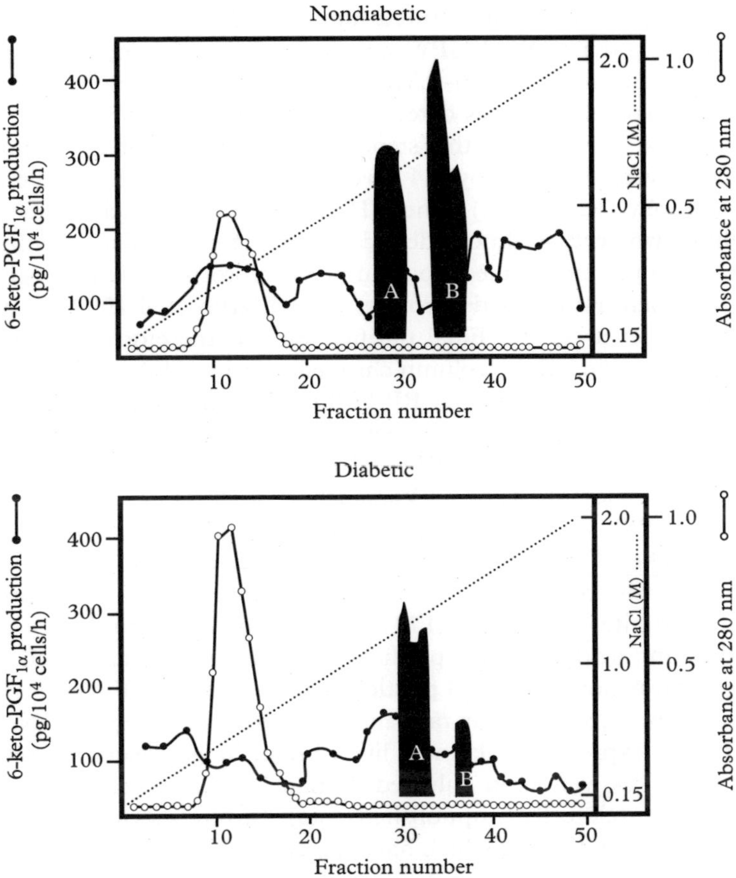

Fig. 2.5 Heparin agarose affinity chromatography of plasma-derived serum (PDS). Individual PDS samples were equally mixed from nondiabetic control subjects (n = 11) or diabetic patients (n = 240). Dialyzed, mixed PDS was then applied to the column. Cultured bovine aortic endothelial cells were incubated in eluted buffer for 60 min and 6-keto-PGF$_{1\alpha}$ concentration in the medium was measured by radioimmunoassay. Shaded areas indicate the separate peaks (indicated by A and B) for PGI$_2$-stimulatory activity (PSA). Note decreased PSA peak B in diabetics. Results are shown as means of two determinations. (Reproduced with permission from Umeda et al 1992)

PURIFICATION OF PGI$_2$-STIMULATORY FACTOR

As described above, the PGI$_2$-stimulatory factor (PSF) has not yet been purified. Our group has tried to purify it from human plasma, but only partial purification of PSF was achieved. Human plasma contains many kinds of proteins and lipids which interfere with the purification of PSF. We found that conditioned medium of human diploid fibroblasts contains PSA on bovine aortic endothelial cells (Yamauchi et al 1994). Therefore, purification of PSF was performed using the material of concentrated serum-free conditioned medium of cultured human diploid fibroblasts by a stepwise chromatography: DEAE-5PW anion exchange column, Heparin-5PW affinity column, and Protein-PAK 300 gel chromatography. After gel filtration, a single band at was detected 31 kDa on SDS polyacrylamide gel electrophoresis. However, at this step, two major peaks, at 28% and 31% acetonitrile, were obtained by C4 reverse-phase high performance liquid chromatography (RP-HPLC). The NH_2-terminal amino acid sequence of one of these two peaks is almost identical to that of insulin-like growth factor (IGF) binding protein purified from human cerebrospinal fluid (Roghani et al 1989), human transformed fibroblast cells (Martin et al 1990) or human serum (Kiefer et al 1991). Final purification was therefore performed by IGF-binding protein affinity column chromatography. After this purification, a single peak was detected by C4 RP-HPLC. The molecular weight of PSF is about 31 kDa. The chemical properties of PSF purified from serum free conditioned medium of human diploid fibroblast are quite different from those substances described above (Yamauchi et al 1994).

Cloning of PSF was performed using a cDNA library of human diploid fibroblasts. The cDNA contained an open reading frame which encodes 282 amino acids from the putative first methionine with a potential N-glycosylation site at position 171. Analysis of hydrophobicity of the deduced amino acid sequence predicts that a hydrophobic stretch of the NH_2-terminal region is a signal peptide. Expression of PSF was examined in several organs from Wistar rats and cultured cells using a cDNA as a probe. PSF is expressed in kidney, liver, brain, lung, skeletal muscle and adipose tissue, as well as in cultured human fibroblasts, endothelial cells and smooth muscle cells (unpublished data). Strong message is observed in kidney and lung, both of which have a greater capacity for prostaglandin synthesis (Christ & van Dorp 1972). Moreover, Western blot analysis showed that human plasma contains this PSF (unpublished data). PSF discovered by our group is a novel peptide present in human plasma. Further studies are needed to evaluate the abnormalities of PSF relative to the pathogenesis of diabetic angiopathy.

CONCLUSION

Prostaglandin metabolism in vascular wall and cultured vascular endothelial cells is reviewed. In diabetes mellitus, PGI_2 production by vascular endothelial cells is reduced, whereas TXA_2 production by platelets is enhanced. Therefore, the imbalance of these potent prostaglandins in vascular wall might lead to the development of diabetic vascular complications, including atherosclerosis. The complete mechanism of altered PGI_2 production in diabetes mellitus is complicated and not completely elucidated, but abnormalities in circulating factors which affect PGI_2 production could play a key role in the altered metabolism of vascular endothelial cells. A novel PSF discovered and cloned by our group is a major candidate as a controlling factor in the prostaglandin abnormalities of diabetes mellitus.

REFERENCES

Aanderud S, Krane K, Nordy A 1985 Influence of glucose, insulin and sera from diabetic patients on prostacyclin synthesis *in vitro* in cultured human endothelial cells. Diabetologia 28: 641-644

Baenziger N L, Force L E, Becherer P R 1980 Histamine stimulates prostacyclin synthesis in cultured human umbilical vein endothelial cells. Biochem Biophys Res Comun 92: 1435-1440

Beitz J, Forster W 1980 Influence of human low density and high density lipoprotein cholesterol on the *in vitro* PGI_2 synthetase activity. Biochim Biophys Acta 620: 352-255

Bicknell R Vallee B L 1989 Angiogenin stimulates endothelial cell prostacyclin secretion by activation of phospholipase A_2. Proc Natl Acad Sci USA 86: 1573-1577

Blasko G, Nemesanszky E, Szabo G et al 1980 The effect of PGI_2 and PGI_2 analogues with increased stability on platelet cAMP content and aggregation. Tromb Res 17: 673-681

Boogaerts M A, Van de Broeck, Deckmyn H et al 1984 Protective effect of vitamin E on immune triggered, granulocyte mediated endothelial injury. Thromb Haemost 51: 89-92

Brock T A, Capasso E A 1988 Thrombin and histamine activate phospholipase C in human endothelial cells via a phorbol ester-sensitive pathway. J Cell Physiol 136: 54-62

Brotherton A F A, Hoak J C 1982 Role of Ca^{2+} and cyclic AMP in the regulation of the production of prostacyclin by the vascular endothelium. Proc Natl Acad Sci USA 79: 495-499

Bunting S, Gryglewski R, Moncada S et al 1976 Arterial walls generate from prostaglandin endoperoxides a substance (prostaglandin X) which relaxes strips of mesenteric and coeliac arteries and inhibits platelet aggregation. Prostaglandins 12: 897-913

Bunting S, Moncada S, Vane J R 1977 Anti-thrombotic properties of vascular endothelium. Lancet 2: 1075-1076

Chan A C, Leith M K 1981 Decreased prostacyclin synthesis in vitamin E-deficient rabbit aorta. Am J Clin Nutr 34: 2341-2347

Chang W-C, Murota S-I, Nakao J et al 1980 Age related decrease in prostacyclin biosynthetic activity in rat aortic smooth muscle cells. Biochim Biophys Acta 620:159-166

Chang W P, Dimitriadis E, Allen T et al 1991 The effect of aldose reductase inhibitors on glomerular prostaglandin production and urinary albumin excretion in experimental diabetes mellitus. Diabetologia 34: 225-231

Christ E J, van Dorp D A 1972 Comparative aspects of prostaglandins. Adv Biosc 9: 35-38

Clark M A, Conway T M, Shorr R G L et al 1987 Identification and isolation of a mammalian protein which is antigenically functionally related to the phospholipase A_2 stimulatory peptide melittin. J Biol Chem 262: 4402-4407

Clark M A, Chen M J, Crooke S T 1988 Tumor necrosis factor (cachectin) induces phospholipase A_2 activity and synthesis of a phospholipase A_2-activating protein in endothelial cells. Biochem J 250: 25-32

Clark M A, Ozgur L E, Conway T M 1991 Cloning of a phospholipase A_2-activating protein. Proc Natl Acad Sci USA 88: 5418-5422

Colwell J A, Lopes-Virella M L, Halushka P V et al 1981 Pathogenesis of atherosclerosis in diabetes mellitus. Diabetes Care 4: 121-133

Coughlin S R, Moskowitz M A, Zetter B R 1980 Platelet-dependent stimulation of prostacyclin synthesis by platelet-derived growth factor. Nature 288: 600-602

Crall F, Roberts W C 1978 The extramural and intramural coronary arteries in juvenile diabetes mellitus. Am J Med 64: 221-230

Craven P A, Caines M A, DeRubertis F R 1987 Sequential alterations in glomerular prostaglandin and thromboxane synthesis in diabetic rats: relationship to the hyperfiltration of early diabetes. Metabolism 36: 95-103

Craven P A, DeRubertis F R 1990 Suppression of urinary albumin excretion in diabetic rats by 4" (imidazol-1-ly) acetophenone, a selective inhibitor of thromboxane synthesis. J Lab Clin Med 16: 469-478

Craven P A, Melhem M F, DeRubertis F R 1992 Thromboxane in the pathogenesis of glomerular injury in diabetes. Kidney Int 42: 937-946

De Caterina R, Weksler B B 1986 Modulation of arachidonic acid metabolism in human endothelial cells by glucocorticoids. Thromb Haemost 55: 369-374

DeRubertis F R, Craven PA 1992 Contribution of platelet thromboxane production to enhanced urinary excretion and glomerular production of thromboxane and to the pathogenesis of albuminuria in the streptozotocin diabetic rats. Metabolism 41: 90-96

Dollery C Z, Friedman L A, Nensby C N et al 1979 Circulating prostacyclin may be reduced in diabetes. Lancet 2: 1365

Dusting G J, Moncada S, Vane J R 1977 Disappearance of prostacyclin in the circulation of the dog. Br J Pharmacol 62: 414-415P

Fielding P E, Vlodavsky I, Gospodarowicz D et al 1979 Effect of contact inhibition on the regulation of cholesterol metabolism in cultured vascular endothelial cells. J Biol Chem 254: 749-755

Fleisher L N, Tall A R, Witte L D et al 1982 Stimulation of arterial endothelial cells prostacyclin synthesis by high density lipoproteins J Biol Chem 257: 6653-6655

Galle J, Luckhoff A, Busse R et al 1990 Low-density lipoprotein stimulate internal free calcium and prostacyclin release in endothelial cells. Eicosanoids 3: 81-86

Gerritsen M E 1987 Functional heterogeneity of vascular endothelial cells. Biochem Pharmacol 36: 2701-2711

Gerrard J M, Stuart M J, Rao G H R et al 1980 Alteration in the balance of prostaglandin and thromboxane synthesis in diabetic rats. J Lab Clin Med 5: 950-958

Gimeno M J, Sterin-Morda L, Borda E S 1980 Human plasma transforms prostacyclin (PGI_2) into a platelet antiaggregatory substance which contracts isolated bovine coronary arteries. Prostaglandins 9: 907-916

Glavind J, Hartmann S, Clemmensen J et al 1952 Studies on the role of lipoperoxides in human pathology. 2. The presence of peroxides lipids in the atherosclerotic aorta. APMIS 30: 1-6

Gryglewski R J, Bunting S, Moncada S et al 1976 Arterial walls are protected against deposition of platelet thrombi by a substance (prostaglandin X) which they make from a prostaglandin endoperoxide. Prostaglandins 2: 685-714

Gryglewski R J, Szczeklik A 1981 Prostacyclin and atherosclerosis. In: Lewis P J, O'Grady J (eds) Clinical Pharmacology of Prostacyclin. Raven Press, New York, pp 88-95

Harrison H E, Reece A H, Johnson M 1978 Decreased vascular prostacyclin in experimental diabetes. Life Sci 23: 351-356

Harrison H E, Reece A H, Johnson M 1980 Effect of insulin treatment on prostacyclin in experimental diabetes. Diabetologia 18: 65-68.

Hora K, Oguchi H, Furukawa T et al 1990 Effects of a selective thromboxane synthetase inhibitor OKY-046 on experimental diabetic nephropathy. Nephron 56: 297-305

Huang N, Lineberger B, Stiner M 1988 Alpha tocopherol, a potent modulator of endothelial cell function. Thromb Res 50: 547-557

Ingerman-Wojenski C, Silver M J, Smith J B et al 1981 Bovine endothelial cells in culture produce thromboxane as well as prostacyclin. J Clin Invest 67: 1292-1296

Inoguchi T, Umeda F, Kunisaki M 1989 Abnormality in prostacyclin stimulatory activity in sera from diabetics. Metabolism 38: 837-842

Inoguchi T, Umeda F, Kunisaki M et al 1991 Platelet stimulation for prostacyclin production in aortic endothelial cell culture: alteration in diabetes mellitus. Horm Metab Res 23: 539-544

Jaffe E A, Grulich J, Weksler B B 1987 Correlation between thrombin-induced prostacyclin production and inositol trisphosphate and cytosolic free calcium levels in cultured human endothelial cells. J Biol Chem 262: 8557-8565

Ishii H, Umeda F, Kunisaki M et al 1989 Modification of prostaglandin synthesis in washed human platelets and cultured bovine aortic endothelial cells by glycosylated low density lipoprotein. Diabetes Res 12: 177-182

Jeremy J Y, Mikhalidis D P, Dandona P 1983 Stimulating the diabetic environment modifies *in vitro* prostacyclin synthesis. Diabetes 32: 217-221

Jeremy J Y, Thompson C S, Mikhailidis D P et al 1985 Experimental diabetes mellitus inhibits prostacyclin synthesis by the rat penis: pathological implications. Diabetologia 28: 365-368

Johnson M, Harrison H E, Raftery A Z 1979 Vascular prostacyclin may be reduced in diabetes in man. Lancet 1: 325-326

Karpen C W, Melora A J, Trewyn R W et al 1981 Modulation of platelet thromboxane A_2 and arterial prostacyclin by dietary vitamin E. Prostaglandins 22: 651-661

Karpen C W, Pritchard Jr K A, Arnold J H et al 1982 Restoration of prostacyclin/thromboxane A_2 balance in diabetic rats. Influence of dietary vitamin E. Diabetes 31: 947-951

Kawakami M, Ishibashi S, Ogawa H 1986 Cachectin/TNF as well as interleukin-1 induces prostacyclin synthesis in cultured vascular endothelial cells. Biochem Biophys Res Commun 141: 482-487

Kaya H, Patton G M, Hong S L 1989 Bradykinin-induced activation of phospholipase A_2 is independent of the activation of polyphosphoinositide-hydrolyzing phospholipase C. J Biol Chem 264: 4972-4977

Kiefer M C, Masearz F R, Bauer D M et al 1991 Identification and molecular cloning of two new 30-kDa insulin-like growth factor binding proteins isolated from adult human serum. J Biol Chem 266: 9043-9049

Kunisaki M, Umeda F, Inoguchi T et al 1989 Effect of vitamin E on prostacyclin production from cultured aortic endothelial cells. Adv Exp Med Biol 242: 113-117

Kunisaki M, Umeda F, Inoguchi T et al 1992 Vitamin E restores reduced prostacyclin synthesis in aortic endothelial cells cultured with a high concentration of glucose. Metabolism 41: 613-621

Kunisaki M, Umeda F, Yamauchi T et al 1993 High glucose reduces specific binding for D-α-tocopherol in cultured aortic endothelial cells. Diabetes 42: 1138-1146

Lo W W Y, Fan T P D 1987 Histamine stimulates inositol phosphate accumulation via the H_1-receptor in cultured human endothelial cells. Biochem Biophys Res Commun 48: 47-53

MacIntyre D E, Pearson J D, Gordon J L 1978 Localization and stimulation of prostacyclin production in vascular cells. Nature 271: 549-551

Martin J L, Willetts K E, Baxter R C 1990 Purification and properties of a novel insulin-like growth factor-2 binding protein from transformed human fibroblasts. J Biol Chem 265: 4124-4130

Moncada S, Gryglewski R, Bunting S et al 1976 An enzyme isolated from arteries transforms prostaglandin endoperoxides to an unstable substance that inhibits platelet aggregation. Nature 263: 663-665

Moncada S, Vane J R 1978 Unstable metabolites of arachidonic acid and their role in haemostasis and thrombosis. Br Med Bull 34: 129-135

Moncada S 1982 Biological importance of prostacyclin. Br J Pharmacol 76: 3-31

Myers T O, Messina E J, Rodrigues A M et al 1985 Altered aortic and cremaster muscle prostaglandin synthesis in diabetic rats. Am J Physiol 257: H1438-1445

Mayhan W G 1989 Impairment of endothelium-dependent dilatation of cerebral arterioles during diabetes mellitus. Am J Physiol 256: H621-625

Mayhan W G, Simmons L K, Sharpe G M et al 1991 Mechanism of impaired responses of cerebral arterioles during diabetes mellitus. Am J Physiol 260: H319-326

Nordoy A, Svensson B, Wiebe D et al 1978 Lipoproteins and the inhibitory effect of human endothelial cells on platelet function. Circulation Res 43: 527-534

Okuma M, Takayama H, Uchino H 1980 Generation of prostacyclin-like substance and lipid peroxidation in vitamin E-deficient rats. Prostaglandins 19: 527-536

Ono H, Umeda F, Inoguchi T et al 1988 Glucose inhibits prostacyclin production by cultured aortic endothelial cells. Thromb Haemost 60: 174-177

Orchard M A, Robinson C 1981 Stability of prostacyclin in human plasma and whole blood: studies on the protective effect of albumin. Thromb Haemost 46: 645-647

Paton R C, Guillot R, Passa P H et al 1982 Prostacyclin production by human endothelial cells cultured in diabetic serum. Diabetes Metab Rev 8: 323-328

Pifer D D, Cagen C H, Chesney C M 1981 Stability of prostaglandin I_2. Prostaglandins 21: 165-175

Ristimaki A, Ylikorkala O, Perheentupa J et al 1988 Epidermal growth factor stimulates prostacyclin production by cultured human vascular endothelial cells. Thromb Haemost 59: 248-250

Ristimaki A 1989 Transforming growth factor a stimulates prostacyclin production by cultured human vascular endothelial cells more potently than epidermal growth factor. Biochem Biophys Res Commun 160: 1100-1105

Ritter J M, Ongari M A, Orchard M A 1983 Prostacyclin synthesis is stimulated by a serum factor formed during coagulation. Thromb Haemost 49: 58-60

Robertson P L, Ar D, Goldstein G W 1990 Phosphoinositide metabolism and prostacyclin formation in retinal microvascular endothelium: stimulation by adenine nucleotides. Exp Eye Res 50: 37-44

Roghani M, Hossenlopp P, Lepage P et al 1989 Isolation from human cerebrospinal fluid of a new insulin-like growth factor-binding protein with a selective affinity for IGF-2. FEBS Lett 255: 253-258

Rossi V, Breviario F, Ghezzi P 1985 Prostacyclin synthesis induced in vascular cells by interleukin-1. Science 229: 174-176

Rothhut B, Russo-Marie F, Wood J et al 1983 Further characterization of the glucocorticoid-induced antiphospholipase protein "renocortin". Biochem Biophys Res Commun 117: 878-884

Salmon J A, Smith D R, Flower R J et al 1978 Further studies on the enzymatic conversion of prostaglandin endoperoxide into prostacyclin by porcine aorta microsomes. Biochim Biophys Acta 523: 250-262

Schambelan M, Blake S, Sraer J et al 1985 Increased prostaglandin production by glomeruli isolated from rats with streptozotocin-induced diabetes mellitus. J Clin Invest 75: 404-412

Seid J M, Jones P B B, Russel R G G 1983 The presence in normal plasma, serum and platelets of factors that stimulate the production of prostacyclin (PGI_2) by cultured endothelial cells. Clin Sci 64: 387-394

Silberbauer K, Schernthaner G, Sinzinger H et al 1979 Decreased vascular prostacyclin in juvenile-onset diabetes. N Engl J Med 300: 366-367

Sinzinger H, Feigl W, Silberbauer K 1979 Prostacyclin generation in atherosclerotic arteries. Lancet 2: 469

Subbiah M T R, Deitemeyer D 1980 Altered synthesis of prostaglandins in platelet and aorta from spontaneously diabetic Wistar rats. Biochem Med Metab Biol 23: 231-235

Sugimoto H, Matsumoto M, Kimura T et al 1980 The effect of vitamin E on prostaglandin metabolism: plasma lipoperoxide and aortic prostacyclin production in vitamin E deficient rats. Journal of the Japanese Atherosclerosis Society 8: 575-578

Tran K, Chan A C 1990 R,R,R-α-tocopherol potentiates prostacyclin release in human endothelial cells. Evidence for structural specificity of the tocopherol molecule. Biochim Biophys Acta 1043: 189-197

Umeda F, Kunisaki M, Inoguchi T et al 1990 Vitamin E enhances prostacyclin production by cultured aortic endothelial cells. J Clin Biochem Nutr 8: 269-277

Umeda F, Inoguchi T, Nawata H 1989 Reduced stimulatory activity on prostacyclin production by cultured endothelial cells in serum from aged and diabetic patients. Atherosclerosis 75: 61-66.

Umeda F, Yamauchi T, Inoguchi T 1992 Partial purification of serum prostacyclin stimulatory activity by heparin-agarose column: abnormality detected in diabetics. Diabetes Res Clin Prac 16: 109-115

Valentovic M A, Lubawy W C 1985 Elevated glucose *in vivo* and *in vitro* adversely alters prostaglandins generation in rat aortas and platelets. Prostaglandins Leukot Med 19: 271-277

van Hinsbergh V W M, Havekes L, Emes J J et al 1983 Low density lipoprotein metabolism by endothelial cells from human umbilical cord arteries and veins. Atherosclerosis 3: 547-559

Watanabe J, Umeda F, Inoguchi T et al 1985 Decreased prostacyclin production and platelet abnormalities in diabetes mellitus. Journal of the Japanese Diabetes Society 28: 1229-1334

Weksler BB, Ley CW, Jaffe EA 1978 Stimulation of endothelial cell prostacyclin production by thrombin, trypsin, and the ionophore A23187. J Clin Invest 62: 923-930

Wey H E, Jakubowski J A, Deykin D 1986 Effect of streptozotocin-induced diabetes on prostaglandin production by rat cerebral microvessels. Thromb Res 42: 527-538

Wu K K, Hatzakis H, Lo S S et al 1988 Stimulation of *de novo* synthesis of prostaglandin G/H synthase in human endothelial cells by phorbol ester. J Biol Chem 263: 3022-3028

Wynalda M A, Fitzpatrick FA 1980 Albumins stabilize prostaglandin I_2. Prostaglandins 20: 853-861

Yamauchi T, Umeda F, Inoguchi T 1989 Antithrombin 3 stimulates prostacyclin production by cultured aortic endothelial cells. Biochem Biophys Res Commun 163: 1404-1411

Yamauchi T, Umeda F, Masakado M et al 1994 (in press) Purification and molecular cloning of prostacyclin-stimulating factor from serum-free conditioned medium of human diploid fibroblast cells. Biochem J

Yui Y, Aoyama T, Morishita H et al 1988 Serum prostacyclin stabilizing factor is to identical apoprotein A-1 (Apo A-1): a novel function of Apo A-1. J Clin Invest 82: 803-807

3

Abnormal antithrombogenic function on endothelial cells in diabetes mellitus

K. Oida, H. Maeda, T. Nakai

INTRODUCTION

Patients with diabetes mellitus have an increased risk of cardiovascular disease, especially myocardial infarction, cerebrovascular disease and peripheral vascular disease, which are major causes of death in them. Such vascular complications are less pronounced in patients who are well-controlled metabolically, and it is therefore assumed that they are not primarily associated with diabetes itself but are rather consequent to associated metabolic disorders. Several components have been investigated as being possibly involved in the generation of these vascular lesions. Among them, an alteration in haemostasis has been extensively studied, including abnormalities in platelet function, increase in blood coagulability and an altered fibrinolytic system. Under basal conditions, the endothelial cell plays an important role in anticoagulation (Fig. 3.1). Once perturbation of the endothelial cell occurs, its surface displays procoagulant function. The endothelial cell synthesizes both prostacyclin (PGI_2) and endothelium-derived relaxing factor (EDRF, identified as nitric oxide), which inhibit platelet activation and vasoconstriction. Plasminogen activator, which initiates blood clot lysis, is synthesized and released constitutively from the endothelium. On the cell surface, heparin-containing proteoglycans function to accelerate antithrombin III-dependent neutralization of many of the serine proteases in the coagulation cascade. Thrombomodulin, a thrombin binding protein on the endothelium, neutralizes thrombin clotting activity and acts as a cofactor for thrombin-catalyzed activation of anticoagulant protein C (Table 3.1).

In this article, we will summarize studies concerning abnormal antithrombogenic function of endothelial cells in diabetes mellitus.

PGI_2 SYNTHESIS IN ENDOTHELIAL CELLS

PGI_2 is potent vasodilator and inhibitor of platelet aggregation. In contrast to PGI_2, thromboxane A_2 (TXA_2) is a vasoconstrictor and potent stimulator of platelet aggregation. A reduction in PGI_2 production and an increase in TXA_2 production have been noted in diabetes mellitus

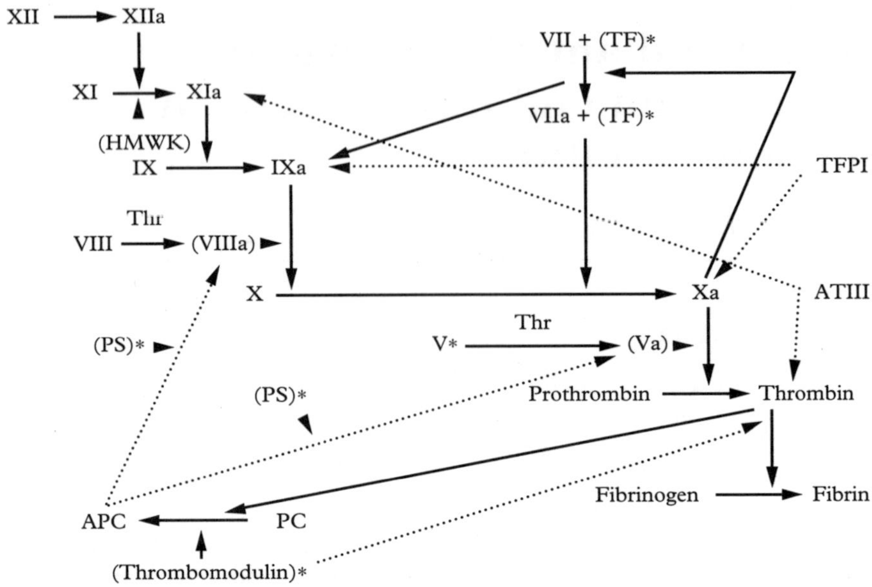

Fig. 3.1 The coagulation cascade showing the intrinsic (factor XII) and the extrinsic pathway (VII + TF), converging on Xa generation. Constituents that are made by vascular endothelium are marked with an asterisk (*). Cofactors are shown in brackets. The natural anticoagulant system in shown with dashed lines. *Abbreviations:* AT III = antithrombin III; APC = activated protein C; PC = protein C; PS = protein S; TF = tissue factor; TFPI = tissue factor pathway inhibitor.

Table 3.1 Antithrombotic and thrombotic factors of endothelial cells.

	Antithrombotic factors	Thrombotic factors
Blood coagulation	Heparin-like compounds (glycosaminoglycan) Antithrombin III (AT III) Thrombomodulin (TM) Protein C (PC) Protein S (PS) Tissue factor pathway inhibitor (TFPI)	Binding of Xa, IXa, Va and fibrinogen Tissue factor (TF) von Willebrand factor (vWF)
Fibrinolysis	Tissue-type plasminogen activator (tPA)	Plasminogen activator inhibitor-1 (PAI-1)
Platelet aggregation	Prostaglandin I_2 (PGI_2) Endothelium-derived relaxing factor (EDRF)	Platelet-activating factor (PAF) Thrombospondin
Vascular tone	PGI_2 EDRF	Endothelin (ET) Angiotensin II (AII)

(Gilbert et al 1983; Harrison et al 1978; Karpen et al 1982; Silberbauer et al 1979; Subbiah & Deitemeyer 1980). However, the precise mechanism of decreased endothelial PGI_2 synthesis in diabetics has not been fully elucidated. The stimulated production of PGI_2 and other prostaglandins by cultured bovine aortic endothelial cells in response to histamine, A23187 (a Ca^{2+} ionophore) or human plasma-derived serum is reduced by the addition of a high glucose concentration (300 mg/dl) [Kunisaki et al 1992]. In addition, supplementation of the culture medium with vitamin E restores the production of PGI_2, prostaglandin E_2 (PGE_2) and TXA_2, products of the cyclooxygenase pathway, but not the production of 15-hydroxyeicosatetraenoate, a product of the lipoxygenase pathway (Kunisaki et al 1992). This suggests that vascular accumulation of lipid peroxides may be a major factor responsible for decreased PGI_2 synthesis in diabetes mellitus (Kunisaki et al 1992). However, there are also several reports in which there is either no change or an increased production of PGI_2 by vascular endothelium exposed to high concentrations of glucose or by isolated vessels from diabetic animals (Aanderud et al 1985; Fujii et al 1986; Jeremy et al 1983). Altered prostaglandin metabolism in the diabetic endothelium is described in detail in another article in this book.

EDRF (NITRIC OXIDE) SYNTHESIS IN ENDOTHELIAL CELLS

The endothelial cell layer is now established as being an important modulator of vascular smooth muscle tone (Fuchgott & Zawadzski 1980). There is one human study in which a defect in endothelium-dependent relaxation of the smooth muscle of the corpora cavernosa from diabetic men has been implicated in the high incidence of impotence associated with diabetes mellitus (De Tejada et al 1989). In chemically-induced diabetes in animals, several studies have demonstrated reduced endothelium-dependent relaxation (Abiru et al 1990; Chang & Stevens 1992; Durante et al 1988; Kamata et al 1989; Mayhan 1989; Mayhan et al 1991; Oyama et al 1986; Pieper & Gross 1988; Tanz et al 1989; Taylor et al 1992; Tesfamariam et al 1991), but others have found no impairment of this response (Head et al 1987; Mulhern & Docherty 1989; Wakabayashi et al 1987; White & Carrier 1986). The reduction of endothelium-dependent relaxation in diabetes can be explained by: 1) a decrease in EDRF release; 2) the release of an endothelium-derived constricting factor arising from the cyclooxygenase pathway; 3) a decreased sensitivity of diabetic vascular smooth muscle to EDRF; 4) an interruption of the diffusion transport/transit time of EDRF from endothelium to the underlying vascular smooth muscle cells; or 5) an increased inactivation of released EDRF by oxygen-derived free radicals. Recent studies by Pieper et al (1992) and Langenstroer and Pieper (1992) demonstrated that diabetic rats release more spontaneous EDRF or similar levels of EDRF in response to acetylcholine compared with control rats, but the activity of EDRF on vascular smooth muscle tone is masked by increased destruction by oxygen-derived free radicals. Since nitric oxide exerts significant inhibitory effects on platelet function (De Graaf et al 1992; Radomski et al 1987) and smooth muscle cell proliferation (Garg & Hassid 1989; O'Connor et al 1991), reduced EDRF activity may contribute to abnormal platelet function and atherosclerosis in diabetes mellitus. Altered vascular tone in diabetes is described in detail in other articles in this book.

FIBRINOLYTIC ACTIVITY

The fibrinolytic system plays a role in several biological phenomena, e.g. tissue repair, malignant transformation, ovulation, embryo implantation. It also plays an important role in the dissolution of blood clots and in the maintenance of a patent vascular system. The fibrinolytic system contains an inactive enzyme, plasminogen, which can be converted to the active enzyme plasmin, which in turn degrades fibrin into soluble fibrin degradation products. Two immunologically distinct types of physiological plasminogen activator have been identified in the blood: tissue-type plasminogen activator (tPA) and urokinase-type plasminogen activator (uPA). uPA, which is derived from pro-urokinase, a single-chain precursor,

Table 3.2 Characteristics of diabetic patients compared with healthy control subjects. All values are given as means ± SD. *Abbreviations:* BMI = body mass index; DBP = diastolic blood pressure; HbA_1 = glycosylated haemoglobin A_1; IDDM = insulin-dependent diabetes mellitus; NIDDM = noninsulin-dependent diabetes mellitus; PAI = plasminogen activator inhibitor; PAP = plasmin-α_2-antiplasmin; SBP = systolic blood pressure; tPA = tissue-type plasminogen activator. *Statistical significance:* *p <0.001; §p <0.01; †p <0.05 comparing IDDM and NIDDM. ‡p <0.001 comparing diabetics with controls. (Reproduced with permission from Auwerx et al 1988)

	Control subjects	All diabetics	IDDM	NIDDM
No.	57	62	29	33
Men/women	31/26	35/27	17/12	18/15
Age (y)	52 ± 12	52.7 ± 15.8	40.8 ± 13.1	63.1 ± 9.4*
BMI (kg/m²)	-	25.8 ± 3.7	23.8 ± 2.6	27.6 ± 3.6*
SBP (mmHg)	-	147.7 ± 20.9	137.7 ± 16.2	156.6 ± 20.7
DBP (mmHg)	-	86.4 ± 10.5	84.1 ± 9.6	88.4 ± 10.9
Diabetes duration (y)	-	11.0 ± 8.9	13.4 ± 9.7	8.8 ± 7.6†
Insulin dosage (U/day)	-	29.9 ± 20.9	40.6 ± 17.3	20.4 ± 19.4*
PAP (nmol/l)	-	1.2 ± 0.5	1.2 ± 0.5	1.2 ± 0.5
HbA_1 (%)	6.8 ± 0.6	10.5 ± 1.9‡	10.4 ± 2.1‡	10.5 ± 1.7‡
Fibrinogen (g/l)	1.5 ± 0.3	2.2 ± 0.5‡	2.1 ± 0.4‡	2.3 ± 0.6‡
Euglobulin fibrinolytic activity (ng/ml)	1.7 ± 1.2	1.2 ± 0.7‡	1.4 ± 0.8	0.9 ± 0.5§,‡
tPA (ng/ml)	6.6 ± 2.9	15.7 ± 8.4‡	10.7 ± 5.2‡	20.0 ± 8.3*,‡
PAI (IU/ml)	1.5 ± 0.7	2.6 ± 1.3‡	1.8 ± 0.9‡	3.3 ± 1.2*,‡

Table 3.3 Multiple regression analysis of plasminogen activator inhibitor activity. The independent variables included in the regression model were: age, BMI, SBP, DBP, diabetes duration, insulin dosage, HbA_1, PAP, fibrinogen and fibrin plate assay. *Abbreviations:* b = partial regression coefficient; BMI = body mass index; DBP = diastolic blood pressure; HbA_1 = glycosylated haemoglobin A_1; IDDM = insulin-dependent diabetes mellitus; NIDDM = non-insulin-dependent diabetes mellitus; PAP = plasmin-α_2-antiplasmin; r_p = partial correlation coefficient; R^2 = coefficient of determination (percent variance explained by the model); SBP = systolic blood pressure. *Statistical significance:* *p <0.001; †p <0.01 for regression slopes. (Reproduced with permission from Auwerx et al 1988)

	Total group (n = 62)		IDDM (n = 29)		NIDDM (n = 33)	
	b	r_p	b	r_p	b	r_p
Constant	-1.49		-2.81		-0.55	
BMI	0.19	0.59*	-	-	0.17	0.59*
Fibrin plate assay	-6.11	-0.42*	-	-	-9.91	-0.51†
DBP	-	-	0.05	0.59†	-	-
R^2	0.50		0.35		0.49	

mediates extravascular proteolysis associated with inflammation and cell migration. tPA, which is produced in endothelium, mediates intravascular fibrinolysis. Inhibition of the fibrinolytic system may occur at the level of either plasminogen activator by specific plasminogen activator inhibitors (PAI-1 and PAI-2) or at the level of plasmin by α_2-antiplasmin. PAI-1 is the primary inhibitor of tPA and uPA. A dynamic equilibrium exists between tPA and PAI-1 on the luminal surface of vessels that determines net local fibrinolytic activity. PAI-1, a serine protease synthesized by the liver and endothelium, is released from activated platelet α-granules. Platelets contain about 90% of the immunoreactive PAI-1 present in plasma. PAI-1 activity is rapidly cleared from circulation by the liver (half-life is 7 min in the rabbit). An increase in PAI-1 expression, a decrease in the tPA expression or both lead to decreased net fibrinolytic activity and predispose to thrombosis (Collen & Lijnen 1991).

Spontaneous fibrinolytic activity is reported to be normal or low in diabetic patients (Almer & Nilsson 1974; Almer et al 1982; Sharma 1981), while release of plasminogen activator from the endothelium is abnormal in some cases (Almer & Nilsson 1975; Fearnly et al 1963). It has been shown that elevated tPA antigen levels in poorly-controlled diabetic patients can be decreased by insulin administration (Juhan-Vague et al 1984). Auwerx et al (1988) examined various fibrinolytic parameters, including euglobulin fibrinolytic activity, tPA antigen, PAI activity and plasmin-α_2-antiplasmin complex in 62 patients with either insulin-dependent (IDDM) or noninsulin-dependent (NIDDM) diabetes mellitus (Table 3.2). Diabetic patients had a significantly lower euglobulin fibrinolytic activity but significantly higher tPA antigen and PAI levels than healthy controls. Body mass index (BMI) was significantly correlated with

PAI activity in the total diabetic population and in the NIDDM group. However, the altered concentrations of tPA and PAI were not correlated with the HbA_1 level, suggesting their independence from diabetic control (Table 3.3). Because of the strong correlation of BMI with PAI activity in NIDDM patients, they argued that hyperinsulinism rather than insulin deficiency may be associated with the decreased fibrinolytic activity, and that the same mechanism might be operative in insulin-treated IDDM patients because they are in a state of therapeutic hyperinsulinism. In addition to diabetes, diminished plasma fibrinolytic activity has also been found in obesity (Juhan-Vague et al 1987; Landin et al 1990; Vague et al 1986), hypertension (Jansson et al 1991) and hypertriglyceridaemia (Juhan-Vague et al 1987; Landin et al 1990; Vague et al 1986). In these other conditions, consistent increases in both PAI-1 protein and functional PAI-1 activity have been associated with increased plasma immunoreactive insulin (IRI) [Juhan-Vague et al 1991]. Both the administration of metformin, a biguanide that decreases peripheral insulin resistance, and fasting have been found to decrease plasma IRI and PAI-1 in nondiabetic obese and in hypertensive patients (Juhan-Vague et al 1987; Vague et al 1987). However, a study by Landin et al (1991) found that treating insulin

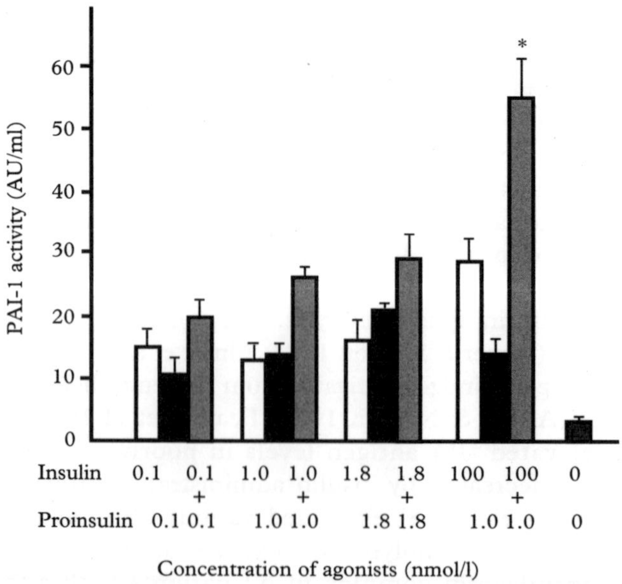

Fig. 3.2 Expression of PAI-1 activity in 24-h conditioned media of porcine aortic endothelial cells after exposure to various concentrations insulin and/or proinsulin. Values are given as means ± SEM. *Statistical significance:* * $p < 0.02$ compared with both insulin alone and proinsulin alone. (Reproduced with permision from Schneider et al 1992)

Table 3.4 Activation of plasminogen from healthy subjects by tissue-type plasminogen activator (tPA) from healthy subjects and by tPA from diabetic patients in the presence of CNBr fragments of fibrinogen (55 μg/ml). Kinetic constants were calculated for the period of maximal and constant plasmin formation, which occurred with controls and with tPA from diabetic patients after improvement of metabolic parameters after a 'lag period' of slow and increasing plasmin formation. *Symbol*: 1 = diabetic tPA before and after normalisation of metabolic parameters. (Reproduced with permission from Geiger & Binder 1988)

	Control tPA	Diabetic tPA	
		before[1]	after[1]
Km (μmol/l)	0.09	7.5	0.048
K_{cat} (sec^{-1})	0.05	0.05	0.03
K_{cat}/Km ($mmol/l^{-1} \cdot sec^{-1}$)	0.55	0.007	0.62
'Lag period' (min)	5-15	>120	pt 1: 53-88 pt 2: 12-18 pt 3: 89-161

resistance in hypertensive patients with metformin increased tPA activity without affecting PAI-1.

In vitro experiments have shown that secretion of PAI-1 protein and PAI-1 mRNA are increased in human hepatoma (HepG2) cells exposed to insulin concentrations similar to or higher than those found in plasma of patients with insulin resistance, such as NIDDM (Alessi et al 1988; Kooistra et al 1989; Schneider & Sobel 1991). Insulin increases PAI-1 mRNA expression by decreasing its degradation without affecting the rate of transcription (Fattal et al 1992). It also has been found that insulin increased PAI-1 secretion in porcine aortic endothelial cells without being accompanied by an increase in PAI-1 mRNA (Fig. 3.2). This appears to be mediated through the insulin receptor and tyrosine kinase. Proinsulin also increased secretion of PAI-1 but this was not accompanied by an increase in PAI-1 mRNA (Schneider & Sobel 1993; Schneider et al 1992). It is possible that increased plasma insulin and/or proinsulin levels may account for the impairment of fibrinolytic activity in NIDDM.

In another recent clinical study, coagulation and fibrinolytic parameters were assessed in 40 IDDM patients (Carmassi et al 1992). Diabetic patients had lower tPA activity than healthy controls. Activated partial thromboplastin time, prothrombin time and functional activities of antithrombin III (AT III), protein C, plasminogen and α_2-antiplasmin were in the normal range, whereas concentrations of fibrinogen, factor VII, thrombin-antithrombin complexes and PAI-1 activity were increased. It is possible that nonenzymatic glycosylation of tPA reduces its activity in IDDM. Geiger and Binder (1988) compared the activation of plasminogen (from healthy subjects) by tPA from healthy subjects versus tPA from metabolically-uncontrolled IDDM patients. The activity of tPA from uncontrolled diabetic patients was decreased (Table 3.4). Decreased plasminogen activity (activity as a substrate for tPA) was also observed for diabetic patients. Since decreased activity of diabetic tPA and plasminogen was much more pronounced than that of tPA and plasminogen from healthy subjects which were glycosylated *in vitro*, they argued that additional events may be important *in vivo*, e.g. different metabolism of the glycosylated and nonglycosylated forms. This result supports the findings that improved glycaemic control in diabetic patients corrects abnormal tPA activity as well as abnormal plasmin levels (Small et al 1987).

uPA mediates the focal proteolysis of extracellular components, consisting of collagen, laminin, fibronectin, elastin, vitronectin and fibrinogen. uPA and plasmin are the primary catalytic activators of latent metalloproteinases, such as collagenase, which are responsible for the proteolysis of extracellular matrix proteins (Kwann 1992). Through activation of collagenase, uPA might modulate collagen deposition, resulting in capillary basement membrane thickening, which is a characteristic of diabetic microangiopathy. Miskin et al (1990) generated a transgenic mouse with selective organ-specific expression of human uPA by introducing a fusion gene of a 2.4-kb fragment of human uPA cDNA and a 409-bp fragment of the murine ocular lens protein α A-crystallin. The presence of the lens α A-crystallin gene resulted in the selected enhanced expression of uPA in the retina, brain and bone marrow, but not in other organs, such as the kidney. The transgenic mice revealed increased fibrinolytic activity in the eye but not in the kidneys. When experimental diabetes was induced in these mice with streptozotocin, microvascular changes of basement membrane thickening took place in the renal glomerular capillaries but not in the retinal vessels (Miskin & Levinger 1991). These results support the concept that local uPA activity, especially in the capillaries, intervenes in the development of diabetic microangiopathy.

Browlee et al (1983) demonstrated that nonenzymatic glycosylation reduced the susceptibility of fibrin to degradation by the specific fibrinolytic enzyme, plasmin. Experimental conditions that increased the rate of nonenzymatic glycation (higher concentration of glucose or glucose-6-phosphate) were associated with correspondingly greater degrees of resistance to degradation by plasmin. They argued that such reduced degradation of nonenzymatically glycosylated proteins *in vivo* may contribute to the accumulation of fibrin and several other proteins observed in those tissues which are most frequently affected by diabetic complications.

HEPARIN-AT III SYSTEM

AT III, synthesized by the liver, is a glycoprotein inhibitor that functions by neutralizing coagulation proteases by forming a 1:1 complex with inhibitors. The reaction probably accounts for the major mechanism of inhibition of thrombin and factor XIa, but the reaction is slow without heparin. Heparin accelerates the reaction about 1,000 fold. As a result, AT III must be present for its function as an effective anticoagulant. With thrombin, optimal rates of inactivation require the simultaneous interaction of heparin with AT III and thrombin. However, naturally-occurring heparin is only found at low levels in blood, whereas the vascular endothelium is rich in heparin-containing proteoglycans. These heparin-containing proteoglycans may contribute to the accelerated inhibition of some coagulation proteases (Comp & Esmon 1991).

Alteration of AT III has been implicated in the development of diabetic vascular complications (Banerjee et al 1974). Inhibition of AT III *in vitro* by nonenzymatic glycation has been demonstrated (Browlee et al 1984; Busby & Ingham 1984; Ceriello et al 1984). Clinical studies on AT III in diabetic patients have provided evidence for a reduction in the biological activity of AT III despite normal plasma AT III concentrations (Ceriello et al 1983). It is reported that the degree of reduction in AT III activity is related to the level of the HbA_1, fasting plasma glucose or glycated proteins, suggesting a role for nonenzymatic glycosylation in determining this effect *in vivo* (Sowers et al 1980). Moreover, there is an increase of AT III activity when good long-term glycaemic control is maintained in diabetic patients (Ceriello et al 1986).

Recently Witmer et al (1992) have examined the distribution and behavior of the rabbit plasma proteins, such as albumin, fibrinogen and AT III (isoforms α and β), by injecting intravenously radiolabelled preparations in groups of alloxan-induced diabetic rabbits and control rabbits. The fractional catabolic rates of both AT III-α and AT III- β were similar in diabetic and control rabbits, but fibrinogen and albumin were catabolized more slowly in diabetic than in control rabbits. At 12 h after injection, the quantities of fibrinogen and albumin associated with endothelium, and particularly the subendothelium, of the diabetic aorta were increased, whereas AT III-α and AT III-β were decreased, resulting a 2- to 3-fold increase of the fibrinogen to AT III ratio compared with controls (Table 3.5) They argued that the increased ratio of fibrinogen to AT III in the acrostic wall may be characteristic of the prothrombotic state that is conspicuous in IDDM.

De Feo et al (1993) examined the synthesis of hepatic proteins, including leucine kinetics and fractional synthetic rates of albumin, fibrinogen, AT III and apolipoprotein B-100 (apo B-100). A 3- to 4-fold increment in basal plasma insulin concentration increased albumin synthesis (+1.0%), did not affect apo B-100 synthesis, and decreased fibrinogen (-5%), AT III synthesis (-12%) and the estimates of whole-body protein synthesis (nonoxidative leucine disposal) [-18%] in humans. They argued that the reduction in fibrinogen and AT III synthesis could be

Table 3.5 Plasma thrombomodulin concentration in control subjects and diabetic patients. *Abbreviations:* NDR = nondiabetic retinopathy; NPDR = nonproliferative diabetic retinopathy; PDR = proliferative diabetic retinopathy; PPDR = pre-proliferative diabetic retinopathy. *Statistical significance:* a, p <0.005; b, p <0.001. (Reproduced with permission from Oida et al 1990)

	Number	Thrombomodulin (ng/ml)
Control subjects	45	32.8 ± 6.5
Diabetic patients	106	40.1 ± 22.4
Proteinuria		
without proteinuria	81	33.6 ± 9.5
with proteinuria	25	61.0 ± 36.0
Retinopathy in all diabetic patients		
NDR	50	32.4 ± 8.9
NPDR	27	33.5 ± 12.9
PPDR	10	63.4 ± 28.9
PDR	19	57.4 ± 34.7
Retinopathy in diabetic patients without proteinuria		
NDR	47	32.2 ± 8.8
NPDR	20	31.9 ± 7.8
PPDR	4	41.5 ± 4.4
PDR	10	41.0 ± 12.8

(Significance brackets: Control vs Diabetic, a; without vs with proteinuria, a; Control vs with proteinuria, a; all diabetic patients: NDR vs PPDR, b; NPDR vs PPDR, b; NDR vs PDR, b; NPDR vs PDR, a; without proteinuria: NDR vs PPDR, a; NPDR vs PPDR, a; NDR vs PDR, a; NPDR vs PDR, a)

caused directly by a negative effect of insulin on protein synthesis or indirectly by insulin-induced changes in amino acid availability. They also speculated that during insulin deficiency the AT III fractional synthesis rate probably increases, which is compensated by protein overconsumption in diabetics, and accounts for the normal plasma concentrations of AT III found in these patients.

THROMBOMODULIN-PROTEIN C REACTION

Thrombomodulin is an endothelial cell membrane glycoprotein, which forms a 1:1 complex with thrombin. This complex activates protein C catalytically, and activated protein C dissociates rapidly from the activation complex. Activated protein C is selectively inactivated by coagulation cofactors Va and VIIIa. For activated protein C to function effectively, it must interact with protein S bound to cell surfaces. This interaction facilitates activated protein C binding to platelets and endothelial cell surfaces. Then, cell-surface-bound protein C-protein S complex inactivates factors Va and VIIIa. Thrombomodulin also directly inhibits the procoagulant activities of thrombin, which include cleavage of fibrinogen to fibrin and platelet activation (Comp & Esmon 1991).

Decreased protein C levels in patients with diabetes (IDDM) has been reported (Vukovich & Schernthaner 1986). Recently, Ceriello et al (1990) examined both protein C antigen level and its biological activity in 30 IDDM patients. Both protein C antigen (0.86 IU/ml *vs* 1.12 IU /ml, p

<0.001) and activity (85.73% *vs* 105.4%, p <0.001) were significantly lower than those of matched controls. An inverse correlation between fasting plasma glucose and both protein C concentration and activity was present. Moreover, induction of hyperglycaemia in diabetic patients and healthy subjects decreased both protein C mass and activity. On the contrary, euglycaemia obtained by insulin infusion in diabetic patients restored depressed protein C levels to normal. These results stress the major role of hyperglycaemia in determining protein C decrease in diabetic patients, although the mechanism is obscure.

At present, there are no studies concerning altered expression of endothelial thrombomodulin in diabetes. The expression of thrombomodulin in endothelial cells is reported to be influenced by various stimuli. Endotoxin (Moor et al 1989), interleukin-1 (Hirokawa & Aoki 1991; Nawroth et al 1986), tumour necrosis factor-α (Conway & Rosenberg 1988; Ishii et al 1992; Lentz et al 1991; Nawroth & Stern 1986) decrease thrombomodulin antigen levels in endothelium. In contrast, up-regulation of thrombomodulin antigen in endothelial cells is obtained when the cells are incubated with phorbol ester for more than 6 hours (Dittman et al 1988; Hirokawa & Aoki 1990), dibutyryl cyclic AMP (Hirokawa & Aoki 1990; Ishii et al 1990a), histamine (Hirokawa & Aoki 1991) or tretinoin (retinoic acid) [Horie et al 1992; Ishii et al 1992].

We have examined the effect of insulin and high glucose concentration on thrombomodulin antigen levels in endothelial cells. Cultured human umbilical vein endothelial cells were incubated with insulin (10 μmol/l), (insulin-like growth factor) IGF-1 (100 nmol/l) or high glucose concentration (29 mmol/l) for 18 h. The amount of thrombomodulin antigen of the cells was then determined by a sandwich enzyme immunoassay on 96-well microtitre plates using purified placental thrombomodulin as a standard (Ishii et al 1990b). However, no significant changes of thrombomodulin levels were observed (Fig. 3.3). Incubation with high glucose concentration may induce nonenzymatic glycosylation of thrombomodulin, resulting its altered biological activity, but this possibility has not yet been examined.

PLASMA SOLUBLE THROMBOMODULIN LEVELS IN DIABETES

Thrombomodulin is an integral membrane protein and does not dissociate from the cell surface under normal physiological conditions. It is detectable in culture medium when endothelial cells are damaged by endotoxin during *in vitro* experiments (Ishii et al 1991). Various soluble forms of thrombomodulin have been found with different electrophoretic mobilities (Ishii & Majerus 1985; Yamamoto et al 1993). Although the physiological significance of circulating thrombomodulin has not yet been sufficiently evaluated, it may reflect the release of soluble thrombomodulin into the circulation from damaged endothelial cells.

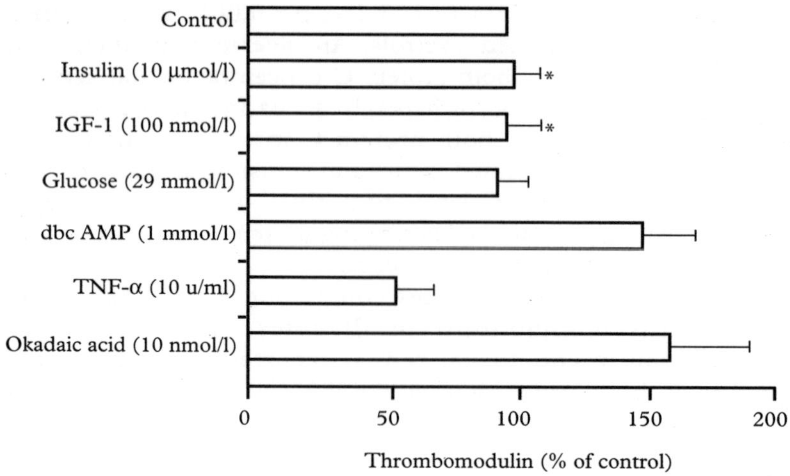

Fig. 3.3 Effects of various agents on thrombomodulin content in human umbilical vein endothelial cells. Values are given as means ± SEM. *Statistical significance:* * p <0.05 *vs* untreated control.

Increased concentrations of plasma thrombomodulin have been reported in diabetic patients by several laboratories including ourselves (Iwashima et al 1990; Oida et al 1990; Tanaka et al 1991), as well as in patients with collagen disease and disseminated intravascular coagulation (Takahashi et al 1992). From our results, elevated plasma thrombomodulin levels in diabetes primarily reflect the presence and degree of nephropathy, because they were especially elevated in diabetic patients with renal failure (Table 3.5) and were strongly positively correlated with serum creatinine levels ($r = 0.78$, $p < 0.001$), urinary albumin excretion ($r = 0.68$, $p < 0.001$) and urinary β_2-microglobulin ($r = 0.64$, $p < 0.001$). Moreover, thrombomodulin clearance (expressed as urinary thrombomodulin concentration × urine volume/plasma thrombomodulin) shows a strong positive correlation with creatinine clearance, suggesting plasma thrombomodulin excretion. Even after excluding the patients with proteinuria, a slight but significant increase of thrombomodulin was still present in patients with preproliferative and proliferative retinopathy. This increase may reflect endothelial damage and/or early-stage nephropathy. Elevation of plasma thrombomodulin is also found in diabetic patients with microalbuminuria but not in those without microalbuminuria (Iwashima et al 1990).

TISSUE FACTOR PATHWAY INHIBITOR

Initiation of blood coagulation via the extrinsic pathway occurs when tissue factor (TF) is exposed to plasma. The resulting factor VIIa-TF complex then proteolytically activates factors IX and X. Physiological regulation of this pathway is mediated by a specific factor Xa-dependent inhibitor of the factor VIIa-TF complex, which has been termed lipoprotein-associated coagulation inhibitor (LACI), extrinsic pathway inhibitor (EPI) or tissue factor inhibitor (TFI). This factor is now denoted as tissue factor pathway inhibitor (TFPI). Normal plasma TFPI concentration is about 2.5 nmol/l, which is a quarter of the plasma concentration of factor VII and almost 1/1,000th the concentration of antithrombin. However, plasma TFPI is not the major intravascular pool of TFPI. A larger intravascular pool has been identified on the luminal surface of vascular endothelium. A bolus injection of heparin releases TFPI from this pool and causes plasma TFPI levels to rise transiently by 2- to 10-fold. Cultured endothelial cells secrete TFPI, and vascular endothelium is thought to be the primary site of synthesis of plasma TFPI. TFPI circulates in human plasma associated with lipoproteins.

TFPI seems to function as a natural anticoagulant to protect humans from potential thrombotic complications of common experiences of living

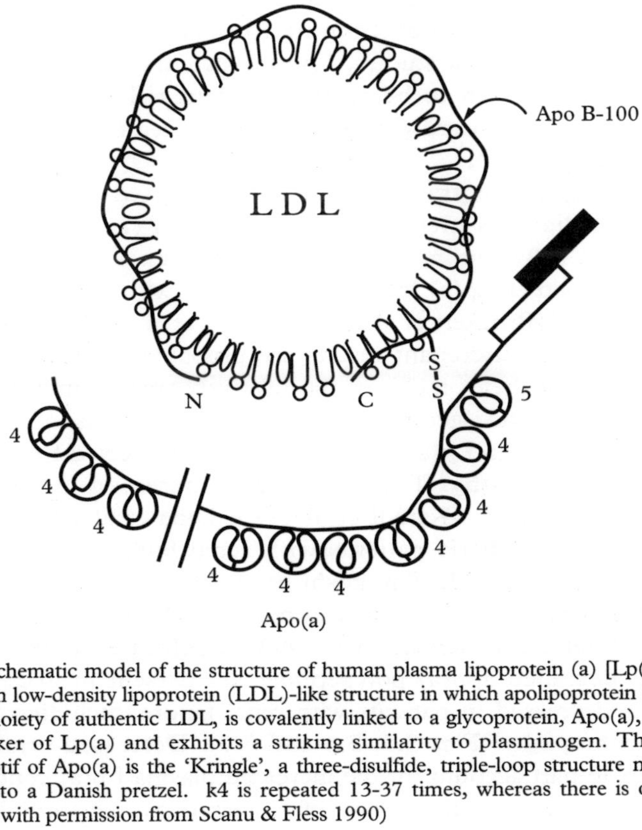

Fig. 3.4 Schematic model of the structure of human plasma lipoprotein (a) [Lp(a)]. Lp(a) is made up of an low-density lipoprotein (LDL)-like structure in which apolipoprotein (Apo) B100, the protein moiety of authentic LDL, is covalently linked to a glycoprotein, Apo(a), which is the specific marker of Lp(a) and exhibits a striking similarity to plasminogen. The dominant structural motif of Apo(a) is the 'Kringle', a three-disulfide, triple-loop structure named for its resemblance to a Danish pretzel. k4 is repeated 13-37 times, whereas there is only one k5. (Reproduced with permission from Scanu & Fless 1990)

that may cause the circulating blood to be exposed to low concentration of tissue factor, e.g. moderate illness that stimulates cytokine production, transient Gram-negative bacteraemia after cytoscopy or other endoscopic procedures, normal birth (Rapaport & Rao 1992). So far, there have been no studies on TFPI in diabetes mellitus.

LIPOPROTEIN(A)

Lipoprotein(a) [Lp(a)] has been shown to be associated with coronary atherosclerosis. Lp(a) is composed of one low-density lipoprotein particle to which one molecule of apolipoprotein(a) [Apo(a)] is covalently linked to the Apo B moiety. Apo(a) shares extensive homology with plasminogen, and the gene for Apo(a) is located adjacent to that of plasminogen. Thus, Lp(a) can compete with plasminogen in impairing several fibrinolytic functions, including binding with fibrin, with plasminogen receptors on the endothelial surface, and with heparin-bound tPA (Figure 3.4). Plasma concentrations of Lp(a) and the molecular mass of Apo(a) vary between individuals and appear to be largely determined genetically, in part because of increased copies of Kringle IV-like domains within the Apo(a) gene. However, the Apo(a) gene accounts for only 40% of plasma Lp(a) concentrations. In several studies, Lp(a) concentrations exceeding 20-30 mg/dl have been shown to be an independent risk factor for coronary atherosclerosis and myocardial infarction (Rader & Brewer 1992; Scanu & Fless 1990; Scott 1991).

Plasma Lp(a) concentrations have been reported to be increased in patients with diabetes mellitus in some studies (Levitsky et al 1991; Winocour et al 1991) but not in others (Klausen et al 1992; Schernthaner et al 1983). Whether Lp(a) levels are correlated with glycaemic control is also controversial (Bruckert et al 1990; Haffner et al 1991, 1992b; Ramirez et al 1992). These discrepant results are probably due to the metabolic heterogeneity of diabetes mellitus, the relatively small number of patients examined, and the wide-genetically determined variations in plasma Lp(a) concentrations. Plasma Lp(a) levels are especially affected by the presence of diabetic nephropathy. They are clearly increased in patients with impaired renal function (Karádi et al 1989; Oida et al 1992; Parra et al 1987), including diabetic patients with renal failure and/or nephrosis (Guillausseau et al 1992; Takegoshi et al 1990). Moreover, increased plasma Lp(a) levels was also found in both IDDM and NIDDM patients with microalbuminuria (Jenkins et al 1992; Kapelrud et al 1991). We have found that degraded apo(a) polypeptides are present in urine and their excretion is decreased in patients with renal failure, including those with diabetic nephropathy (Figs 3.5, 3.6 and 3.7). Decreased urinary loss of Apo(a) may in part account for the increased plasma Lp(a) concentrations seen in renal failure, as in the case of increased plasma thrombomodulin

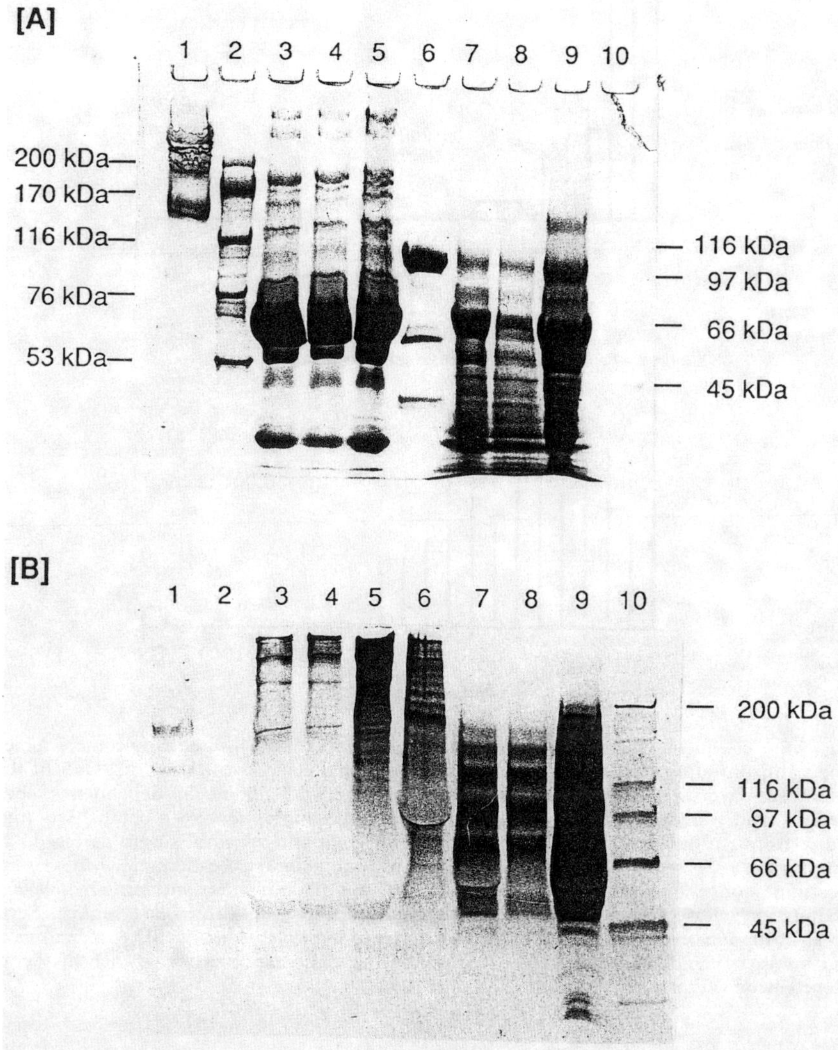

Fig. 3.5 Detection of apolipoprotein(a) [Apo(a)] by Western blotting. Samples were electrophoretically separated under reducing conditions on 4-12% gradient polyacrylamide gels. [**A**], gel stained with Coomassie Brilliant Blue R-250; [**B**], immunoblotting of identical nitrocellulose-paper transfers incubated with anti-Apo(a) antibodies after immunodetection with the Vectastain system. Lane 1, 10 μg of low-density lipoprotein; lane 2, Pharmacia HMW-SDS calibration kit as negative control; lanes 3-5, serum; lane 6, plasminogen; lanes 7-9, urine dialyzed against saline and concentrated ~80 fold; lane 10, Bio-Rad Biotinylated SDS-PAGE standards (high range) as markers. Samples in lanes 3 and 7, 4 and 8, and 5 and 9 are from the same person. Plasminogen (lane 6, from Sigma) contained immunodetectable Apo(a). (Reproduced with perssion from Oida et al 1992)

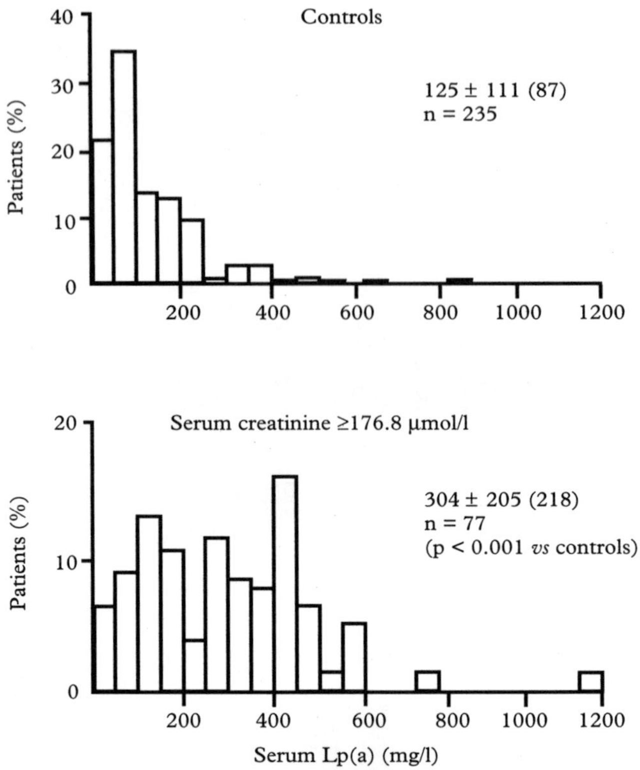

Fig. 3.6 Frequency distribution of serum lipoprotein(a) [Lp(a)] in healthy control subjects (top) and patients with renal dysfunction (bottom). As control subjects, 235 healthy volunteers were used. Blood samples from 43 patients with noninsulin-dependent diabetes mellitus who were admitted to our hospital and 111 samples sent to a clinical laboratory centre from various hospitals for measurement of creatinine clearance were assessed. The samples were separated into two groups: those with obvious renal dysfunction whose serum creatinine concentrations were ≥176.8 μmol/l (2 mg/dl) and those without obvious renal dysfunction whose serum creatinine concentrations were ≤88.4 μmol/l (1 mg/dl). Serum Lp(a) of the former group was compared with that of controls. Mean ± SD (median) values and number of individuals are indicated in the top right-hand corner of each histogram. (Reproduced with permission from Oida et al 1992)

levels in renal failure. Recently, it has been shown that Apo(a) isoform frequencies were apparently the same in both IDDM and NIDDM patients compared with controls (Császár et al 1993). These findings do not exclude the possibility that Lp(a) may be increased in patients with nephropathy, in whom coronary artery disease frequently co-exists, or that Lp(a) at a given concentration is more atherogenic in diabetic patients than in those without diabetes mellitus. However, it has been reported that there was no association between Lp(a) concentrations and coronary heart disease mortality in diabetes (Haffner et al 1992a).

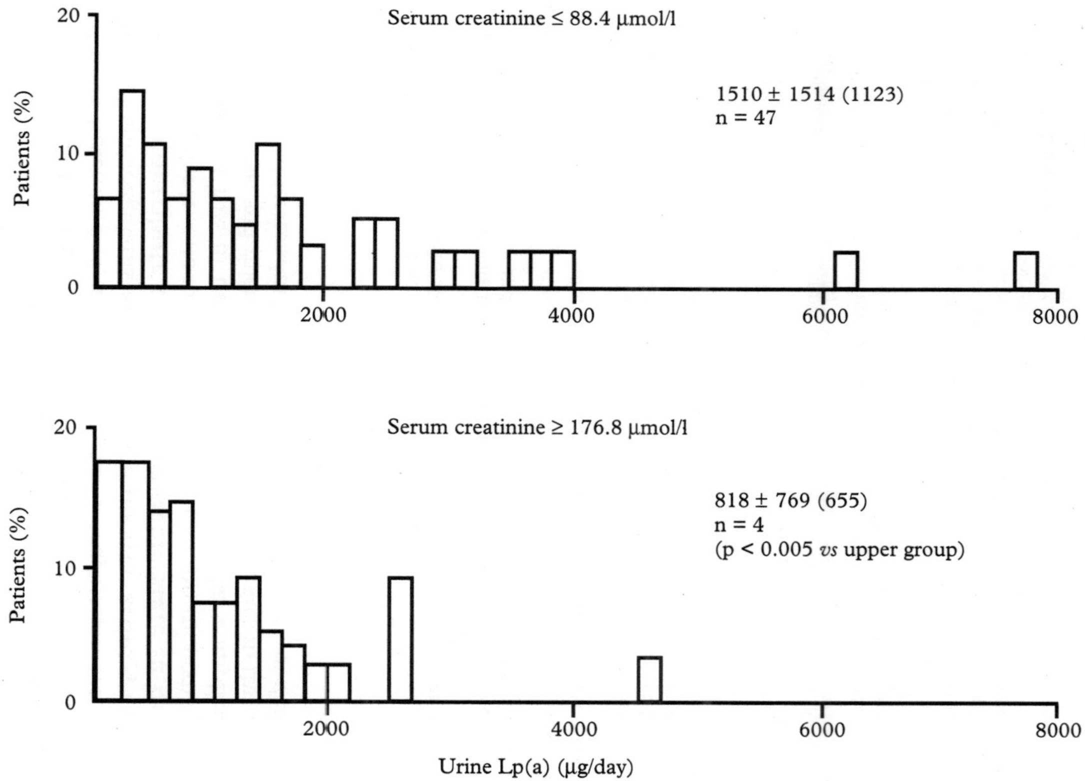

Fig. 3.7 Frequency distribution of daily urinary lipoprotein(a) [Lp(a)] excretion in patients with serum creatinine ≤88.4 µmol/l (top) and ≥176.8 µmol/l (bottom). The patients are the same as described in figure 3.6. Mean ± SD (median) values and number of individuals are indicated in the top right-hand corner of each histogram. (Reproduced with permission from Oida et al 1992)

CONCLUSION

The endothelial cell has multiple mechanisms for controlling its coagulant status. These are under tight control, with the cell being capable of sustaining reciprocal changes in function that work synergistically. The vascular endothelium, which is an anticoagulant surface under basal conditions, may change its state and provide a potent template for the generation of thrombin in people with diabetes. In addition to abnormal platelet function and increases in several coagulation factors, decreases in natural anticoagulants and impaired fibrinolytic activity, as described here, possibly contribute to a hypercoagulable state in diabetes. Such a hypercoagulable state may cause the increased thromboembolic risk and play an important role in the pathogenesis of vascular complications, including atherosclerosis and microangiopathy. Further studies in this field may lead to our better understanding of these major complications of diabetes.

REFERENCES

Aanderud S, Krane H, Nordoy A 1985 Influence of glucose, insulin and sera from diabetic patients on prostacyclin synthesis *in vitro* in cultured human endothelial cells. Diabetologia 28: 641-644

Abiru T, Kamata K, Miyata N et al 1990 Differences in vascular responses to vasoactive agents of basilar artery and aorta from rabbits with alloxan-induced diabetes. Can J Physiol Pharmacol 68: 882-888

Alessi M C, Juhan-Vague I Kooistra T et al 1988 Insulin stimulates the synthesis of plasminogen activator inhibitor 1 by the human hepatocellular cell line HepG2. Thromb Haemost 60: 491-494

Almer L O, Nilsson I M 1974 Fibrinolytic activity and treatment of diabetes. Lancet 1: 1342

Almer L O, Nilsson I M 1975 On fibrinolysis in diabetes mellitus. Acta Med Scand 198: 101-106

Almer L O, Sundkvist G, Lilja B 1982 Endothelial factors, toe temperature and leg circulation in diabetics with and without autonomic neuropathy. Thromb Res 26: 119-128

Auwerx J, Bouillon R, Collen D et al 1988 Tissue-type plasminogen activator antigen and plasminogen activator inhibitor in diabetes mellitus. Arteriosclerosis 8: 68-72

Banerjee R N, Sahani A L, Kumar U et al 1974 Antithrombin III deficiency in maturity onset diabetes mellitus and atherosclerosis. Thromb Diath Haemorrh 31: 339-345

Browlee M, Vlassara H, Cerami A 1984 Inhibition of heparin-catalyzed human antithrombin III activity by nonenzymatic glycosylation. Diabetes 33: 532-535

Browlee M, Vlassara H, Cerami A 1983 Nonenzymatic glycosylation reduces the susceptibility of fibrin to degradation by plasmin. Diabetes 32: 680-684

Bruckert E, Davidoff P, Grimaldi A et al 1990 Increased serum levels of lipoprotein(a) in diabetes melitus and their reduction with glycemic control. JAMA 263: 35-36

Busby F T, Ingham K C 1984 Thermal stabilization of antithrombin III by sugars and sugars derivates and the effects of nonenzymatic glycosylation. Biochem Biophys Acta 799: 80-89

Carmassi F, Morale M, Puccetti R et al 1992 Coagulation and fibrinolytic system impairment in insulin dependent diabetes mellitus. Thromb Res 67: 643-654

Ceriello A, Curcio F, Dello Russo P et al 1984 Non-enzymatic glycosylation reduces antithrombin III activity. Thromb Haemost 52: 363

Ceriello A, Dello Russo P, Zuccotti C et al 1983 Decreased antithrombin III activity in diabetes may be due to non-enzymatic glycosylation: a preliminary report. Thromb Haemost 50: 633-634

Ceriello A, Giugliano D, Quatraro A et al 1986 Metabolic control may alter antithrombin III activity but not its plasma concentration in diabetes: a possible role for nonenzymatic glycosylation. Diabetes Care 9: 32-35

Ceriello A, Quatraro A, Dello Russo P et al 1990 Protein C deficiency in insulin-dependent diabetes: a hyperglycemia-related phenomenon. Thromb Haemost 64: 104-107

Chang K S, Stevens W C 1992 Endothelium-dependent increase in vascular sensitivity to phenylephrine in long-term streptozotocin diabetic rat aorta. Br J Pharmacol 107: 983-990

Collen D, Lijnen H R 1991 Molecular and cellcular basis of fibrinolysis. In: Hoffman R et al (eds) Hematology: Basic Priciples and Practice. Churchill Livingstone, New York, pp 1232-1242

Comp PC, Esmon C T 1991 Regulatory mechanisms in hematosis: natural anticoagulants. In: Hoffman R et al (eds) Hematology: Basic Priciples and Practice. Churchill Livingstone, New York, pp 1243-1251

Conway E M, Rosenberg R D 1988 Tumor necrosis factor suppresses transcription of the thrombomodulin gene in endothelial cells. Mol Cell Biol 8: 5588-5592

Csaszar A, Dieplinger H, Sandholzer C et al 1993 Plasma lipoprotein(a) concentration and phenotypes in diabetes mellitus. Diabetologia 36: 47-51

De Feo P, Volpi E, Lucidi P et al 1993 Physiological increments in plasma insulin concentrations have selective and different effects on synthesis of hepatic proteins in normal humans. Diabetes 43: 995-1002

De Graaf J C, Banga J D, Moncada S et al 1992 Nitric oxide functions as an inhibitor of platelet adhesion under flow conditions. Circulation 85: 2284-2290

De Tejada I S, Goldstein I, Azadzoi K et al 1989 Impaired neurogenic and endothelium-mediated relaxation of penile smooth muscle from diabetic men with impotence. N Engl J Med 320: 1025-1030

Dittman W A, Kumada T, Sadler J E et al 1988 The structure and function of mouse thrombomodulin: phorbol myristate acetate stimulates degradation and synthesis of thrombomodulin without affecting mRNA levels in hemangioma cells. J Biol Chem 263: 15815-15822.

Durante W, Sen A K, Sunahara F A 1988 Impairment of endothelium-dependent relaxation in aortae from spontaneously diabetic rats. Br J Pharmacol 94: 463-468

Fattal P G, Schneider D J, Sobel B E et al 1992 Post-transcriptional regulation of expression of plasminogen activator inhibitor type 1 mRNA by insulin and insulin-like growth factor 1. J Biol Chem 267: 12412-12415

Fearnly G R, Chakrabarti R, Avis P R 1963 Blood fibrinolytic activity in diabetes mellitus and its bearing on ischaemic heart disease and obesity. Br Med J 1: 921-923

Fuchgott R F, Zawadzski J V 1980 The obligatory role of endothelial cells in the relaxation of arterial smooth muscle by acetylcholine. Nature 288: 373-376

Fujii K, Soma M, Huang Y H et al 1986 Increased release of prostaglandins from the mesenteric vascular bed of diabetic animals: the effect of glucose and insulin. Prostoglandins Leukot Med 24: 151-161

Garg U C, Hassid A 1989 Inhibition of rat mesangial cell mitogenesis by nitric oxide-generating vasodilators. Am J Physiol 257: F60-F66

Geiger M, Binder B R 1988 Plasminogen activation in diabetes mellitus. Enzyme 40: 149-157

Gilbert V A, Zebrowski E J, Chan A C 1983 Differential effects of megavitamin E on prostacyclin and thromboxane synthesis in streptozotocin-induced diabetic rats. Horm Metab Res 15: 320-325

Guillausseau P-J, Poupon J, Peynet J et al 1992 Lipoprotein(a) in diabetic patients with and without chronic renal failure. Diabetes Care 15: 976-979

Haffner S M, Moss S E, Klein B E K et al 1992a Lack of association between lipoprotein(a) concentrations and coronary heart disease mortality in diabetes: the Wisconsin epidemiologic study of diabetic retinopathy. Metabolism 41: 194-197

Haffner S M, Tuttle K R, Rainwater D L 1991 Decrease of lipoprotein(a) with improved glycemic control in IDDM subjects. Diabetes Care 14: 302-307

Haffner S M, Tuttle K R, Rainwater D L 1992b Lack of change of lipoprotein(a) concentration with improved glycemic control in subjects with type II diabetes. Metabolism 41: 116-120

Harrison H E, Reece A H, Johnson M 1978 Decreased vascular prostacyclin in experimental diabetes. Life Sci 23: 351-356

Head R J, Longhurst P A, Panek R L et al 1987 A contrasting effect of the diabetic state upon the contractile responses of aortic preparations from diabetic rats. Eur J Pharmacol 91: 275-287

Hirokawa K, Aoki N 1991 Up-regulation of thrombomodulin by activation of histamine H_1-receptors in human umbilical vein endothelial cells *in vitro*. Biochem J 276: 739-743

Hirokawa K, Aoki N 1990 Up-regulation of thrombomodulin in human umbilical vein endothelial cells *in vitro*. J Biochem 108: 839-845

Horie S, Kizaki K, Ishii H et al 1992 Retinoic acid stimulates expression of thrombomodulin, a surface anticoagulant glycoprotein, on human endothelial cells: differences between up-regulation of thrombomodulin by retinoic acid and cyclic AMP. Biochem J 281: 149-154

Ishii H, Horie S, Kizaki K et al 1992 Retinoic acid counteracts both the downregulation of thrombomodulin and the induction of tissue factor in cultured human endothelial cells exposed to tumor necrosis factor. Blood 80: 2556-2562

Ishii H, Kizaki K, Uchiyama H et al 1990a Cyclic AMP increases thrombomodulin expression on membrane surface of cultured human umbilical vein endothelial cells. Thromb Res 59: 841-850

Ishii H, Majerus P W 1985 Thrombomodulin is present in human plasma and urine. J Clin Invest 76: 2178-2181

Ishii H, Nakano M, Tsubouchi J et al 1990b Establishment of enzyme immunoassay of human thrombomodulin in plasma and urine using monoclonal antibodies. Thromb Haemost 63: 157-162

Ishii H, Uchiyama H, Kazama M 1991 Soluble thrombomodulin antigen in coditioned medium is increased by damage of endothelial cells. Thromb Haemost 65: 618-623

Iwashima Y, Sato T, Watanabe K et al 1990 Elevation of plasma thrombomodulin level in diabetic patients with early diabetic nephropathy. Diabetes 39: 983-988

Jansson J H, Johansson B, Boman K et al 1991 Hypo-fibrinolysis in patients with hypertension and elevated cholesterol. J Intern Med 229: 309-316

Jenkins A J, Steele J S, Janus E D et al 1992 Plasma apolipoprotein(a) is increased in type 2 (non-insulin-dependent) diabetic patients with microalbuminuria. Diabetologia 35: 1055-1059

Jeremy J Y, Mikhailidis D P, Dandona P 1983 Simulating the diabetic environment modifies *in vitro* prostacyclin synthesis. Diabetes 32: 217-221

Juhan-Vague I, Alessi M C, Vague P 1991 Increased plasma plasminogen activator inhibitor 1 levels: a possible link between insulin resistance and atherothrombosis. Diabetologia 34: 457-462

Juhan-Vague I, Vague P, Alessi M C et al 1987 Relationships between plasma insulin, triglyceride, body mass index, and plasminogen activator inhibitor 1. Diabete Metab 13: 331-336

Juhan-Vague I, Vague P, Poisson C et al 1984 Effect of 24 hours of normoglycemia on tissue-type plasminogen activator plasma levels in insulin-dependent diabetes. Thromb Haemost 51: 97-98

Kamata K, Miyata N, Kasuya Y 1989 Impairment of endothelium-dependent relaxation and changes in levels of cyclic GMP in aorta from streptozotocin-induced diadetic rats. Br J Pharmacol 97: 614-618

Kapelrud H, Bangstad H-J, Dahl-Jørgensen K et al 1991 serum Lp(a) lipoprotein concentration in insulin dependent diabetic patients with microalbuminuria. Br Med J 303: 675-678

Karádi I, Romics L, Pálos G et al 1989 Lp(a) lipoprotein concentration in serum of patients with heavy proteinuria of different origin. Clin Chem 35: 2121-2123

Karpen C W, Pritchard Jr K A, Arnold J H et al 1982 Restoration of prostacyclin/thromboxane A_2 balance in diabetic rat: influence of dietary vitamin E. Diabetes 31: 947-951

Klausen I C, Schmidt E B, Lervang H H et al 1992 Normal lipoprotein(a) concentrations and apolipoprotein(a) isoforms in patients with insulin-dependent diabetes mellitus. Eur J Clin Inv 22: 538-541

Kooistra T, Bosma P J, Tons H A M et al 1989 Plasminogen activator inhibitor 1: biosynthesis and mRNA level are increased by insulin in cultured human hepatocytes. Thromb Haemost 62: 723-728

Kunisaki M, Umeda F, Inoguchi T et al 1992 Vitamin E restores reduced prostacyclin synthesis in aortic endothelial cells cultured with a high concentration of glucose. Metabolism 41: 613-621

Kwaan H C 1992 Changes in blood coagulation, platelet function, and plasminogen-plasmin system in diabetes. Diabetes 41 (suppl): 32-35

Landin K, Stigendal L, Eriksson E et al 1990 Abdominal obesity is associated with an impaired fibrinolytic activity and elevated plasminogen activator inhibitor-1. Metabolism 39: 1044-1048

Landin K, Tengborn L, Smith U 1991 Treating insulin resistance in hypertension with metformin reduces both blood pressure and metabolic risk factors. J Intern Med 229: 181-187

Langenstroer P, Pieper G M 1992 Regulation of spontaneous EDRF release in diabetic rat aorta by oxygen free radicals. Am J Physiol 263: H257-265

Lentz S R, Tsiang M, Sadler J E 1991 Regulation of thrombomodulin by tumor necrosis factor-α: comparison of transcriptional and posttranscriptional mechanisms. Blood 77: 542-550

Levitsky L L, Scanu A M, Gould S H 1991 Lipoprotein(a) levels in black and white children and adolescents with IDDM. Diabetes Care 14: 283-287

Mayhan W G, Simmons L K, Sharpe G M 1991 Mechanism of impaired responses of cerebral arterioles during diabetes mellitus. Am J Physiol 260: H319-326

Mayhan W G 1989 Impairment of endothelium-dependent dilatation of cerebral arterioles during diabetes mellitus. Am J Physiol 56: H621-625

Miskin R, Axelrod J H, Griep A E et al 1990 Human and murine urokinase cDNAs linked to the murine A-crystallin promoter exhibit lens and non-lens expression in transgenic mice. Eur J Biochem 190: 31-38

Miskin R, Levinger S 1991 Diabetic mice expressing transgenic urokinase in retina: limited thickening of retinal capillary basement membrane. In: Proceedings of the International Workshop on Molecular and Cellular Biology of Plasminogen Activation. Elsinore, Denmark, p 71

Moor K L, Esmon C, Esmon N L 1989 Tumor necrosis factor leads to the internalization and degradation of thrombomodulin from the surface of bovine aortic endothelial cells in culture. Blood 73: 159-165

Mulhern M, Docherty J R 1989 Effects of experimental diabetes on the responsiveness of rat aorta. Br J Pharmacol 97: 1007-1012

Nawroth P P, Handley D A, Esmon C et al 1986 Interleuken 1 induces endothelial cell procoagulant while suppressing cell-surface anticoagulant activity. Proc Natl Acad Sci USA 83: 3460-3464

Nawroth P P, Stern D M 1986 Modulation of endothelial cell hemostatic properties by tumor necrosis factor. J Exp Med 163: 740-745

O'Connor K J, Knowles R G, Patel K D 1991 Nitrovasodilators have proliferative as well as antiproliferative effects. J Cardiovasc Pharmacol 17 (suppl 3): 100-103

Oida K, Takai H, Maeda H et al 1990 Plasma thrombomodulin concentration in diabetes mellitus. Diabetes Res Clin Pract 10: 193-196

Oida K, Takai H, Maeda H, et al 1992 Apolipoprotein(a) is present in urine and its excretion is decreased in patients with renal failure. Clin Chem 38: 2244-2248

Oyama Y, Kawasaki H, Hattori Y et al 1986 Attenuation of endothelium-dependent relaxation in aorta from diabetic rats. Eur J Pharmacol 131: 75-78

Parra H J, Mezdour H, Cachera C et al 1987 Lp(a) lipoprotein in patients with chronic renal failure treated by hemodialysis. Clin Chem 33: 721

Pieper G M, Gross G J 1988 Oxygen free radicals abolish endothelium dependent relaxation in diabetic rat aorta. Am J Physiol 255: H825-833

Pieper G M, Mei D A, Langenstroer P et al 1992 Bioassay of endothelium-derived relaxing factor in diabetic rat aorta. Am J Physiol 263: H676-680

Rader D J, Brewer Jr H B 1992 Lipoprotein(a): clinical approach to a unique atherogenic lipoprotein. JAMA 267: 1109-1112

Radomski M W, Palmer R M J, Moncada S 1987 The anti-aggregating properties of vascular endothelium: interactions between prostacyclin and nitric oxide. Br J Pharmacol 92: 639-646

Ramirez L C, Arauz-Pacheco C, Lackner C et al 1992 Lipoprotein(a) levels in diabetes mellitus: relationship to metabolic control. Ann Intern Med 117: 42-47

Rapaport S I, Rao L V M 1992 Initiation and regulation of tissue factor-dependent blood coagulation. Arterioscler Thromb 12: 1111-1121

Scanu A M, Fless G M 1990 Lipoprotein(a): heterogeneity and biological relevance. J Clin Invest 85: 1709-1715

Schernthaner G, Kostner G M, Dieplinger H et al 1983 Apolipoproteins (A-I, A-II, B), Lp(a) lipoprotein and lecithin:cholesterol acyltransferase activity in diabetes mellitus. Atherosclerosis 49: 277-293

Schneider D J, Nordt T K, Sobel B E 1992 Stimulation by proinsulin of expression of plasminogen inhibitor type-1 in endothelial cells. Diabetes 41: 890-895

Schneider D J, Sobel B E 1993 Attenuated fibrinolysis and accelerated atherogenesis in type II diabetic patients. Diabetes 42: 1-7

Schneider D J, Sobel B E 1991 Augmentation of synthesis of plasminogen activator inhibitor type-1 by insulin and insulin-like growth factor type-1: implication for vascular disease in hyperinsulinemic states. Proc Nat Acad Sci USA 88: 9959-9963

Scott J 1991 Lipoprotein(a): thrombotic and atherogenic. Br Med J 303: 663-664

Sharma S C 1981 Platelet adhesiveness, plasma fibrinogen and fibrinolytic adtivity in juvenile onset and maturity onset diabetes mellitus. J Clin Pathol 34: 501-503

Silberbauer K, Schernthaner G, Sinzinger H et al 1979 Decreased vascular prostacyclin in juvenile-onset diabetes. N Engl J Med 300: 366-367

Small M, Lowe G D O, MacCuish A C et al 1987 Thrombin and plasmin activity in diabetes mellitus and their association with glycemic control. Q J Med 65: 1025-1031

Sowers J R, Tuck M L, Sowers D K 1980 Plasma antithrombin III and thrombin generation time: correlation with hemoglobin A_1 and fasting serum glucose in young diabetic women. Diabetes Care 3: 655-658

Subbiah M T R, Deitemeyer D 1980 Altered synthesis of prostaglandins in platelet and aorta from spontaneously diabetic Wistar rats. Biochem Med 23: 231-235

Takahashi H, Ito S, Hanano M et al 1992 Circulating thrombomodulin is a novel endothelial cell marker: comparison of its behavior with von Willebrand factor and tissue-type pasminogen activator. Am J Hematol 41: 32-39

Takegoshi T, Haba T, Hirai J et al 1990 Alterations of lipoprotein(a) in patients with diabetic nephropathy. Atherosclerosis 83: 99-100

Tanaka A, Ishii H, Hiraishi S et al 1991 Increased thrombomodulin values in plasma of diabetic men with microangiopathy. Clin Chem 37: 269-272

Tanz R D, Chang K S K, Weller T S 1989 Histamine relaxation of aortic rings from diabetic rats. Agents Actions 28: 2-8

Taylor P D, McCarthy A L, Thomas C R 1992 Endothelium-dependent relaxation and noradrenaline sensitivity in mesenteric resistance arteries of streptozotocin-induced diabetic rats. Br J Pharmacol 107: 393-399

Tesfamariam B, Brown M L, Cohen R A 1991 Elevated glucose impaires endothelium-dependent relaxation by activating protein kinase C. J Clin Invest 87: 1643-1648

Vague P, Juhan-Vague I, Aillaud M F et al 1986 Correlation between blood fibrinolytic activity, plasminogen activator inhibitor level, plasma insulin level and relative body weight in normal and obese subjects. Metabolism 35: 250-253

Vague P, Juhan-Vague I, Alessi M C et al 1987 Metformin decreases the high plasminogen activator inhibition capacity, plasma insulin and triglyceride levels in non-diabetic obese subjects. Thromb Haemost 57: 326-328

Vukovich T C, Schernthaner G 1986 Decreased protein C levels in patients with insulin-dependent type I diabetes mellitus. Diabetes 35: 617-619

Wakabayashi I, Hataka N, Kimura E et al 1987 Modulation of vascular tonus by the endothelium in experimental diabetes. Life Sci 40: 643-648

White RE, Carrier GO 1986 Supersensitivity and endothelium dependency of histamine-induced relaxation in mesenteric arteries from diabetic rats. Pharmacology 33: 34-38

Winocour P H, Bhatnagar D, Ishola M et al 1991 Lipoprotein(a) and microvascular disease in type1 (insulin-dependent) diabetes. Diabetic Med 8: 922-927

Witmer M R, Hadcock J H, Peltier S L et al 1992 Altered levels of antithrombin III and fibrinogen in the aortic wall of the alloxan-induced diabetic rabbit: evidence of a prothrombotic state. J Lab Clin Med 119: 221-230

Yamamoto S, Mizoguchi T, Tamaki T et al 1993 Urinary thrombomodulin, its isolation and characterization. J Biochem 113: 433-440

SECTION 2

New Approach of Pathogenesis of Diabetic Vascular Complications

4

Protein kinase C activation in the pathogenesis of diabetic vascular complications

T. Inoguchi, F. Umeda, H. Nawata, G.L. King

INTRODUCTION

Hyperglycaemia seems to be an important aetiological factor in the development of micro- and macrovascular diseases in diabetic patients. Since glucose is metabolized by numerous pathways, hyperglycaemia may cause a variety of metabolic abnormalities in vascular cells via multiple mechanisms. Several theories have been proposed to explain the adverse effects of hyperglycaemia, such as polyol pathway activation (Greene et al 1987) and nonenzymatic glycation (Brownlee et al 1988).

Recently, the possible activation of the enzyme of protein kinase C (PKC) by diabetes and hyperglycaemia has been reported in retina (King GL 1990), aorta (Inoguchi et al 1992a), heart (Inoguchi et al 1992a; Tanaka et al 1991; Xiang & McNeill 1992) and renal glomeruli (Craven & DeRubertis 1989) in parallel with the increased level of total diacylglycerol (DAG) in those vascular tissues. PKC is a serine/threonine-specific protein kinase which is dependent on DAG, Ca^{2+} and phospholipids (Nishizuka 1986). The activation of PKC involves translocation of the enzyme to the membrane, which leads to phosphorylation of target proteins, thereby regulating important intracellular processes. These processes include many vascular functions such as cell growth (Kariya et al 1987), contraction (Jiang et al 1987; Rasmussen et al 1984), permeability (Lynch et al 1990), hormone and growth factor receptor turnover (Hachiya et al 1987), and basement membrane synthesis (Huhtala et al 1990). Therefore, it is likely that the alteration of this enzyme activity could cause a number of vascular function abnormalities.

Since DAG is an activator of PKC (Berridge et al 1987), the activation of PKC in diabetic vascular tissues is probably due to an increased level of DAG. DAG is formed in response to extracellular signals by turnover of phosphoinositides and other membrane phospholipids as well as by *de novo* synthesis from glycolytic intermediates (dihydroxyacetone phosphate and glycerol-3-phosphate) by means of a stepwise acylation into DAG (Berne 1975; Dunlop & Larkins 1985). Our group and other investigators have shown that elevated glucose levels can increase DAG levels in cultured vascular cells (Inoguchi et al 1992a) and tissues (Craven et al 1990; Wolf et al 1991). The mechanism responsible for the increased level of DAG induced by high glucose concentrations has been suggested to be caused by increased *de novo* synthesis. Additional mechanisms are discussed in this article. We further review recent evidence with respect to the hypothesis of PKC activation in diabetic vasculature, including our original data (published and unpublished). In addition, the pathophysiological meaning of PKC activation is also discussed.

PKC ACTIVATION IN AORTA AND HEART BY DIABETES

Cardiovascular disease is the major cause of mortality and morbidity in diabetic patients (Kannel & McGree 1979; Kessler 1971). Pathological studies have shown an increased rate of atherosclerotic lesions. In addition, cardiomyopathy has also been ascribed to diabetes (Fein & Sonnenblick 1985). The risk factors for atherosclerosis in diabetic patients are multiple, such as hypercholesterolaemia, hypertension and possibly hyperglycaemia (Fuller et al 1980).

There are several hypotheses for explaining how the effects of hyperglycaemia on vascular cells might be involved in the process of atherosclerosis. We measured PKC activities in aorta and heart of streptozotocin-induced (STZ)-diabetic rats (2 weeks' duration) and genetically-induced diabetic BB rats (4 weeks' duration) compared with age-matched control rats (Inoguchi et al 1992a). Briefly, PKC in both the membranous and cytosolic fractions were partially purified from aorta and heart. The specific activity of PKC was measured by its ability to transfer ^{32}P from ^{32}P-ATP into a specific octapeptide substrate (RKRTLRRL) [corresponding to the threonine phosphorylation sites of the epidermal growth factor receptor] in the presence of Ca^{2+}, phosphatidylserine and DAG. PKC activity in the membranous fraction from the aorta was significantly increased in both STZ-diabetic rats and BB diabetic rats compared with controls (Inoguchi et al 1992a) [Fig. 4.1]. There was no significant difference in PKC activity in the cytosolic fraction between BB diabetic rats and controls as well as between STZ-diabetic rats and controls. Furthermore, for hearts, PKC activity in the membranous fraction was also significantly increased in STZ-diabetic rats and BB diabetic rats compared with controls (Fig. 4.1). No significant difference was found in the cytosolic fraction. Similar results on PKC activation in diabetic heart have been reported by two other groups (Tanaka et al 1991; Xiang & McNeill 1992).

Recent biochemical and immunohistochemical analyses have revealed that PKC is represented by a large family of proteins with multiple subspecies, which may present different distributions in particular cell types and even within the cell (Nishizuka 1989). The subspecies also exhibit distinctly different modes of activation, kinetic properties and

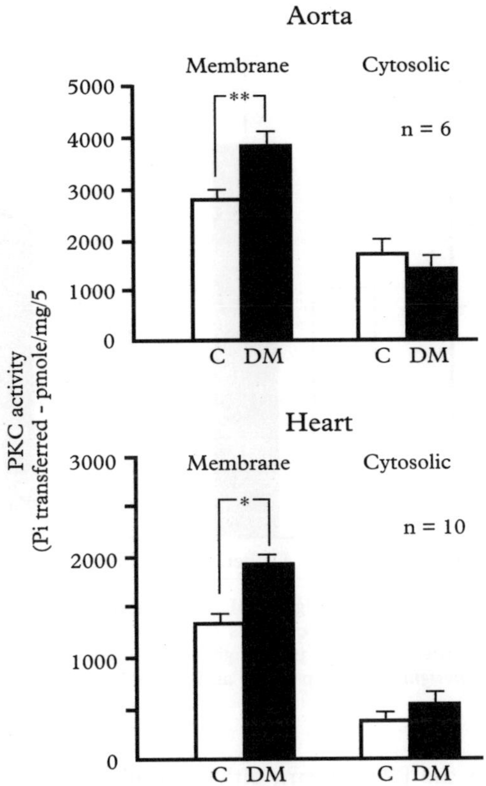

Fig. 4.1 Effect of diabetes on protein kinase C (PKC) activity in rat aorta and heart. PKC specific activities were measured in both membranous and cytosolic fractions from age-matched controls (C) and BB diabetic rats (DM). *Abbreviation:* n = number of preparations. For aorta, two rats were used for each preparation. For heart, one rat was used for each preparation. Values are given as means ± SEM. *Statistical significance:* * $p < 0.05$ and ** $p < 0.01$.

substrate specificities. We therefore characterized the alteration in PKC isoforms in aorta and heart from STZ-diabetic rats. The characterization of isoforms in aorta and heart was first performed using monospecific polyclonal antibodies against α, β1, β2, and γ PKC isoforms. Western blot analysis showed that only α and β2 isoforms were detected in rat aorta and heart. The β2 isoform in the membranous fraction was preferentially increased in both aorta and heart of STZ-diabetic rats rather than the α isoform (Inoguchi et al 1992a). There was no change in the amounts of α and β2 isoforms in the cytosolic fraction of both aorta and heart. These data suggest that the mechanism for the increase in PKC activity is probably due to an increased amount of PKC, chiefly the β2 isoform in the membranous fraction. In the retina of both STZ- and BB diabetic rats, PKC activity in the membrane fraction was increased. The most increased

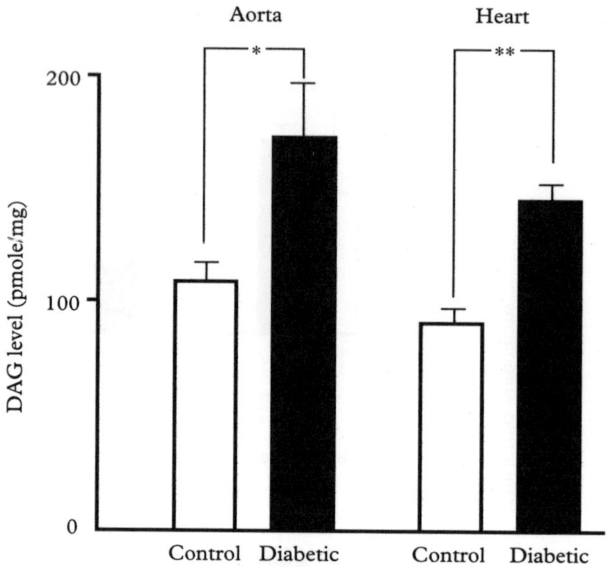

Fig. 4.2 Effect of diabetes on diacylglycerol (DAG) levels in rat aorta and heart. DAG levels were measured in age-matched controls (Control) and BB diabetic rats (Diabetic). DAG content is represented as pmole per weight (mg) of dried tissue. Values are given as means ± SEM. *Statistical significance:* * $p < 0.05$ and ** $p < 0.01$.

isoform was again the β2 isoform, although all PKC isoforms (α, β1, β2, and ε) were increased (Shiba et al 1993). The possible mechanism for the predominant increase in β2 isoform is that the various PKC isoforms may respond to DAG, Ca^{2+} and phospholipid differently. There is evidence that the β2 isoform rather than the α isoform may be more sensitive to DAG (Nishizuka 1989). Another possible mechanism is that the diabetic state might induce an increase in the DAG level at specific subcellular sites. This might account for the preferential activation of the β2 isoform, since PKC isoforms may have different subcellular distribution, with the a isoform mainly in the plasma membrane and the β2 isoform in intracellular bodies (Nishizuka 1989).

The source of increased membranous PKC could be due to an increase in translocation despite a lack of decrease in cytosolic PKC. The assay used might not be sensitive enough to detect small changes in the amount and activity of PKC in the cytosol. Only a small change in the cytosol fraction would be expected, since 80% of PKC is found in cytosol (Inoguchi et al 1992a). Thereby, a small change in the cytosol is magnified several fold in the membrane. However, the possibility of an increase in PKC synthesis should also be investigated.

TOTAL DAG LEVEL IN AORTA AND HEART IN DIABETES

One of the possible mechanisms for the increase in membranous PKC activity might be related to an elevation of DAG levels in vascular tissues. Total DAG in extracted lipids from aorta and heart was measured by the method of Pries et al (1987) using DAG kinase. Total DAG levels were significantly increased in aorta and heart of both STZ-diabetic rats and BB diabetic rats compared with controls (Fig. 4.2). Other investigators have also reported that total DAG levels are increased in the heart of diabetic rats (Okumura et al 1988), but a decrease has been noted in the aorta (Okumura et al 1991). The different result for the aorta is probably due to the fact that in those studies with the aorta, but not the heart, the DAG extraction procedure involved preincubation for 25 min at 37°C under mechanical stimulation of shaking. Mechanical stimulation during the preincubation step might nullify the effect of the diabetic milieu on aortic DAG levels.

Since DAG is a physiological activator of PKC translocation, the findings of increased DAG levels in aorta and heart also support the hypothesis of PKC activation in these vascular tissues during diabetes.

EFFECT OF PREVENTIVE INSULIN TREATMENT ON PKC ACTIVITY AND DAG LEVEL

We have examined the effect of preventative insulin treatment in STZ-diabetic rats (unpublished observations). Osmotic minipumps were implanted intraperitoneally 24 h after STZ injection and regular insulin 10 U/kg/day was delivered. Insulin treatment completely prevented the increase in the total DAG level and the increase in membranous PKC activity in both aorta and heart from diabetic rats. This result differed from that of a previous report showing a sustained elevation of the DAG level in heart from STZ-diabetic rats in response to subcutaneous insulin treatment (Okumura et al 1988). One possible explanation for the difference is that insulin administration in our study constitutes a more physiological route than subcutaneous insulin injection, which might induce peripheral hyperinsulinaemia. This is supported by the finding that insulin itself may stimulate DAG synthesis in the heart (Farese et al 1987). Another report also showed that the increase in membranous PKC activity in retina of diabetic rats was only partially normalized by subcutaneous insulin treatment (Shiba et al 1993).

INCREASED DAG LEVEL AND PKC ACTIVATION IN RETINA, RENAL GLOMERULUS AND PERIPHERAL NERVE

The results of The Diabetes Control and Complications Trial (1993) have confirmed those of earlier clinical trials on the reduction in the development or progression of retinopathy (Klein et al 1988) and nephropathy (Reichard et al 1991) consequent to a reduction in hyperglycaemia. A large amount of experimental evidence also suggests that hyperglycaemia induces a variety of biochemical and functional changes in vascular cells. All of these epidemiological and biochemical studies have suggested that the causal factor for retinopathy and nephropathy is probably hyperglycaemia, which includes increased polyol pathway activity (Greene et al 1987) and advanced glycosylation end-product accumulation (Brownlee et al 1988). Increased membrane PKC activity has also been shown in retina (King et al 1990; Shiba et al 1993) and glomeruli (Craven & DeRubertis 1989) of diabetic rats in parallel with increased DAG levels. Taken together with the previously mentioned aorta and heart studies, this evidence suggests that PKC might be activated in response to increased DAG levels in both micro- and macrovascular tissue during diabetes. With respect to peripheral nerves, previous reports have suggested that total PKC was reduced in diabetic nerve (Kim et al 1988). It has been proposed that reduced nerve myo-inositol content in diabetes leads to a reduction in inositol phospholipids or their turnover, with a resultant diminished generation of DAG and lessened PKC activity (Green et al 1987). However, these authors showed that the reduction in PKC activity was due to a decrease in soluble activity alone. Membranous PKC activity, which is probably an index of enzyme activation, might be increased. This is supported by a report that the phosphorylation of

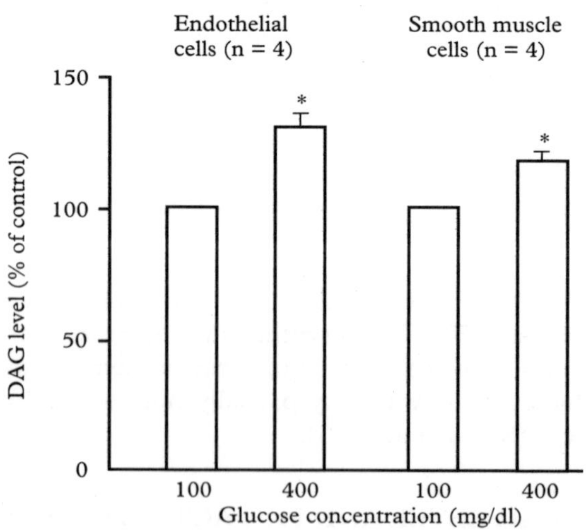

Fig. 4.3 Effect of glucose concentration on diacylglycerol (DAG) levels in cultured rat aortic endothelial cells and smooth muscle cells. Confluent cultured cells were incubated with medium containing either 100 or 400 mg/dl glucose with 2% serum, which was changed every day. After 4 days' incubation, the DAG level was measured. *Abbreviation:* n = number of preparations. Values are given as means ± SEM. *Statistical significance:* * $p < 0.05$. (Reproduced with permission from Inoguchi et al 1992a)

specific nerve proteins, which are thought to be substrates for PKC, are increased during diabetes (Schrama et al 1987). This is supported by the finding that PKC inhibitors completely restore the abnormality of Na^+, K^+-ATPase activity in the sciatic nerve of diabetic mice (Hermenegildo et al 1993). With respect to other tissues, no significant change was found in the PKC activity and DAG level in the brain of diabetic rats (Shiba et al 1993). It is possible that diabetes or high glucose concentration alters the metabolism of DAG and PKC activity in a different manner depending on the tissues involved.

INCREASED DAG LEVEL AND PKC ACTIVATION INDUCED BY HIGH GLUCOSE CONCENTRATION

One of the causal factors for the increases in the DAG level in vascular tissues of diabetes is probably due to hyperglycaemia, although other changes in hormonal and nutritional factors could be responsible. This hypothesis is supported by the finding that elevated glucose levels can stimulate DAG synthesis in cultured aortic endothelial cells and smooth muscle cells (Fig. 4.3). Elevating glucose concentration from 5.5 to 22 mmol/l significantly increased the DAG in both types of vascular cells after only 2 days' incubation, which persisted for at least 7 days. The high glucose concentration did not immediately induce an increase in DAG levels. A similar effect of high glucose concentrations on DAG was also noted in cultured capillary endothelial cells derived from bovine retina and rat epididymal fat (unpublished observations). Other investigators have demonstrated that DAG was increased in response to high glucose concentrations in vascular tissues, such as renal glomeruli (Craven et al 1990) and granulation tissue (Wolf et al 1991).

In parallel with the increases in DAG levels, PKC is activated *in vitro* by high glucose concentrations in various kinds of vascular cells (Ayo et al 1991; Inoguchi et al 1992a; Shiba et al 1993; Studer et al 1993; Williams & Schrier 1992) and tissues (Craven et al 1990). Using cultured smooth muscle cells, we examined the effect of high glucose concentration on PKC activity and phosphorylation of MARCKS protein, which is well documented as a specific substrate for PKC and as a parameter for the *in situ* measurement of activity of the PKC system (Witters & Blackshear 1987). As shown in figure 4.4, PKC activity in the membranous fraction was significantly increased after 4 days' exposure to high glucose concentration (20 mmol/l), which is consistent with our observations in diabetic rats. MARCKS protein phosphorylation was also increased under these conditions, which clearly demonstrated the persistent activation of PKC by high glucose concentration (Fig. 4.5). Using another assay in digitonin-permeabilized vascular smooth muscle cells, Williams and Schrier (1992) confirmed the sustained activation for up to 48 h by

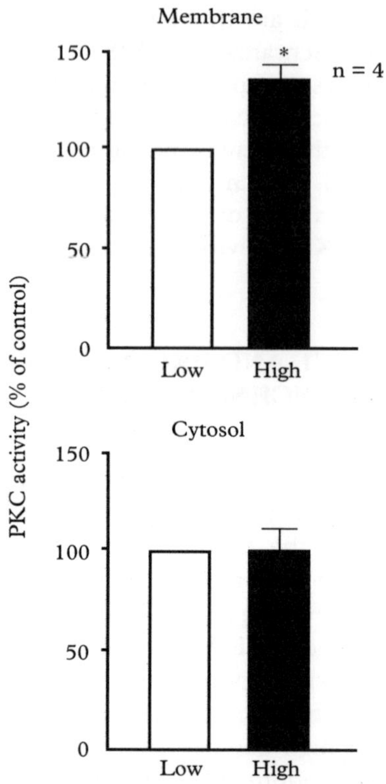

Fig. 4.4 Effect of elevated glucose concentration on protein kinase C (PKC) activity in membrane and cytosolic fractions in cultured rat smooth muscle cells after 4 days' incubation with glucose 400 mg/dl (High) and 100 mg/dl (Low). *Abbreviation:* n = number of preparations. Values are given as means ± SEM. *Statistical significance:* * $p < 0.05$

continued exposure to high glucose concentration (20 mmol/l), while PKC activation in response to angiotensin II and vasopressin was short lived and returned to the baseline within minutes. Another group also demonstrated the sustained increases in MARCKS protein phosphorylation by high glucose concentration using mesangial cells (Studer et al 1993). Several reports have suggested that high glucose concentration and diabetes might induce an increase in cyotsolic Ca^{2+} in vascular tissues (Heyliger et al 1987) and cells (Graier et al 1993) as well as pancreatic islets (Nilsson et al 1988). Tanaka et al (1991) have reported that Ca^{2+} antagonism could prevent the activation of PKC in heart of STZ-diabetic rats. Since an increase in cytosolic Ca^{2+} is another important activator of PKC, the possibility that hyperglycaemia-induced increases in cytosolic Ca^{2+} contributes to the activation of PKC in vasculature remains to be examined in more detail.

DE NOVO SYNTHESIS OF DAG BY HIGH GLUCOSE CONCENTRATION

The mechanism responsible for the stimulatory effect of high glucose concentration on DAG levels has not been established. DAG can be derived from multiple pathways. It is formed from the phosphodiesteratic cleavage of phosphatidylinositol-4,5-disphosphate or other membrane phospholipids stimulated by a wide variety of receptor agonists. Alternatively, it can be synthesized *de novo* from the glycolytic intermediate, dihydroxyacetone phosphate and glycerol-3-phosphate, by means of step-wise acylation (Berne 1975; Dunlop & Larkins 1985). This pathway of DAG synthesis has been reported in islet cells as a possible signal for glucose-stimulated insulin release (Berne 1975; Dunlop & Larkin 1985; Peter-Riesch et al 1988).

Studies in pancreatic islets and adipose tissue have demonstrated that high glucose concentration can increase DAG production by stimulating *de novo* synthesis (Berne 1975; Dunlop & Larkins 1985; Ishizuka et al 1989) as well as by enhancing phospholipase C-induced hydrolysis of inositol phospholipids (Biden et al 1987). In vascular cells, the mechanism for the increases in DAG level induced by elevated glucose concentration has been suggested as occurring via the *de novo* synthesis pathway. Craven et al (1990) reported that glucose increases DAG production in glomeruli by the *de novo* synthesis pathway rather than by stimulating hydrolysis of inositol phospholipids. This was implied by observations that glucose did not increase the production of inositol phosphates which were prelabelled

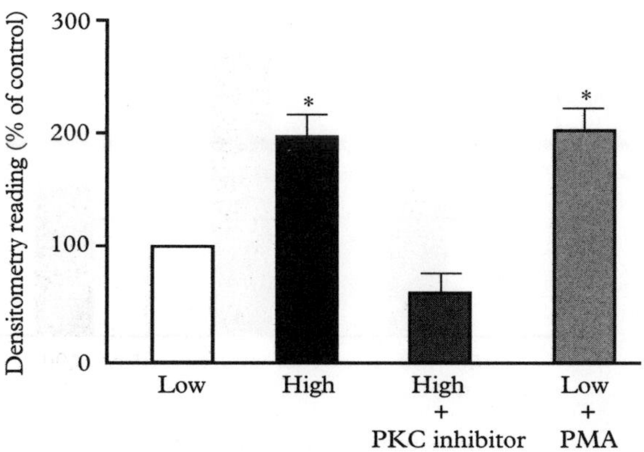

Fig. 4.5 Effect of elevated glucose concentration on *in situ* phosphorylation of MARCKS protein in cultured rat smooth muscle cells after 4 days' incubation with glucose 400 mg/dl (High) and 100 mg/dl (Low). Measurement of MARCKS protein was made after 3 hours' incubation with 0.5 mCi/ml ^{32}P, immunoprecipitatation, and quantitation using scanning densitometry and autoradiography following SDS polyacrilamide gel separation. Values are given as means ± SEM. *Statistical significance:* * $p < 0.05$.

with ^{3}H-inositol, while ^{14}C-glucose was labelled into DAG in glomeruli. Furthermore, in radioactive labelling studies using aortic endothelial cells, we found that high glucose concentration did not affect labelled DAG when cells were incubated with ^{3}H-arachidonate, whereas the labelled DAG level was significantly increased when incubated with ^{3}H-palmitate and ^{3}H-oleic acid (Fig. 4.6). These data suggest that the increased DAG induced by high glucose concentration has a palmitate- and oleic acid-enriched fatty acid composition.

The *de novo* synthesis of DAG requires a step-wise acylation catalyzed by glycerol-3-phosphate acyltransferase and monoacylglycerol-3-phosphate acyltransferase (Fig. 4.7). The first enzyme is selective for saturated fatty acyl-coenzyme A, whereas the latter has selectivity for unsaturated fatty acyl-coenzyme A. Although the particular fatty acids incorporated might depend on their availability, it should be noted that in pancreatic islets studies, analysis of the fatty acid composition of DAG induced by high glucose concentration also showed a predominance of palmitic acid and oleic acid in good agreement with our observations (Wolf et al 1989). This fatty acid composition is clearly different from that of DAG generated by hydrolysis of phosphatidylinositol, which has the specific composition of 1-stearoyl-2-arachidonyl-sn-glycerol (Holub & Kuksis 1986). Most DAG that contains both saturated and unsaturated fatty acids, including 1-

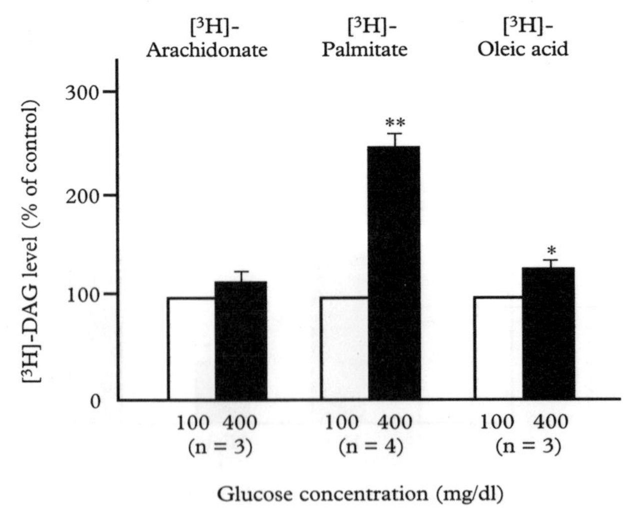

Fig. 4.6 The effect of high glucose concentration on radiolabelled fatty acid incorporation into diacylglycerol (DAG). After 3 days' incubation with high glucose (400 mg/dl) or low glucose (100mg/dl), ^{3}H-arachidonate, ^{3}H-palmitate or ^{3}H-oleic acid was added at the concentration of 20 μCi/ml. After 16 hours' incubation, DAG was extracted and separated by thin layer chromatography and its radioactivity was counted. *Abbreviation:* n = number of preparations. Values are given as means ± SEM. *Statistical significance:* * $p < 0.05$ and ** $p < 0.01$.

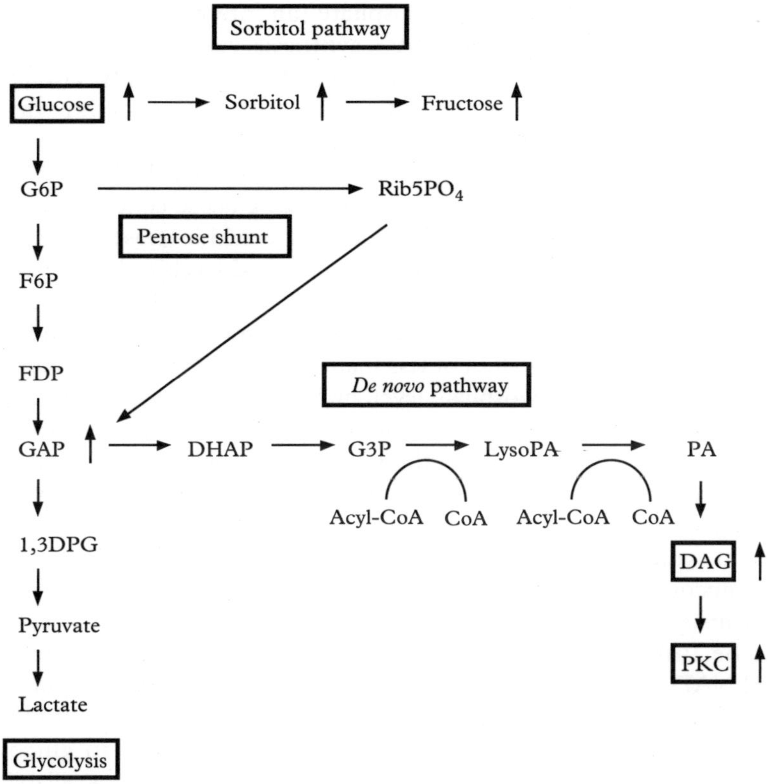

Fig. 4.7 Pathways of glucose metabolism linked to hyperglycaemia and effects on DAG and PKC. Sorbitol pathway and glycolytic *de novo* synthesis pathway may be activated by hyperglycaemia. *Abbreviations:* Acyl-CoA = acyl coenzyme A; CoA = coenzyme A; DAG = diacylglycerol; DHAP = dihydroxyacetone phosphate; 1,3DPG = 1,3-disphosphoglycerate; FDP = fructose-1,6-disphosphate; F6P = fructose-6-phosphate; GAP = glyceradehyde-3-phosphate; G3P = glycerol-3-phosphate; G6P = glucose-6-phosphate; LysoPA = lysophosphatidate; PA = phosphatidate; PKC = protein kinase C; $Rib5PO_4$ = ribose 5-phosphate.

palmitoyl-2-oleoyl-sn-glycerol, seems to be active in stimulating PKC activity, although 1-stearoyl-2-arachidonyl-sn-glycerol may be the most powerful activator of PKC (Go et al 1987). Therefore, DAG generated via the *de novo* pathway is capable of activating PKC.

Furthermore, we have noted no significant increase in DAG labelled with ^{3}H-glycerol despite the increased DAG level, again indicating that phosphatidylinositol hydrolysis contributed very little to DAG synthesis (unpublished observations). This finding indicates that the source of the glycerol backbone of increased DAG might be mostly derived from an increased amount of unlabelled glycerol due to enhanced flux derived from the glycolytic *de novo* pathway. In pancreatic islets, glyceraldehyde, which is converted to glyceraldehyde-3-phosphate (an intermediate of glycolysis), has been reported to stimulate DAG synthesis via the *de novo* pathway (Wollheim et al 1988). We have also confirmed that glyceraldehyde increased DAG levels in cultured aortic endothelial cells, which is consistent with the concept that high glucose concentration increases DAG levels via the glycolytic *de novo* synthesis pathway (Inoguchi et al 1992b).

Sustained exposure of endothelial cells to high glucose concentration from 5.5 to 22 mmol/l has been reported to induce a 3-fold increase in the level of glucose-6-phosphate (Lorenzi et al 1987). Increased levels of lactate in retina and nerve of diabetic rats may also support the possibility of enhanced glycolysis in these tissues (Paulson et al 1983). Despite the saturation kinetics of hexokinase having Km values of less than 0.4 mmol/l with down-regulation depending on glucose-6-phosphate level, high glucose concentrations seem to induce enhanced flux in glycolysis. The possible mechanisms responsible for the increase in glycolysis might be the release of hexokinase inhibition by the high glucose concentration (Fujii & Beutler 1985), the presence of hexokinase with a higher Km for glucose (Grossbard & Schimke 1966), or the induction of protein synthesis of hexokinase or other enzyme(s) by long-term exposure to high glucose concentration.

Williamson et al (1993) have suggested that increased *de novo* synthesis might be linked to increased polyol pathway activity via increased $NADH/NAD^+$ produced by sorbitol oxidation to fructose. Namely, increased cytosolic $NADH/NAD^+$ might favour increased *de novo* synthesis of DAG by both enhanced reduction of dihydroxyacetone phosphate to glucose-3-phosphate (the first step of *de novo* pathway) and by enhancing availability of dihydroxyacetone phosphate due to impaired oxidation of glyceraldehyde-3-phosphate to 1,3-diphosphoglycerate. Our preliminary data (Inoguchi et al 1992b) demonstrated that the aldose reductase inhibitor, sorbinil, at a fairly high concentration did not prevent the increase in DAG induced by high glucose concentration, although flux through the polyol pathway rather than through sorbitol levels remains to be evaluated.

Preliminary studies by our group have shown that galactose can increase the DAG level, possibly via glycolysis and the *de novo* synthesis pathway (Xia et al 1993). Galactose can be metabolized by other pathways including glycolysis, besides the conversion into galactitol by aldose reductase, which is thought to mimic the effect of sorbitol. The increased DAG levels were found in aorta, heart and retina in this galactose-fed dog model (Xia et al 1993).

CONCLUSION - POSSIBLE BIOCHEMICAL AND PHYSIOLOGICAL CONSEQUENCES OF PKC ACTIVATION IN DIABETES

PKC activation induced by diabetes and hyperglycaemia may cause many of vascular function abnormalities which have been found in diabetes, since PKC has been shown to modulate smooth muscle growth (Kariya et al

1987) and contraction (Jiang & Morgan 1987; Rasmussen et al 1984), endothelial cell permeability (Lynch et al 1990), hormone receptor turnover (Hachiya et al 1987) and cardiomyocyte contraction (Leatherman 1987).

Several lines of evidence have implied that PKC activation may alter vascular functions in macro- and microvessels in diabetes. Testfamariam et al (1991) have reported that high glucose concentration induces an impairment of endothelium-dependent relaxation of rabbit aorta similar to that observed in the diabetic rabbit, and that this functional change can be blocked by a PKC inhibitor. Elevated glucose-induced increases in the levels of mRNA specific for matrix components in cultured endothelial cells have been partially mimicked by PKC agonists (Cagliero et al 1991). In mesangial cells, elevated glucose-induced accumulation of fibronectin was mimicked by phorbol ester and was abolished when PKC was down-regulated (Studer et al 1993). Wolf et al (1991) have also reported that PKC activation by high glucose concentration is associated with enhanced vascular permeability and flow in the skin chamber model. Shiba et al (1993) found that PKC activation by vitreous injection of phorbol ester can mimic the abnormal retinal blood circulation of diabetic rats.

PKC has been implicated in the modulation of prostaglandin synthesis in glomeruli and mesangial cells (Craven et al 1988). Enhanced production of vasodilatory prostaglandins has been reported to be linked with increases in the glomerular filtration rate (Esmatjes et al 1985; Jensen et al 1986). Therefore, it has been suggested that the PKC activation in diabetic glomeruli may contribute to the increase in glomerular filtration rate which is characteristic of early diabetes (Craven & DeRubertis 1989). In addition, the elevation of DAG level itself may cause alteration of cellular functions without mediating the effect via PKC activation. A recent report has shown that DAG can stimulate actin polymerization and control cytoskeletal assembly, which might modulate cellular growth, cellular movement or signal transduction by hormones (Shariff & Luna 1992).

ACKNOWLEDGMENTS

The authors wish to express their appreciation for the artwork preparation of Mrs Diana King. Financial support was provided by the American Diabetes Association Mentor Based Fellowship (Toyoshi Inoguchi) and National Institutes of Health Grant EY05110, DERC grant DK 36836, with supplemental funding from Massachusetts Lions' Eye Research.

REFERENCES

Ayo S H, Radnik R, Garoni J A et al 1991 High glucose increases diacylglycerol mass and activate protein kinase C in mesangial cell cultures. Am J Physiol 261: F571-577

Berne C 1975 The metabolism of lipids in mouse pancreatic islets. The biosynthesis of triacylglycerol and phospholipids. Biochem J 152: 667-673

Berridge M J 1987 Inositol trisphosphate and diacylglycerol: two interacting second messengers. Annu Rev Biochem 56: 159-193

Biden T J, Peter-Riesch B, Schlegel W et al. 1987 Ca^{++}-mediated generation of inositol 1,4,5-triphosphate and inositol 1,3,4,5-tetrakisphosphate in pancreatic islets. J Biol Chem 262: 3567-3571

Brownlee M, Cerami A, Vlassara H 1988 Advanced glycosylation end products in tissue and the biochemical basis of diabetic complications. N Engl J Med 318: 1315-1321

Cagliero E, Roth T, Roy S et al 1991 Expression of genes related to the extracellular matrix in human endothelial cells. J Biol Chem 266: 14244-14250

Craven P A, DeRubertis F R 1989 Protein kinase C is activated in glomeruli from streptozotocin diabetic rats. J Clin Invest 83: 1667-1675

Craven P A, Davidson M C, DeRubertis F R 1990 Increase in diacylglycerol mass in isolated glomeruli by glucose from *de novo* synthesis of glycerolipids. Diabetes 39: 667-674

Craven P A, Patterson M C, DeRubertis F R 1988 Role for protein kinase C in the modulation of glomerular PGE_2 production by angiotensin II. Biochem Biophys Res Commun 152: 1481-1489

Dunlop M E, Larkins R G 1985 Pancreatic islets synthesize phospholipids *de novo* from glucose via acyl-dihydroxyacetone phosphate. Biochem Biophys Res Commun 132: 467-473

Esmatjes E, Fernandez M R, Halperin I et al 1985 Renal hemodynamic abnormalities in patients with short term insulin-dependent diabetes mellitus: role of renal prostaglandins. J Clin Endocrinol Metab 60: 1231-1236

Farese R V, Konda T S, Davis J S et al. 1987 Insulin rapidly increases diacylglycerol by actvating *de novo* phosphatidic acid synthesis. Science 236: 586-589

Fein F S, Sonnenblick E H 1985 Diabetic cardiomyopathy. Prog Cardiovasc Dis 27: 255-270

Fujii S, Beutler E 1985 High glucose concentrations partially release hexokinase from inhibition by glucose 6-phosphate. Proc Natl Acad Sci USA 82: 1552-1554

Fuller J H, Shipley M J, Rose G et al 1980 Coronary heart disease and impaired glucose tolerance. The Whitehall Study. Lancet 1: 1371-1376

Go M, Sekiguchi K, Nomura H et al 1987 Further studies on the specificity of diacylglycerol for protein kinase C activation. Biochem Biophys Res Commun 144: 598-605

Graier W F, Wascher T C, Lackner L et al 1993 Exposure to elevated D-glucose concentrations modulates vascular endothelial cell vasodilatory response. Diabetes 42: 1497-1505

Green D A, Lattimer S A, Sima A F 1987 Sorbitol, phosphoinositides, and sodium-potassium-ATPase in the pathogenesis of diabetic complications. N Engl J Med 316: 599-606

Grossbard L, Schimke R T 1966 Multiple hexokinases of rat tissues: purification and comparison of soluble forms. J Biol Chem 241: 3546-3560

Hachiya H L, Takayama S, White M F et al 1987 Regulation of insulin receptor internalization in vascular endothelial cells by insulin and phorbol ester. J Biol Chem 262: 6417-6424

Hartwig J H, Thelen M, Rosen A et al 1992 MARCKS is an actin filament crosslinking protein regulated by protein kinase C and calcium-calmodulin. Nature 356: 618-622

Hermenegildo C, Felipo V, Minana M-D et al 1993 Sustained recovery of Na^+-K^+-ATPase activity in sciatic nerve of diabetic mice by administration of H7 or calphostin C, inhibitors of PKC. Diabetes 42: 257-262

Heyliger C E, Prakash A, McNeill J H 1987 Alterations in cardiac sarcolemmal Ca pump activity during diabetes mellitus. Am J Physiol 252: H540-547

Holub B J, Kuksis A 1986 Metabolism of molecular species of diacylglycerol phospholipids. Adv Lipid Res 16: 1-125

Huhtala P, Chow L T, Tryggvason 1990 Structure of the human type IV collagenase gene. J Biol Chem 265: 11077-11082

Inoguchi T, Battan R, Handler E et al. 1992a Preferential elevation of protein kinase C isoform βII and diacylglycerol levels in the aorta and heart of diabetic rats: differential reversibility to glycemic control by islet cell transplantation. Proc Natl Acad Sci USA 89: 11059-11063

Inoguchi T, Battan R, King G L 1992b Characterization of the mechanism of hyperglycemia's effect on the elevation of diacylglycerol (DAG) and protein kinase C (PKC) in macrovascular tissues and cells in culture. Diabetes 41 (suppl 1): 17A

Ishizuka T, Hoffman J, Copper D R et al 1989 Glucose-induced synthesis of diacylglycerol *de novo* is associated with translocation (activation) of protein kinase in rat adipocyte. FEBS Lett 249: 234-238

Jensen P K, Steven K, Blaehr H et al. 1986 Effects of indomethacin on glomerular hemodynamics in experimental diabetes. Kidney Int 29: 490-495

Jiang M J, Morgan K G 1987 Intracellular calcium levels in phorbol ester-induced contractions of vascular muscle. Am J Physiol 253: H1365-1371

Kannel W B, McGree D L 1979 Diabetes and cardiovascular disease: the Framingham Study. Diabetes Care 2: 920-926

Kariya K-I, Fukumoto Y, Tsuda T at al 1987 Inhibition of DNA synthesis by phorbol esters through protein kinase C in rabbit aortic smooth muscle. FEBS Lett 217: 69-73

Kessler I I 1971 Mortality experience of diabetic patients - a twenty-six year follow-up study. Am J Med 51: 715-724

King G L, Johnson S, Wu G 1990 Possible growth modulators involved in the pathogenesis of diabetic proliferative retinopathy. In: Westermark B et al (eds) Growth Factors in Health and Diseases. Excerpta Medica, New York, pp 303-317

Kim J, Agranoff B, Ueda T et al. 1988 Dietary myo-inositol prevents decreased native protein kinase C activity in diabetic rat nerve. Clin Res 36: 586a

Klein R, Klein B E R, Moss S E et al 1988 Glycosylated hemoglobin predicts the incidence and progression of diabetic retinopathy. JAMA 260: 2864-2871

Leatherman G F, Kim D, Smith T W 1987 Effect of phorbol esters on contractile state and calcium flux in cultured chick heart cells. Am J Physiol 253: H205-209

Lorenzi M, Toledo S, Boss G R et al 1987 The polyol pathway and glucose 6-phosphate in human endothelial cells culyured in high glucose concentrations. Diabetologia 30: 222-227

Lynch J S, Ferro T J, Blumenstock F A et al 1990 Increased endothelial albumin permeability mediated by protein kinase C activation. J Clin Invest 85: 1991-1998

Nilsson T, Arkhammer P, Berggren P 1988 Dual effects of glucose on cytoplasmic free Ca^{++} concentration and insulin release reflects the B-cell being deprived of fuel. Biochem Biophys Res Commun 153: 984-991

Nishizuka Y 1986 Studies and perspectives of protein kinase C. Science 233: 305-312

Nishizuka Y 1989 The family of protein kinase C for signal transduction. JAMA 262: 1826-1833

Okumura K, Akiyama N, Hashimoto H et al 1988 Alteration of 1,2-diacylglycerol content in myocardium from diabetic rats. Diabetes 37: 1168-1172

Okumura K, Nishiura T, Awaji Y et al 1991 1,2-diacylglycerol content and its fatty acid composition in thoracic aorta of diabetic rats. Diabetes 40:820-824

Paulson R, Mirrlees D J, Earl D C N et al 1983 The effects of an aldose reductase inhibitor upon the sorbitol pathway, fructose-1-phosphate and lactate in the retina and nerve of streptozotocin-diabetic rats. Exp Eye Res 36: 751-760

Peter-Riesch B, Fathi M, Schlegel W et al 1988 Glucose and carbachol generate 1,2-diacylglycerols by different mechanisms in pancreatic islets. J Clin Invest 81: 1154-1161

Priess J E, Loomis C R, Bell R M et al 1987 Quantitative measurement of sn-1, 2-diacylglycerols. Methods Enzymol 141: 294-300

Pu X, Inoguchi T, King G L 1993 Characterization of the mechanism for the chronic activation of DAG-PKC pathway in diabetes and hypergalactosemia. Diabetes 42 (suppl 1): 96A

Rasmussen H, Forder J, Kozimo I et al 1984 TPA-induced contraction of isolated rabbit vascular smooth muscle. Biochem Biophys Res Commun 122: 776-784

Reichard P, Berglund B, Britz A et al. 1991 Intensified conventional insulin treatment retards the microvascular complications in insulin-dependent diabetes mellitus (IDDM) after 5 years: the Stockholm Diabetes Intervention Study (SDIS). J Intern Med 230: 101-108

Schariff A, Luna E 1992 Diacylglycerol-stimulated formation of actin nucleation sites at plasma membranes. Science 256: 245-247

Schrama L H, Berti-Mattera L N, Eichberg J 1987 Altered protein phosphorylation in sciatic nerve from rats with streptozotocin induced diabetes. Diabetes 36: 1254-1260

Shiba T, Inoguchi T, Sportsman J R et al 1993 Correlation of diacylglycerol level and protein kinase C activity in rat retinal circulation. Am J Physiol 265: E783-793

Studer R K, Craven P A, DeRubertis F R 1993 Role for protein kinase C in the mediation of increased fibronectin accumulation by mesangial cells grown in high-glucose medium. Diabetes 42: 118-126

Tanaka Y, Kashiwagi A, Ogawa T et al 1991 Effect of verapamil on cardiac protein kinase C activity in diabetic rats. Eur J Pharmacol 200: 353-356

Tesfamarian B, Brown M L, Cohen R A 1991 Elevated glucose impairs endothelium-dependent relaxation by activating protein kinase C. J Clin Invest 87: 1643-1648

The Diabetes Control and Complications Trial (DCCT) 1993 N Engl J Med 329: 683-689

Williams B, Schrier R W 1992 Characterization of glucose-induced *in situ* protein kinase C activity in cultured vascular smooth muscle cells. Diabetes 41: 1464-1472

Williamson J R, Chang K, Frangos M et al 1993 Hyperglycemiic pseudohypoxia and diabetic complications. Diabetes 42: 801-813

Witters L A, Blackshear P J 1987 Protein kinase C-mediated phosphorylation in intact cells. Methods Enzymol 141: 412-424

Wolf B A, Williamson J R, Easom R A et al. 1991 Diacylglycerol accumulation and microvascular abnormalities induced by elevated glucose levels. J Clin Invest 87: 31-38

Wolf B A, Easom R A, Hughes J H et al 1989 Secretagogue-induced diacylglycerol accumulation in isolated pancreatic islets: mass spectrometric characterization of the fatty acyl content indicates multiple mechanisms of generation. Biochemistry 28: 4291-4301

Wollheim C B, Dunne MJ , Peter-Riesch B et al 1988 Activators of protein kinase C depolarize insulin-secreting cells by closing K channels. EMBO J 7: 2443-2449

Xiang H, McNeill J H 1992 Protein kinase C activity is altered in diabetic rat heart. Biochem Biophy Res Commun 187: 703-710

5

Regulation of gene expression in vascular cells by glucose and its relationship to diabetic vascular complications

Y. Nishio, G. L. King

INTRODUCTION

Diabetes mellitus causes both micro- and macrovascular complications, and sustained periods of hyperglycaemia appear to play a major pathogenic role in the initiation and progression of the diabetic vascular complications (Krolewkski et al 1987; Pirat 1978; Siperstein 1983). Many epidemiological studies have shown that the development of diabetic microvascular diseases is strongly associated with the duration and magnitude of hyperglycaemia (Krolewkski et al 1987; Pirat 1978; Siperstein 1983; Skyler 1990). Hyperglycaemia is probably also one of the major independent risk factors for macrovascular diseases, although data for this are not as clear (Siger et al 1992). It is likely that many metabolic factors present in diabetic patients, such as hypertension, hyperlipidaemia and hyperinsulinaemia, contribute to the clinical course of vascular complications. The results of the recently reported Diabetes Complication Control Trial (DCCT) clearly documented the clinical course of vascular complications and relationship between development of complications and hyperglycaemic levels (The Diabetes Control and Complications Trial Research Group 1993).

The consistent features of diabetic vascular complications are the requirement of chronicity for their development and difficulty of reversibility by euglycaemic control once the diseases have been established. Indeed, most studies have reported that normalisation of blood glucose slowed the progression of, but did not reverse, the vascular complications of diabetes. Furthermore, nonproliferative retinopathy developed in the histologically normal eyes of diabetic dogs during the 2.5-year period of normalised blood glucose that followed 2.5 years of hyperglycaemia (Engerman & Kern 1987). This implies that hyperglycaemia induces significant biochemical changes which can become irreversible after a certain period of time, possibly due to alterations in gene expression in vascular cells. In addition, recent studies have indicated that susceptibility to the progression of diabetic complications might be genetically determined (Krolewkski et al 1987), suggesting the involvement of an alteration of gene expression in the pathogenesis of diabetic vascular complications. Considerable interest has therefore been focused on the identification of genes in vascular cells and tissues which are altered by diabetes or hyperglycaemia. In the following, we will review reports on the expression of various genes which are affected by diabetes or hyperglycaemia as well as the effector mechanism of hyperglycaemia.

METHODS OF IDENTIFYING GLUCOSE-INDUCED GENE EXPRESSION IN VASCULAR CELLS

The identification of hyperglycaemia or diabetes-induced alterations in gene expression has been undertaken primarily by the 'candidate gene' approach. Since thickening of capillary basement membrane has been recognised as a clinical characteristic of diabetic microangiopathy, the main components of basement matrix have been targeted by various groups for gene expression studies. Numerous reports have shown that elevation of glucose levels will affect the expression of collagen and fibronectin (Ayo et al 1990a; Cagliero et al 1988; Wakisaka et al 1994). This method can be easily performed and provides information about gene expression under steady-state conditions. The limitation of this approach is that it only permits screening of known molecules on an individual basis, such as type IV collagen or fibronectin. In order to avoid this limitation, several techniques have been used to identify multiple and unknown genes differentially. Some of the standard techniques are subtractive and differential hybridisation, which have been used to identify a diabetes-related gene, RAD (Reynet & Kahn 1993), a member of the *Ras* family, which is only expressed in the skeletal muscle of diabetic patients and animals.

However, since these methods need substantial amounts of mRNA to construct a subtractive library and it take more than a year to screen the library, they have not been used widely to identify new genes regulated by elevated glucose conditions in vascular tissues or cultured vascular cells. Recently, a new technique called mRNA differential display was developed, originally to identify novel oncogenes in tumour cells (Liang & Pardee 1992; Liang et al 1992). We have modified this technique and demonstrated that it is very useful for identifying changes in gene expression induced by metabolic alterations (Aiello et al 1994; Nishio et al 1994). The main difference between identifying new oncogenes and metabolically-regulated genes is that the magnitude of the changes are much smaller in glucose-induced compared with hormone-induced gene expression.

The general outline of the method of mRNA differential display is schematically drawn in figure 5.1. Briefly, after replicating the cDNA by reverse transcription from mRNA using either $T_{12}NG$, $T_{12}NA$, $T_{12}NT$ or $T_{12}NC$ oligonucleotide as primer, where N is the 3-fold degenerate for G,

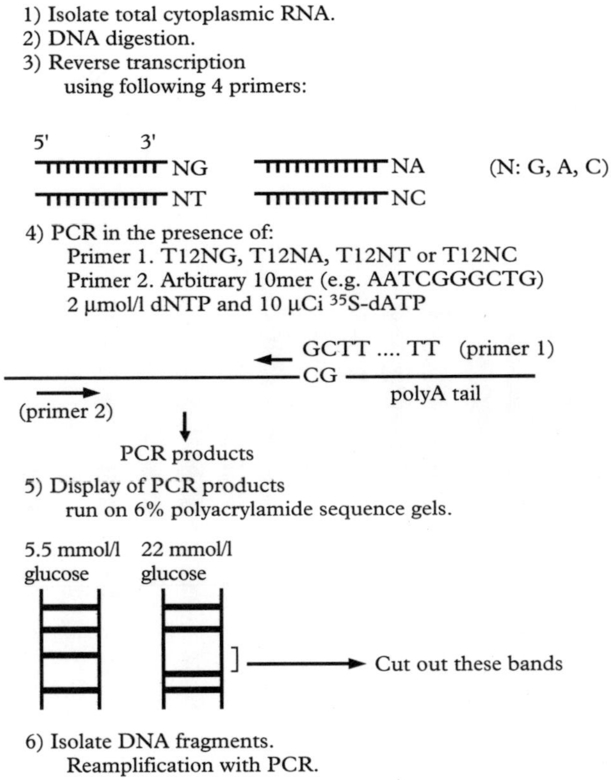

Fig. 5.1 Outline of mRNA differential display method. *Abbreviation:* PCR = polymerase chain reaction.

A and C, each clone of cDNA is amplified in the presence of ^{35}S-dATP by polymerase chain reaction (PCR) using an artificial 10-mer and the same primer as that for reverse transcription. Each amplified clone is visualised on a sequence gel as a band and can be compared under different conditions. These bands can be extracted from the gel and used as a probe for Northern blot analysis. After ligating these clones to a sequence vector, the clone can be identified by searching its sequence in a gene bank.

Figure 5.2 shows a representative result of this differential display comparing gene expression by cultured bovine retinal endothelial cells exposed to 5.5 or 22 mmol/l glucose conditions. As we reported previously (Nishio et al 1994; Aiello et al 1994), this new method provides the following merits compared with standard subtractive and differential hybridization. Firstly, it does not need polyA$^+$ RNA and requires only small amounts of total RNA from a small amount of tissue or cultured cells for the initial screening. In addition, the results can be obtained and

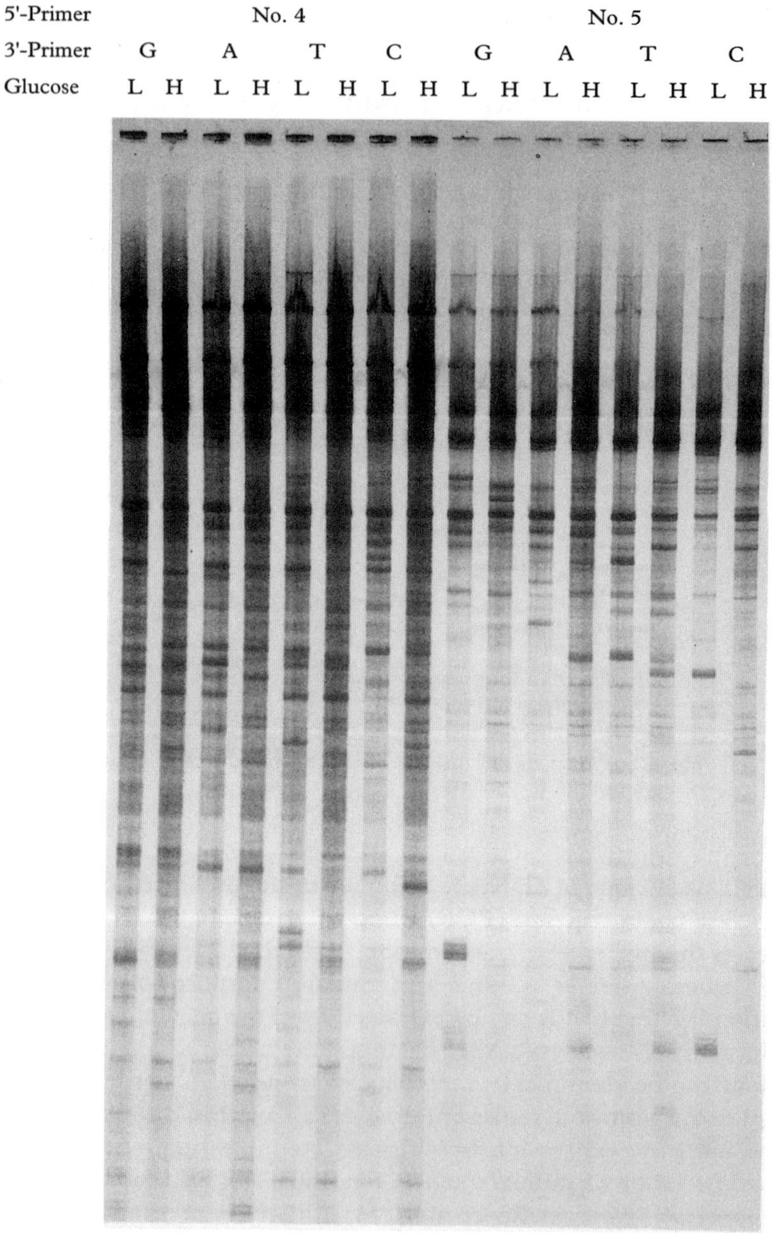

Fig. 5.2 Representative result of mRNA differential display. Total cellular RNA was isolated from bovine retinal endothelial cells exposed to either 5.5 mmol/l (L) or 22 mmol/l (H) glucose for 5 days.

confirmed very rapidly: it usually takes only 1-2 months for screening, confirmation of the results with Northern blot analysis, and identification of the clone's sequence. It is also very easy to compare gene expression induced by multiple conditions on a single gel with side-by-side analysis. Lastly, the sensitivity of the assay is high since the differences are amplified by PCR, which enables detection of changes in the 50-200% range. In contrast, subtractive hybridisation requires at least a 5-fold change in message level to recognise a difference between conditions (Dworkin & Dawid 1980). Thus, these advantages of the mRNA differential display method allow the user to screen most known or unknown glucose-regulated genes in a relatively short period of time in either cultured vascular cells or tissues.

EFFECT OF HIGH GLUCOSE CONDITIONS ON GENE EXPRESSION

EFFECTS OF HIGH GLUCOSE CONDITIONS ON DNA

Analogous to the reaction observed with proteins, the amino groups of DNA bases are also thought to be able to react nonenzymatically with reducing sugars. Bucala et al (1984) reported that *in vitro* incubation of DNA or nucleotides with glucose-6-phosphate (G6P) showed increases in absorbance in the 300-400 nm range which were similar to those of nonenzymatically glycated proteins. However, there was no significant reaction of the reducing sugar with thymidine, which indicates the requirement for a free amino group on the nucleotide for the reaction to occur. Furthermore, they demonstrated the biological effect of the reaction of glycated DNA by studying the capacity of f1 phage DNA to transfect *E. coli*. The incubation of f1 phage DNA with either glucose or G6P resulted in a time- and concentration-dependent decrease in transfection capability of the phage DNA. Similar results were obtained when plasmid pBR322 DNA was incubated with G6P, which led to a time- and concentration-dependent loss in transformation efficiency (Bucala et al 1985). In addition, incubation of plasmid DNA with G6P caused plasmid DNA mutations when it was transformed into a repair-proficient *E. coli* host but not when it transformed into repair-deficient host (*uvrC*$^-$).

The frequency of this mutation of plasmid DNA has also been investigated using two glycolytic mutant strains of *E. coli*, with which lack phosphoglucose isomerase or phosphoglucose isomerase and G6P-dehydrogenase, respectively. Lee and Cerami (1987) reported that G6P accumulated in these respective glycolytic strains 20 and 30 times more, and the frequency of *lac*$^+$ to *lac*$^-$ mutation of transformed plasmid increased 7 and 13 fold compared with the control strain. These results indicate that the high concentration of reducing sugar alters not only the physical property of DNA but also its biological properties, resulting in a higher DNA mutation frequency.

Although the above results were obtained from a prokaryote cell system, DNA damage induced by high glucose conditions has also been reported in eukaryote cells. DNA from human umbilical endothelial cells, but not from fibroblasts, exposed to glucose 30 mmol/l for more than 7 days manifested an accelerated rate of unwinding in alkali, which is indicative of an increased number of single-strand DNA breaks. An increased amount of hydroxyurea-resistant thymidine incorporation was also noted, which was indicative of increased DNA repair synthesis (Lorenzi et al 1986). Although the significance of glycation on the property of DNA in the pathogenesis of diabetic vascular complications is not clear, these results provide one of the possible mechanisms through which high glucose levels can affect gene expression.

EFFECT OF HIGH GLUCOSE CONDITIONS ON GENE EXPRESSION IN CULTURED CELLS

The effects of elevated glucose levels on gene expression have been investigated using several kinds of cultured vascular cells. In human umbilical endothelial cells, Cagliero et al (1988) reported that cells exposed to glucose 30 mmol/l for 11 days expressed increased levels of type IV collagen (138%) and fibronectin (121%) mRNA compared with control cells cultured in glucose 5 mmol/l, while type I collagen and *c-myc* mRNA levels remained unchanged. In addition, they characterised the overexpression of the basement membrane component induced by high glucose conditions as follow (Cagliero et al 1991a; Roy et al 1990): the glucose-induced overexpression of fibronectin and collagen IV persists after replating and several cell doublings in physiological glucose medium, and susceptibility to glucose is very different between different cultures. These results may explain the variability of the characteristics of diabetic vascular complication, but they could also be the results of variation of the culture conditions on endothelial cells.

Recently, Roth et al (1993) reported that in human umbilical endothelial cells, high glucose (30 mmol/l) conditions induced increases in the levels of mRNA encoding fibronectin-specific integrin receptor $\alpha 5\ \beta 1$ and $\alpha 3\beta 1$, which are polyspecific receptors for fibronectin, laminin and collagen. These data clearly showed that alterations of extracellular matrix gene expression were induced by high glucose conditions in endothelial cells. However, all the studies were performed using endothelial cells which had undergone primary culture from large vessels. Therefore the effect of high glucose conditions on capillary vascular cells, which are thought to be the most important lesion for diabetes-specific microangiopathy, remains unclear.

Extracellular matrix proteins are also overexpressed in cultured glomerular mesangial cells exposed to elevated glucose concentrations for 3-

4 days. Ayo et al (1990a) reported higher levels of type IV collagen, laminin and fibronectin mRNA on exposure to glucose 30 mmol/l compared with 10 mmol/l. Similarly, Wakisaka et al (1994) reported increases in the expression of type IV and type VI collagen in cultured glomerular mesangial cells when exposed to glucose 20 mmol/l. However, they did not find any increase in fibronectin expression under elevated glucose conditions. With respect to the mechanism of glucose's effect on the expression of collagen genes, Ziyadeh et al (1990) demonstrated that high glucose conditions increased the transcription rate of type I and type IV collagen genes. They found that glucose 450 mg/dl increased the steady-state mRNA level of type I and type IV procollagen 2.2 and 2.6 fold over control, respectively. Nuclear run-off studies showed that the transcription rate of procollagen genes was increased by up to 150% of control levels. Furthermore, using chloramphenicol-acetyltransferase reporter gene constructs, they demonstrated that an enhancer for type I procollagen gene, which had been identified in the first intron of the genomic sequence from +418 to +1524, responded to high glucose conditions by a 5-fold increase compared with low glucose (100mg/dl) conditions. Although these results were obtained from renal proximal tubule cells and not from vascular cells, it suggested the involvement of a transacting factor providing one of the possible mechanisms through which high glucose conditions induce the overexpression of extracellular matrix genes.

We have recently identified new sets of glucose-induced genes in retinal pericytes (Aiello et al 1994) and aortic smooth muscle cells (Nishio et al 1994) using the mRNA differential display method. In cultured bovine aortic smooth muscle cells, we showed a 2-fold decrease in the expression of a clone, which is highly homologous to human elongation factor 2, and 2- to 3-fold changes in novel sequences in cells exposed to glucose 22 mmol/l for 5 days compared with cells exposed to glucose 5.5 mmol/l. Elongation factor 2 is an essential modulator of polypeptide chain synthesis in eukaryotic cells and belongs to the GTPase family of proteins (Bourne et al 1991). It has homology to other GTP-binding proteins including *Ras* proteins, initiation factors, transducin and G proteins. The pathophysiological significance of a change in elongation factor 2 expression with regard to vascular abnormalities in diabetics currently remains unclear. It has been reported that translation of mRNA was less efficient because peptide chain elongation and termination were impaired in diabetic animals (Jefferson 1980), suggesting the presence of an abnormality of elongation factors *in vivo*. In addition, abnormalities of other GTP-binding proteins have been reported in diabetic animals and patients (Gawler et al 1986; Nishio et al 1988; Reynet & Kahn 1993).

In bovine retinal pericytes, we found decreases in the expression of fibronectin, caldesmon, Rieske FeS reductase and a novel tyrosine kinase-like molecule and increases in 27S and 28S ribosomal proteins and human antigen homologous molecule expression when cells were exposed to glucose 22 mmol/l for 7 days compared with glucose 5.5 mmol/ (Aiello et al 1994). In contrast to the results of human umbilical vein endothelial cells (Cagliero et al 1988) or mesangial cells (Ayo et al 1990a), fibronectin gene expression decreased in retinal pericytes under high glucose conditions. Although basement membrane thickening is reported in all vascular tissues, including retinal capillaries (Siperstien 1988), quantitative increases in fibronectin protein are often not observed. Indeed, alteration of fibronectin in diabetic human glomerular basement membrane and calf glomerular epithelial or endothelial cells were reported not to increase despite thickening of basement membrane (Danne et al 1993; Shimomura & Spiro 1987). Fibronectin can be deposited from circulation as well as secreted from microvascular cells including pericytes. Therefore, it is possible to have a decrease in fibronectin synthesis and secretion in pericytes, even when basement membrane is thickened.

Fibronectin stimulates cell growth through its specific receptor, integrin, which can activate intracellular tyrosine kinase activities (e.g. focal adhesion kinase). The difference of response to high glucose levels between pericytes and other vascular cells may provide the possible reason for explaining the selective loss of pericytes in diabetic retinal microvessels. We have found that pericytes exposed to glucose 22 mmol/l for 7 days reduced the expression of a novel gene with homology to known tyrosine kinases and proto-oncogenes by at least 16 fold (Aiello et al 1994). Tyrosine kinases are well known as mediating in the activity of growth factors and cytokines. Thus, the dramatic reduction of this gene induced by elevated glucose levels suggests that it may have an important role in the pathophysiology of the pericyte loss found in diabetic retinopathy. Further characterisation of this gene including full sequence cloning and expression are currently underway in our laboratory to determine its functional role in the pericyte. Expression of caldesmon is also reduced by elevated glucose levels in pericytes (Aiello et al 1994). Caldesmon is a regulatory protein of smooth muscle cell contractility via inhibition of actomyosin ATPase activity. Protein kinase C can phosphorylate caldesmon, which inhibits the activity of caldesmon and restores actomyosin ATPase activity, thereby leading to an increase in smooth muscle cell contractility (Hettasch & Sellers 1991). A decrease in the expression of caldesmon in pericytes may cause an increase in retinal microvessel contractility, resulting in the decrease of retinal blood flow which has been reported in both diabetic patients and animals in the early stages of diabetes (Bursell et al 1993; Shiba et al 1993).

THE EFFECT OF HIGH GLUCOSE CONDITIONS ON GENE EXPRESSION *IN VIVO*

The identification of diabetes-induced alterations in vascular tissue gene expression has been primarily studied using the 'candidate gene' approach, especially for extracellular matrix genes. Using glomeruli from rats with 4 weeks of diabetes induced by streptozotocin injection, Fukui et al (1992) reported that the steady-state level of mRNA encoding for the alpha 1 chains of type I, III and IV collagen and laminin B1 and B2 chains increased significantly. In contrast, expression of heparan sulphate proteoglycan gene in glomeruli was decreased after 4 weeks of diabetes compared with control rats. These abnormalities of extracellular matrix gene expression were ameliorated after 4 weeks of insulin treatment . This study suggests the important role of hyperglycaemic conditions on the abnormal regulation of extracellular matrix genes in cultured vascular cells. Another study proposed increases in circulating transforming growth factor (TGF)-β1 concentration and its mRNA expression in glomeruli are the possible cause of overexpression of collagen in diabetic rats (Bollineni & Reddi 1993). In this study, TGF-β1 increased collagen synthesis in normal glomeruli but not diabetic glomeruli. Furthermore, antibody to TGF-β1 prevented an increase in basal collagen synthesis in diabetic glomeruli. However, Silbiger et al (1993) reported that the mRNA level for TGF-β in cultured mesangial cells grown for 4 weeks at elevated glucose concentrations was similar to that cultured with normal glucose concentrations.

In vivo studies on diabetes-induced genes are very limited so far. The levels of type IV collagen alpha 1 chain and laminin B1 chain mRNA were tested using rat retinal tissue isolated from long-term (28-week) diabetic rats and galactosaemic rats (Polsuom et al 1990). Both groups of animals exhibited no significant changes in mRNA expression for either of these molecules compared with controls, while both groups showed a significant decrease in laminin B1 chain mRNA expression in lens. Recently, Roy et al (1994) reported an overexpression of type IV collagen in human diabetic retina. Using the quantitative reverse transcriptase PCR method, they investigated the level of mRNA for alpha 1 chain of type IV collagen as a ratio of β-actin mRNA level in human retinal tissue obtained post mortem from 5 patients with diabetes for a mean of 8 years and 6 nondiabetic controls. The ratio of collagen IV mRNA and β-actin mRNA was significantly higher in diabetic patients when compared with control subjects (0.53 *vs* 0.24, respectively). These investigations on extracellular matrix gene expression *in vivo* are preliminary and the results need to be confirmed.

MECHANISM OF THE EFFECT OF HIGH GLUCOSE CONCENTRATION ON GENE REGULATION

ROLE OF THE POLYOL PATHWAY, DIACYLGLYCEROL LEVELS AND PROTEIN KINASE C ACTIVITY

A role for the polyol pathway and the effects of aldose reductase inhibitors, which bind to the key enzyme of polyol pathway, have been extensively studied with respect to the development of diabetic complications. However, the results have not been particularly positive (Green et al 1992). Glucose is converted by aldose reductase to sorbitol in the polyol pathway. Because sorbitol does not pass readily through cell membranes and is relatively slowly metabolised by sorbitol dehydrogenase to fructose, it is postulated that it could accumulate to a high level intracellularly, thereby increasing intracellular osmolarity. In this situation, the intracellular concentration of myo-inositol, which is another organic osmolite, has been reported to decrease. In fact, this reciprocal alteration of sorbitol and myo-inositol was observed in cultured lens epithelial cells (Carper et al 1990). Yorek et al (1989) demonstrated that intracellular myo-inositol depletion induced by high glucose conditions was prevented by an aldose reductase inhibitor. In addition, they found that the cellular depletion of myo-inositol caused diminished incorporation of myo-inositol into inositol phosphate. However, the intracellular increases in sorbitol levels in vascular cells were minimal, only in the nanomolar range. Thus, others have postulated that the metabolism of the sorbitol and not its accumulation could be important.

Recently, we and others have postulated that the activation of protein kinase C (PKC) pathway by hyperglycaemia can explain diverse abnormalities in vascular cell induced by elevated glucose conditions (King et al 1990; Wolf et al 1991). Numerous investigations have subsequently reported that elevated glucose concentrations activate PKC activity in various vascular tissues and cultured cells: heart (Inoguchi et al 1992), renal glomeruli (Craven & DeRubertis 1989), aorta (Inoguchi et al 1992), retina (Shiba et al 1993), skin chamber granulation tissue (Wolf et al 1991), smooth muscle cells (Williams et al 1992) and mesangial cell (Ayo et al 1990b). Furthermore, increased diacylglycerol (DAG) concentrations have also been reported in heart (Inoguchi et al 1992), aorta (Inoguchi et al 1992), retina (Shiba et al 1993) skin chamber granulation tissue (Wolf et al 1991), smooth muscle cells (Inoguchi et al 1992), mesangial cells (Ayo et al 1990b) and endothelial cells (Inoguchi et al 1992). We have shown by that increased DAG levels are the result of *de novo* synthesis from glucose (Inoguchi et al 1992).

Wolf et al (1991) have proposed that there may be an alteration in the cytoplasmic NAD^+/NADH redox couple to the oxidation of sorbitol to fructose by sorbitol dehydrogenase. As a result of an increase in the reduced redox potential, *de novo* synthesis of DAG from triose phosphates is stimulated. Inoguchi et al (1992) investigated the reversibility of the abnormalities in DAG levels and PKC activity *in vivo*. After 2 weeks of diabetes without treatment in streptozotocin-induced diabetic BB rats, blood glucose levels were then normalised for up to 3 weeks by islet cell transplantation. Both elevated DAG levels and PKC activity in membranous fraction were normalised only in the heart but not in the aorta, suggesting persistent activation of DAG levels and PKC activity in macrovascular diabetic tissues. These findings are consistent with the sustained abnormality in vascular function in diabetes and alteration of gene expression even after maintenance of euglycaemia.

PKC is known to alter gene expression by regulating either at transcription or translation levels. For the former mechanism, consensus sequences in the regulatory region of genes, such as TRE or AP-1 binding site, have been identified (Mitchell & Tjian 1989). At present, study on the mechanism of gene regulation by glucose is very limited, partly because the changes in known glucose-inducer genes, such as extracellular matrix proteins, are too small to be precisely analysed for the characterisation of the regulatory mechanism. Cagliero et al (1991b), however, reported a possible role of PKC activity on overexpression of extracellular matrix genes. They studied the effect of phorbol, which stimulates PKC activity, on the mRNA level for type IV collagen using cultured human umbilical vein endothelial cells and found that phorbol significantly increased type IV collagen gene expression by 2-3 fold for 2-48 h. On the other hand, fibronectin expression was not changed for up to 6 h and decreased after exposure for 48 h. This study suggests the important role of PKC activity on type IV collagen expression, although the effect of PKC on expression of fibronectin remains unclear.

ROLE OF GLYCATION ON ALTERING GENE EXPRESSION INDUCED BY GLUCOSE

Another theory which has been postulated to explain glucose-induced vascular changes is nonenzymatic glycation. Glucose irreversibly modifies long-lived macromolecules by advanced glycation end-product (AGE) formation. AGE formation of extracellular matrix proteins can modify their functions by altering cellular functions and gene expression. Crowley et al (1991) reported that AGE modification of mesangial cell matrix decreased the mesangial cell proliferation by 50%, while fibronectin production was increased. However, this is different *in vivo* where no decrease in mesangial cells have been noted in early diabetic nephropathy. Recently, AGE-specific receptors have been identified in various tissues and cells, including mesangial cells (Skolnik et al 1991) and endothelial cells (Esposito et al 1989). Ligand binding to these receptors on macrovascular endothelial cells induces an increase in tissue factor activity and a reduction in thrombomodulin activity (Esposito et al 1989). Furthermore, AGE protein binding to the endothelial cell AGE receptor also induces increased production of the endothelin-1 involving the AP-1 DNA binding site for transcriptional regulatory proteins (Brownlee 1992). In mesangial cells, AGE receptors were reported to increase the production of type IV collagen, laminin and heparan sulphate proteoglycan mediated by platelet-derived growth factor (Doi et al 1992). As mention before, reducing sugars, including glucose and G6P, can also modify DNA and nuclear proteins by glycation, which is thought to injure DNA. However, this possibility needs to be established *in vivo*.

CONCLUSION

The clinical and biochemical characteristics of diabetic vascular complications suggest involvement of alterations of gene expression in vascular cells. A number of investigations using the 'candidate gene' approach have suggested that elevated glucose levels can cause overexpression of selected extracellular matrix genes in vascular cells. Although controversy remains about the mechanism of the effect of glucose, we believe that the main mechanism for causing changes in gene expression is induced by elevated PKC activity, as shown in figure 5.3, since PKC changes can alter the expression of so many genes responsible for vascular cell function. Further screening for glucose-induced genes using more sophisticated methods, such as the recently developed mRNA display method, would provide a whole new set of target genes for studying the effects of high glucose conditions in vascular cells. These studies will increase our understanding about the pathogenesis of diabetic vascular complications.

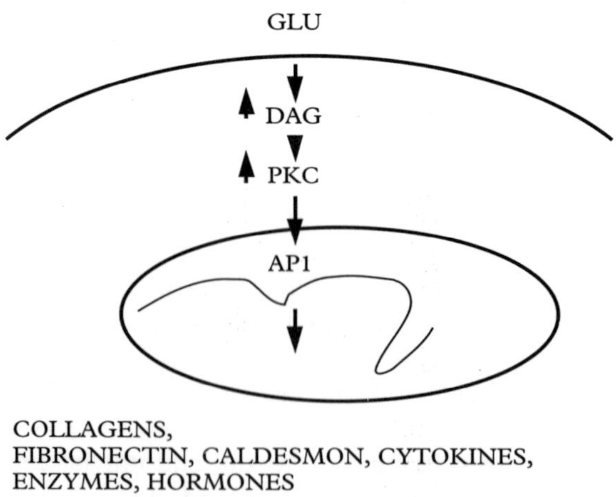

Fig. 5.3 Mechanism of glucose's effect on gene expression. *Abbreviations:* DAG = diacylglycerol; GLU = glucose; PKC = protein kinase C.

ACKNOWLEDGMENTS

The studies presented were supported by grants NIH EY05110, EY09178 and DK36433, Massachusetts University Eye Research Foundation, and grant DK36836, Joslin Diabetes Center in Diabetes Endocrinology Research Center.

REFERENCES

Aiello L P, Robinson G S, Lin Y W et al 1994 Identification of multiple glucose-regulated genes in bovine retinal pericytes by mRNA differential display. Proc Natl Acad Sci USA 91: 6231-6235

Ayo S H, Radink R A, Glass W F I I et al 1990a Increased extracellular matrix synthesis and mRNA in mesangial cells grown in high-glucose medium. Am J Pathol 136: 1339-1348

Ayo S H, Radnik R, Garoni J et al 1990b High glucose increases diacylglycerol mass and activates protein kinase C in mesangial cell cultures. Am J Physiol 260: F185-191

Bollineni J S, Reddi A S 1993 Transforming growth factor-beta 1 enhances glomerular collagen synthesis in diabetic rats. Diabetes 42: 1673-1677

Bourne H, Sanders D A, McComick F 1991 The GTPase superfamily: conserved structure and molecular mechanism. Nature 349: 117-126

Brownlee M 1992 Glycation products and the pathogenesis of diabetic complications. Diabetes Care 15: 1835-1843

Bucala R, Model P, Cerami A 1984 Modification of DNA by reducing sugars: possible mechanism for nucleic acid aging and age-related dysfunction in gene expression. Proc Natl Acad Sci USA 81: 105-109

Bucala R, Model P, Russel M et al 1985 Modification of DNA by glucose-6-phosphate induces DNA rearrangements in an *Escherichia coli* plasmid. Proc Natl Acad Sci USA 82: 8439-8442

Bursell S E, Clermont A, Wald H et al 1993 Decreased retinal blood flow in early stage type I diabetes. Diabetes 42 (suppl): 89A

Cagliero E, Maiello M, Boeri D et al 1988 Increased expression of basement membrane components in human endothelial cells cultured in high glucose. J Clin Invest 82: 735-738

Cagliero E, Roth T, Roy S et al 1991a Characteristics and mechanisms of high-glucose-induced overexpression of basement membrane components in cultured human endothelial cells. Diabetes 40: 102-110

Cagliero E, Roth T, Roy S et al 1991b Expression of genes related to the extracellular matrix in human endothelial cells J Biol Chem 266: 14244-14250

Carper D, Masyuki K, Stark H et al 1990 Increase in aldose reductase mRNA in dog lens epithelial cells under hypertonic conditions. Exp Eye Res 50: 743-749

Craven P A, DeRubertis F R 1989 Protein kinase C is activated in glomeruli from streptozotocin diabetic rats: possible mediation by glucose. J Clin Invest 83: 1667-1675

Crowley S T, Brownlee M, Edelstein D et al 1991 Effects of nonenzymatic glycosylation of mesangial matrix on proliferation of mesangial cells. Diabetes 40: 540-547

Danne T, Spiro M J, Spiro R G 1993 Effect of high glucose on type IV collagen production by cultured glomerular epithelial, endothelial, and mesangial cells. Diabetes 42: 170-177

Doi T, Vlassara H, Kirstein M et al 1992 Receptor specific increase in extracellular matrix productions in mouse mesangial cells by advanced glycosylation end products is mediated via platelet derived growth factor. Proc Natl Acad Sci USA 89: 2873-2877

Dworkin M B, Dawid I B 1980 Use of a cloned library for the study of abundant Poly(A)$^+$ RNA during *Xenopus laevis* development. Dev Biol 76: 449-464

Engerman R L, Kern T S 1987 Progression of incipient diabetic retinopathy during good glycemic control. Diabetes 36: 808-812

Esposito C Gerlach H, Brett J et al 1989 Endothelial receptor-mediated binding of glucose modified albumin is associated with increased monolayer permeability and modulation of cell surfactant coagulant properties. J Exp Med 170: 1387-407

Fukui M, Nakamura T, Ebihara I et al 1992 ECM gene expression and its modulation by insulin in diabetic rats. Diabetes 41: 1520-1527

Gawler D, Milligan G, Spiegel A et al 1986 Abolition of the expression of inhibitory guanine nucleotide regulatory protein Gi activities in diabetes. Nature 323: 182-185

Green D A, Sima A A F, Stevens M J et al 1992 Complications: neuropathy, pathogenetic consideration. Diabetes Care 15: 1902-1925

Hettasch J M, Sellers J R 1991 Caldesmon phosphorylation in intact human platelets by cAMP-dependent protein kinase and protein kinase C. J Biol Chem 266: 19971-19975

Inoguchi T, Battan R, Handler E et al 1992 Preferential elevation of protein kinase C isoform βII and diacylglycerol level in the aorta and heart of diabetic rats: differential reversibility to glycemic control by islet cell transplantation. Proc Natl Acad Sci USA 89: 11059-11063

Jefferson L S 1980 Role of insulin in the regulation of protein synthesis. Diabetes 29: 487-496

King G L, Johnson S, Wu G 1990 Possible growth modulators involved in the pathogenesis of diabetic proliferative retinopathy. In: Westermark B et al (eds) Growth Factors in Health and Diseases, Excerpta Medica, Amsterdam, pp 303-317

Krolewkski A S, Warram J H, Rand L I et al 1987 Epidemiologic approach to the etiology of type 1 diabetes mellitus and its complications. N Engl J Med 317: 1390-1398

Lee A T, Cerami A 1987 Elevated glucose-6-phosphate levels are associated with plasmid mutations *in vivo*. Proc Natl Acad Sci USA 84: 8311-8314

Liang P, Averboukh L, Keyomarsi K et al 1992 Differential display and cloning of messenger RNAs from human breast caner versus mammary epithelial cells. Cancer Res 52: 6966-6968

Liang P, Pardee A B 1992 Differential display of eukaryotic messenger RNA by means of polymerase chain reaction. Science 257: 967-971

Lorenzi M, Montisano D F, Toledo S et al 1986 High glucose and DNA damage in endothelial cells. J Clin Invest 77: 322-325

Mitchell P J, Tjian R 1989 Transcriptional regulation in mammalian cells by sequence-specific DNA binding proteins. Science 245: 371-378

Nishio Y, Aiello L P, King G L 1994 Glucose induced genes in bovine aortic smooth muscle cells identified by mRNA differential display. FASEB J 8: 103-106

Nishio Y, Kashiwagi A, Kida Y et al 1988 Deficiency of cardiac β-adrenergic receptor in streptozotocin-induced diabetic rats. Diabetes 37: 1181-1187

Pirat J 1978 Diabetes mellitus and its degenerative complications: a prospective study of 4,400 patients observed between 1947 and 1973. Diabetes Care 1: 168-188

Polsuom R, Prockop D J, Boot-Handford R P 1990 Effects of long-term diabetes and galactosaemia upon lens and retinal mRNA levels in the rat. Exp Eye Res 51: 33-37

Reynet C, Kahn C R 1993 Rad: a member of the Ras family overexpressed in muscle of type II diabetics. Science 262: 1441-1444

Roth T, Podesta F, Stepp M A 1993 Integrin overexpression induced by high glucose and by human diabetes: potential pathway to cell dysfunction in diabetic microangiopathy. Proc Natl Acad Sci USA 90: 9640-9644

Roy S, Maiello M, Lorenzi M 1994 Increased expression of basement membrane collagen in human diabetic retinopathy. J Clin Invest 93: 438-442

Roy S, Sala R, Cagliero E et al 1990 Overexpression of fibronectin induced by diabetes or high glucose: phenomenon with a memory. Proc Natl Acad Sci USA 87: 404-408

Shiba T, Inoguchi T, Sportsman J R et al 1993 Correlation of diacylglycerol level and protein kinase C activity in rat retina to retinal circulation. Am J Physiol 265: E783-793

Shimomura H, Spiro R G 1987 Studies on macromolecular components of human glomerular basement membrane and alterations in diabetes. Decreased levels of heparan sulfate proteoglycan and laminin. Diabetes 36: 374-381

Siger D E, Nathan D M, Anderson K M et al 1992 Association of HbA_{1c} with prevalent cardiovascular disease in the original cohort of the Framingham Heat Study. Diabetes 41: 202-209

Silbiger S, Crowley S, Shan Z et al 1993 Nonenzymatic glycation of mesangial matrix and prolonged exposure of mesangial matrix to elevated glucose reduces collagen synthesis and proteoglycan charge. Kidney Int 43: 853-864

Siperstein M D 1983 Diabetic macroangiopathy and the control of blood glucose. N Engl J Med 309: 1577-1579

Siperstien M D 1988 Diabetic microangiopathy, genetics, environment, and treatment. Am J Med 85: 119-130

Skolnik E Y, Yang Z, Makita Z et al 1991 Human and rat mesangial cell receptors for glucose-modified proteins: potential role in kidney tissue remodelling and diabetic nephropathy J Exp Med 174: 931-939

Skyler J S 1990 Relation of metabolic control of diabetes mellitus to chronic complications. In: Rifkin H, Porte Jr D (eds) Diabetes Mellitus: Theory and Practice. Elsevier, New York, pp 856-868

The Diabetes Control and Complications Trial Research Group 1993 The effect of intensive treatment of diabetes on the development and progression of long-term complications in insulin-dependent diabetes mellitus. N Engl J Med 329: 977-986

Wakisaka M, Spiro M J, Spiro R G 1994 Synthesis of type VI collagen by cultured glomerular cells and comparison of its regulation by glucose and other factors with that of type IV collagen. Diabetes 43: 95-103

Williams B, Tsai P, Schrier R W 1992 Glucose induced downregulation of angiotensin II and arginine vasopressin receptors in cultured rat aortic vascular smooth muscle cells. J Clin Invest 90: 1992-1999

Wolf B A, Williamson J R, Easom R A et al 1991 Diacylglycerol accumulation and microvascular abnormalities induced by elevated glucose levels. J Clin Invest 87: 31-38

Yorek M A, Dunlap J A, Leeney E M 1989 Effect of galactose and glucose levels and sorbinil treatment on myo-inositol metabolism and Na^+K^+-ATP pump activity in cultured neuroblastoma cells. Diabetes 38: 996-1004

Ziyadeh F N, Snipes E R, Watanabe M et al 1990 High glucose induces cell hypertrophy and stimulates collagen gene transcription in proximal tubule. Am J Physiol 259: F704-714

6

Gene transfection to cultured endothelial cells

Y. Mitsui, N. Ishida, M. Kondo, M. Matsui

INTRODUCTION

Vascular endothelial cells play important roles in permeability of macromolecules into tissue, infiltration of neutrophils and lymphocytes into inflammatory sites, extravasation of cancer cells, induction of blood cell maturation, prevention of coagulation, regulation of vascular tone, and secretion of hormonal factors (Kitayama et al 1993; Mitsui et al 1984; Neichi et al 1982; Okada et al 1994). Dysfunction of these endothelial cells is considered to cause various diseases, such as microangiopathy in diabetes, atherosclerosis, ischaemia and dementia. A change in endothelial cell function is also inevitable during the ageing process, since all somatic cells loose their proliferation potential and alter function with each cell division (Mitsui & Hirokawa 1984). We have previously shown that prostacyclin production and angiotensin-converting enzyme activity decline with *in vitro* cellular ageing (Hasegawa et al 1988). In contrast, endothelin secretion and fibronectin production increase as a function of human age and *in vitro* cellular ageing (Kumazaki et al 1993; Tokunaga et al 1992). Our recent studies indicate that the enhanced production of fibronectin and endothelin is due to up-regulation of their mRNA expression in aged cells (Kumazaki et al 1993; Kumazaki 1994).

Manipulation of endothelial cell function by means of gene transfection and/or their introduction into artificial vascular tubes might be expected to lead to developments that would allow normalisation or improvement of endothelial cell dysfunction and related diseases. However, gene transfection to normal human endothelial cells has not been successful so far. One of the reasons for this might be that the *in vitro* life span of normal human endothelial cells is too short to isolate stable transformants. We have recently established a serum-free culture system of the human endothelial cell line, t-HUE2 (Kobayashi et al 1991). By using this cell line, we succeeded in transfecting preproendothelin cDNA and mp41 cDNA. In this article, we describe these two examples of specific gene introduction and their expression in the human endothelial cell line.

DEVELOPMENT OF ENDOTHELIAL HOST CELLS FOR GENE TRANSFECTION

There are at least three requirements which need to be fulfilled by a host cell line for it to be used for gene transfection. The first is escape from limited division potential, i.e. immortalization. Normal somatic cells have a limited division potential *in vitro*. For instance, human adult skin fibroblasts cease to divide after about a 30 population doubling level (PDL) [Schneider & Mitsui 1976]. Likewise, human aorta endothelial cells loose their division potential at 20-40 PDL depending on the age of donors (Tokunaga et al 1992). Human umbilical cord vein endothelial cells have a longer life span, but still eventually stop dividing at 70-80 PDL (Kumazaki et al 1994). Escape from this proliferation limitation leads to immortalization (Wadhwa et al 1993). Development of an immortal endothelial cell line is therefore crucial for the continuous supply of endothelial cells with specific function.

Endothelial cell lines can be derived from various animals including mouse, rat, pig and cow. Treatment of cells with chemical carcinogens, physical mutagens or oncogenic viruses is the usual way to establish their transformants. The immortalization achieved by this treatment is always accompanied by some genetic changes, e.g. point mutation, gene rearrangement and deletion. In the case of porcine aorta endothelial cells, however, we could obtain spontaneously-transformed cell lines after long-term subcultivations. Among these transformants, the PAE-20 cell line was selected for further use (Imamura & Mitsui 1987; Imamura et al 1991), since it had minimal chromosomal aberration (Mitsui et al 1984), i.e. it showed a normal diploid chromosomal pattern, but had an additive chromosome fragment on chromosome 4. It was originally subcultivated in routine growth medium as used for normal endothelial cells. The growth medium used is MCDM 151 basal medium supplemented with foetal bovine serum (10%) and acidic fibroblast growth factor (aFGF) 2 ng/ml. Later on, we noticed that it can be subcultivated without aFGF on fibronectin-uncoated flasks.

The second requirement for a host cell line is maintenance of the specific function of the original tissue cells. Immortalized cells or cancer cells often loose their differentiated properties. The PAE-20 cell line, however, had preserved certain specific functions of endothelial cells such as the abilities to produce prostacyclin and to produce tube-like structures. They had a cobblestone-like structure with a monolayer sheet. The negative charge of the cell surface was maintained unaltered, and they contained a high amount of heparan sulphate with a trace of hyaluronic acid. Endothelial cell-derived vasoconstrictor, endothelin (ET), was isolated from the conditioned medium of this cell line (Yanagisawa et al 1988).

The third requirement is a high frequency of transformation by exogenous gene transfection. Transformation frequency differs among host cells. Besides this, the expression of the transfected exogenous gene should also be high enough. In some cases, proper processing of precursor protein and its post-translational modification are required. One of the modifications which is difficult to control is protein glycosylation. The sequence for the sugar chain is not coded in the transfected gene. In addition, the site and degree of glycosylation is more or less species specific and tissue origin specific.

For the mass production of bioactive substances, the host cell needs to be cultured in serum-free medium on a large scale. Long-term subcultivation of PAE-20 cells in a gradually decreasing concentration of serum achieved the establishment of PAE-20 clone 1, which can be cultured in serum-free medium. We were able to isolate endothelin, as mentioned above (Yanagisawa et al 1988), from the serum-free conditioned medium of large-scale culture of PAE-20 clone 1.

Using a similar procedure, it has been possible to isolate from ECV-305 a human endothelial cell line, t-HUE2, with the ability to grow in serum-free conditions (Kobayashi et al 1991). t-HUE2 cells can grow in ASF 301, a serum-free medium (Ajinomoto), which contains epidermal growth factor, insulin, transferrin and albumin. This t-HUE-2 cell line was found to have lost the ability to produce endothelin-1 (ET-1) despite its vascular tube origin. In contrast, the PAE-20 cell line secreted ET-1 into culture medium of the same components (ASF 301). In the present manuscript we

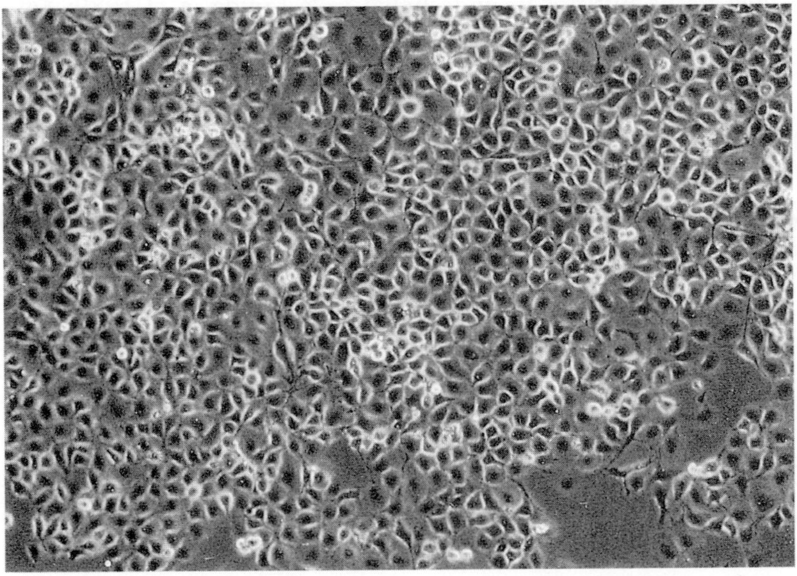

Fig. 6.1 Phase contrast microscopic morphology of t-HUE2 cells. t-HUE2 cells can grow in ASF301 serum-free medium without coating the culture flask and do not secrete ET-1 into culture medium.

used the t-HUE2 cell line (see figure 6.1 for phase contrast morphology) as a host cell for gene transfection to examine endothelial cell-specific expression and its application. Transformed human B lymphocyte (Raji) cells were used as a control cell line.

PREPRO ET cDNA AND MP41 cDNA FOR TRANSFECTION

ENDOTHELIN AND THE PRECURSOR

ET-1 is a potent peptide vasocontrictor originally isolated from serum-free conditioned medium of porcine vascular endothelial cells (Yanagisawa et al 1988). Cloning of human and porcine cDNA for the ET-1 precursor indicated that mature ET-1 is identical for these species (Ito et al 1988). From cDNA sequence analysis, human ET-1 is supposed to be cleaved by a unique ET-1-converting enzyme from its precursor, big ET-1, (37 amino acid residues), which is cleaved from prepro ET-1 (203 amino acid residues) [Inoue et al 1989; Sawamura et al 1990]. Prepro ET-1 cDNA also has a signal sequence. Northern blot analysis has revealed that t-HUE2 and Raji cells do not express prepro ET-1 mRNA (Kondo et al 1992).

Vasoactive intestinal contractor (VIC) has been found in the mouse to be one of the three members of the ET peptide family (Ishida et al 1989, Mitsui & Saida 1991; Saida et al 1989). In the case of humans, endothelin-2 (ET-2) was found to be human type VIC. Human ET-2 differs from murine VIC at only one amino acid. Prepro VIC mRNA is expressed in intestinal tissue but not in endothelial cells (Saida et al 1989; Saida & Mitsui 1991). As a consequence the transformed human endothelial cell line, t-HUE2, did not express ET-2 mRNA.

MP41: A NOVEL SPLEEN-DERIVED cDNA CONTAINING THE *PER* REPEAT SEQUENCE

Screening of a mouse spleen cDNA library with a DNA probe [*Eco*RI-*Eco*RI 2.5-kb fragment from cp2.2] containing *per* repeat sequences has

```
                              30        40        50        60        70
                        STQSTAQHSTAQHSTAQHSTAQHNTAHHSTPQHSTAQHTTAHHSTPQHTTAHYSTG
                           ..  .:: .::. ..:. :.:   .:.. .::. ..:. .::.  .:. ::.. :   (29.4%)
His-rich glycoprotein   DLHPHKHHSHEQHPHGHHPHAHHPHEHDTHRQHPHGHHPHGHHPHGHHPHGHHPHG
      (Human)                   360        370       380        390       400

                              30        40        50        60
                        STQSTAQHSTAQHSTAQHSTAQHNTAHHSTPQHSTAQH-TTAHH
                        :    : :  : :  : :  : :  :::    :  : :  : ::        (40.9%)
His Ala rich glycoprotein SHHDDAHHDGAHHDDAHHDGAHHDGAHHDGAHHDGAHHNATTHH
(Plasmodium faciparum)     180        190        200        210
```

Fig. 6.2 Homologous region between mp41 and His-rich glycoprotein. Two dots (:) and a single dot (.) indicate identical and related amino acids, respectively.

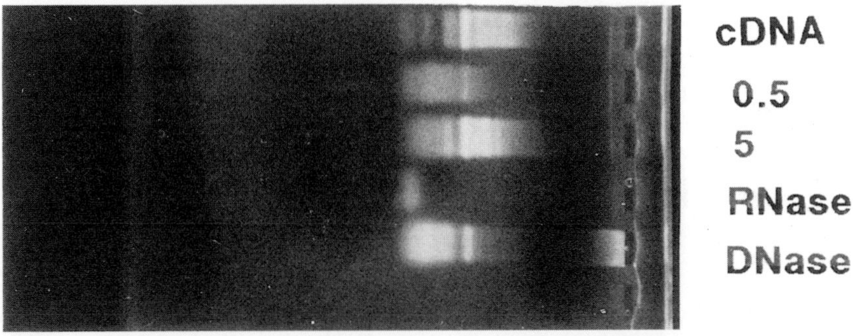

Fig. 6.3 mRNA expression of mp41 gene by direct PCR analysis. mRNA was reverse transcribed and amplified by Taq-polymerase. cDNA indicates mp41 cDNA template 1 ng as a positive control. 0.5 and 5 indicate mouse spleen polyA$^+$ RNA 0.5 and 5 mg. RNase and DNase indicate polyA$^+$ RNA 5 mg treated by RNase 0.2 mg/ml or DNase 2 U/ml at 37 °C for 30 min prior to PCR reaction.

been performed (Ishida et al 1991; Matsui et al 1993; Shin et al 1985). Among the numerous cDNA clones isolated in the screening, clone mp41 contains an open reading frame that consist of 133 amino acids, which has no signal peptide, a (Ser-Thr-Ala-Gln-His)$_{11}$ repetitive sequence region, a CDC25 similarity region, and a C-terminal hydrophobic sequence (Ishida et al 1994). The nucleotide sequence encoding Ser-Thr-Ala-Gln-His, which is tandemly repeated 11 times, showed some similarity with human and plasmodium His-rich glycoprotein (Fig. 6.2). mp41 is unusually rich in serine and threonine residues (26% of the total amino acids).

The cap site of the mp41 transcript was determined by primer extension analysis using polyA$^+$ RNA from normal mouse spleen and found to be 128 bp upstream from the 5' end point of the mp41 cDNA (data not shown). Polymerase chain reaction (PCR) analysis showed that mp41 gene mRNA is expressed in normal mouse spleen (Fig. 6.3). RNase treatment and DNase treatment prior to direct PCR indicate that an amplified product is specific for RNA. The results indicate that mp41 mRNA is expressed in normal mouse spleen (Ishida et al 1994). Sequence comparison of the mp41 translation product with known proteins by the FAST-P computer program and the algorithm of Lipman and Pearson revealed no significant similarities with proteins in the European Molecular Biology Laboratory (EMBL) database, indicating that the mp41 translation product is a novel protein, which showed circadian regulation at the suprachiasmatic nucleus of rat brain (Ishida et al 1994).

CONSTRUCTION OF EXPRESSION VECTOR, DNA TRANSFECTION AND SELECTION OF TRANSFORMANTS

The *Eco*gpt fragment (*Eco*RI-*Pvu*II, 3.2-kb) from pSV2gpt was ligated into the *Sal*I site of pcDL-SP α 296 (designated the pSR α gpt vector) [Mitsui

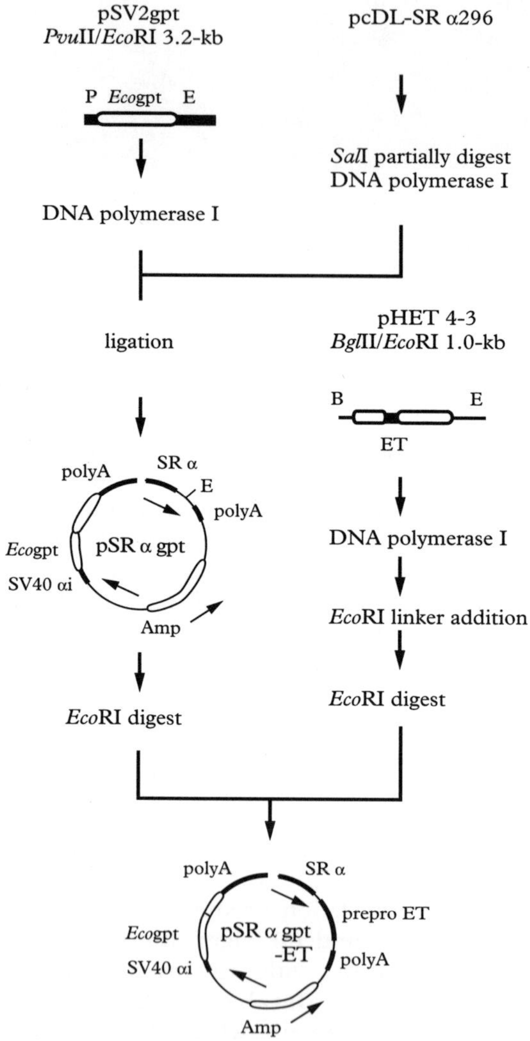

Fig. 6.4 Construction of expression vector for prepro ET and mp41. Vector for prepro ET expression was constructed as above and similarly the mp41 expression vector, pSR α gpt-mp41, was constructed by inserting *Eco*RI-*Eco*RI 2.8 kb fragment. Details are described in text.

et al 1984] The prepro ET-1 expression vector, pSR α gpt-ET, was constructed by inserting prepro ET-1 cDNA, which was obtained from pHET4-3 (*Eco*RI-*Bgl*II, 1.0-kb) [Ito et al 1988], into the *Eco*RI site of pSR α gpt for expressing ET-1 as shown in figure 6.4 (Kondo et al 1991). The mp41 expression vector, pSR α gpt-mp41, was constructed by inserting *Eco*RI-*Eco*RI 2.8-kb fragment (the whole mp41 cDNA) [Ishida et al 1994).

For transfection, cells from a logarithmically growing culture were collected by trypsinisation and centrifugation, and resuspended, at a final concentration of 1×10^7 cells/ml, in Dulbecco's phosphate-buffered saline (PBS). Plasmid DNAs were added, at a final concentration of 80 μg/ml (Raji) or 20 μg/ml (t-HUE2), received 3 electric pulses of 4 kV/cm (Raji) or 2 kV/cm (t-HUE2). The gpt selection medium, which contained xanthine (250 μg/ml), hypoxanthine (13.6 μg/ml), glycine (10 μg/ml), thymidine (11.8 μg/ml), aminopterin (2 μg/ml) and mycophenolic acid (25 μg/ml or 2.5 μg/ml) [Mulligan & Berg 1981], was applied after 48 h of nonselective growth. The cells were then replated into 24-well plates (2×10^2 cells or 2×10^3 cells per well for Raji and t-HUE2, respectively) with selection medium. A few months later, the growing transformants were transferred into growth medium to examine their expression and stability of the inserted DNA.

CLONING OF CELLS TRANSFECTED WITH HUMAN PREPRO ET-1 cDNA AND MP41 cDNA

The pSR α gpt-ET and pSR α gpt-mp41 were transfected by electroporation into two types of human cell lines, Raji and t-HUE2, under the conditions described above. We recommend determining the electric pulse conditions for each cell line by using chloramphenicol acetyl transferase (CAT) assay (Gorman et al 1982). Growing colonies of putative transformants in a selective gpt medium were isolated 14-21 days after seeding and were subcultivated for another few months in a selective medium. They were then cultured in growth medium for further examination. The transformation frequencies of Raji and t-HUE-2 were in the range of 1×10^{-5} and 7.8×10^{-5}, respectively, under the present experimental conditions (Table 6.1). 15 cloned ET expressors and 13 cloned mp41 expressors of the transformed t-HUE2 cells, along with 2 cloned ET expressors and 5 cloned mp41 expressors of the transformed Raji cells were finally selected for further analysis.

EXPRESSION OF EXOGENOUS PREPRO ET-1 mRNA

Several clones of transformants growing in selective medium were isolated and analyzed for prepro ET-1 mRNA expression. Northern blot analysis indicated that all the transformants examined expressed exogenous prepro

Table 6.1 Transformation frequency of human endothelial cell line, t-HUE-2 and B lymphocyte line, Raji. Prepro ET-1 cDNA and mp41 cDNA were transfected by electroporation as described in the text. Transformation frequency of endothelial cells was similar to that of well established cell line, Raji cells.

	Concentration of mycophenolic acid (μg/ml)	Number of total cells	Number of transformants	Frequency of transformation
t-HUE 2	2.5	7.2×10^5	56	7.8×10^{-5}
pSR α gpt-ET	25	7.2×10^5	39	5.4×10^{-5}
Raji	2.5	1.9×10^5	13	6.8×10^{-5}
pSR α gpt-ET	25	1.9×10^5	2	1.0×10^{-5}
t-HUE 2	2.5	2.4×10^5	8	3.3×10^{-5}
pSR α gpt-mp 41	25	2.4×10^5	2	0.8×10^{-5}

ET-1 mRNA, while normal endothelial cells, HUE, expressed endogenous prepro ET-1 mRNA, which was easily distinguishable from the transcript of exogenous DNA (2.0 kb) because of their size differences (Kondo et al 1991; Kondo et al 1992). Levels of prepro ET-1 mRNA were quantified by measuring their radiogram intensity on the Northern blot filters. Seven different clones of transformants (t-HUE2 clones 1 to 7) expressed 288, 247, 234, 225, 81, 19 and 17% of normal human umbilical endothelial cells (HUE). A transformant of the Raji cell line (Raji-1) expressed 50% of prepro ET-1 mRNA (Kondo et al 1992).

PRODUCTION AND SECRETION OF ET-1 AND ITS PRECURSOR

Conditioned media of the transfectant cell lines were examined for their ET-1 and big ET-1 contents. Big ET-1 was separated by HPLC and subjected to analysis by radioimmunoassay. ET-1 levels secreted by these cells were very high compared with normal human cells. The ratio of the amount of ET-1 secreted to the level of prepro ET-1 mRNA expressed in each cell line was 150-550% of normal endothelial cells. Among them, the t-HUE2-1 cell line secreted 9170 fmol per day per 10^6 cells, while the value for normal endothelial cells was 580. In contrast to these t-HUE2 cell transformants, a transfectant of the B lymphocyte transformant, Raji-1, did not secrete any detectable level of ET-1 into culture medium despite its high level of prepro ET-1 mRNA.

Conversion of the precursor to mature ET-1 is essential for expression of biological activity. Determination of ratio of ET-1 (mature ET) to its precursor (big ET-1) also indicated that the Raji-1 cell line does not secrete significant levels of ET-1 precursor. A possibility that the Raji-1

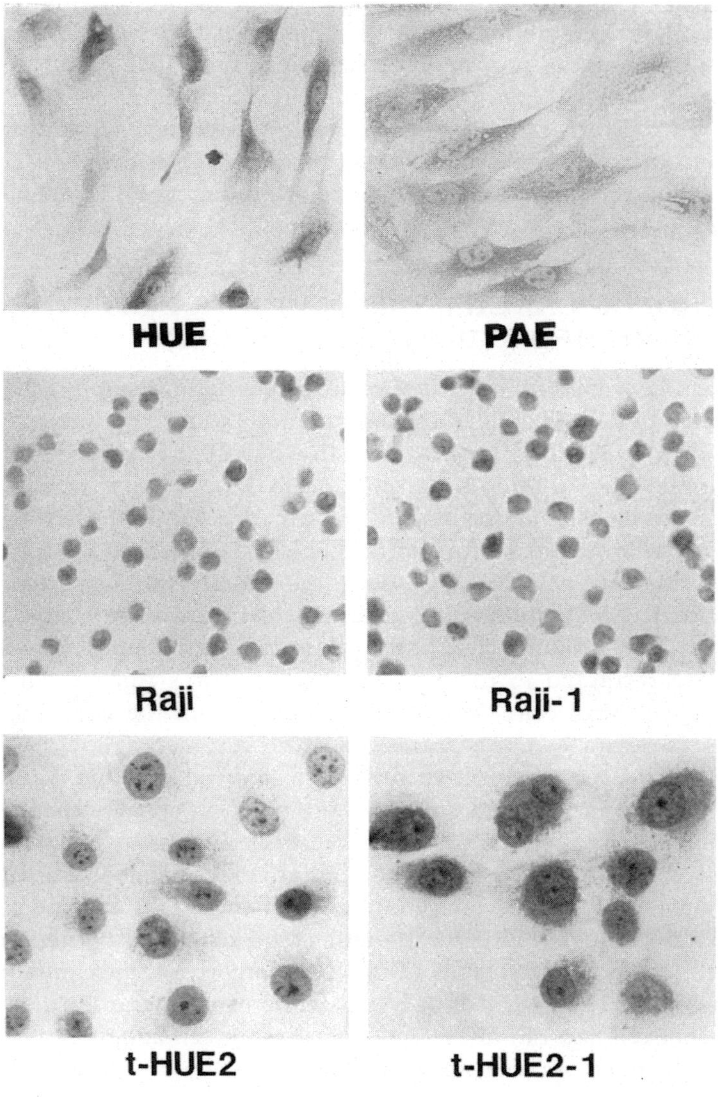

Fig. 6.5 Immunocytochemical analysis of ET-1 production in normal, immortalized and transfected cells. HUE is a normal human umbilical cord vein endothelial cell line. PAE is an immortalized porcine aorta endothelial cell line. Raji is a human B lymphocyte cell strain. Raji-1 is a prepro ET-1 cDNA transfected Raji cell line. t-HUE2-1 is a prepro ET-1 cDNA t-HUE2 cell line. HUE and PAE were used as positive controls for ET-1-producing cells. Raji-1 and t-HUE2-1 have been confirmed as expressing prepro ET-1 mRNA by Northern blot analysis. Note that t-HUE2-1 but not Raji-1 accumulated ET-1 in their cytoplasm.

transformant might accumulate ET-1 or big ET-1 in the cytoplasm was pursued by examining the presence of these peptides using a specific antibody. Results of immunocytological staining of normal endothelial cells (HUE), an immortal porcine endothelial cell line (PAE-20), Raji and its transfectant (Raji-1), and t-HUE2 and its transfectant (t-HUE2-1) are shown in figure 6.5. Strong positive staining was observed in transfectant t-HUE2-1 but not in transfectant Raji-1. Thus, it seems that Raji-1 cell line is expressing prepro ET-1 mRNA but not producing ET-1 precursor nor mature ET-1.

MORPHOLOGICAL CHANGES IN MP41 TRANSFECTION INTO A TRANSFORMED ENDOTHELIAL CELL LINE

To obtain information on the functional properties of the mp41 cDNA, we transfected this cDNA under a strong promoter (a fused promoter between the HTLV-1 LTR sequence and the SV-40 early sequence) to a transformed human endothelial cell line. GPT selection yielded several independent clones that maintained stable expression of the mp41 mRNA. Each of the mp41 transformants displayed the same morphological changes: the cells assumed a raised, three-dimensional shape reminiscent of endothelial cells undergoing an initial tube formation step (Ingber & Folkman 1989), and the edge of the cell islands of the mp41 transformants was more retracted in the transformant cultures than in the vector-transfected control cells. Moreover, consistent with the light microscopic results, the transformants showed a more retraced shape in scanning electron microscopy than the vector-transfected controls (Fig. 6.6).

The mp41 transformants showed morphological changes reminiscent of the initial step in the formation of capillary structures by endothelial cells (Ingber & Folkman 1989). These changes consist of multicellular retraction caused by mechanical interaction between the cell and malleable extracellular matrix, and are thought to be regulated by cell adhesion molecules such as fibronectin. Thus, it is important to examine whether morphological changes in mp41 transfection into a transformed human endothelial cell line can affect the expression of cell adhesion molecule or the growth ability of these transformants.

CONCLUSION

A human immortal endothelial cell line, t-HUE2, seems to be very useful host cell for the production of bioactive substances. It can be cultivated in serum-free medium on a large scale using bead culture. The HUE4 cell line, a new clone of t-HUE2, is capable of growing in completely protein-free medium, which enable us to isolate bioactive peptides or proteins very easily. The results shown in table 6.2 and figure 6.4 indicate that the t-

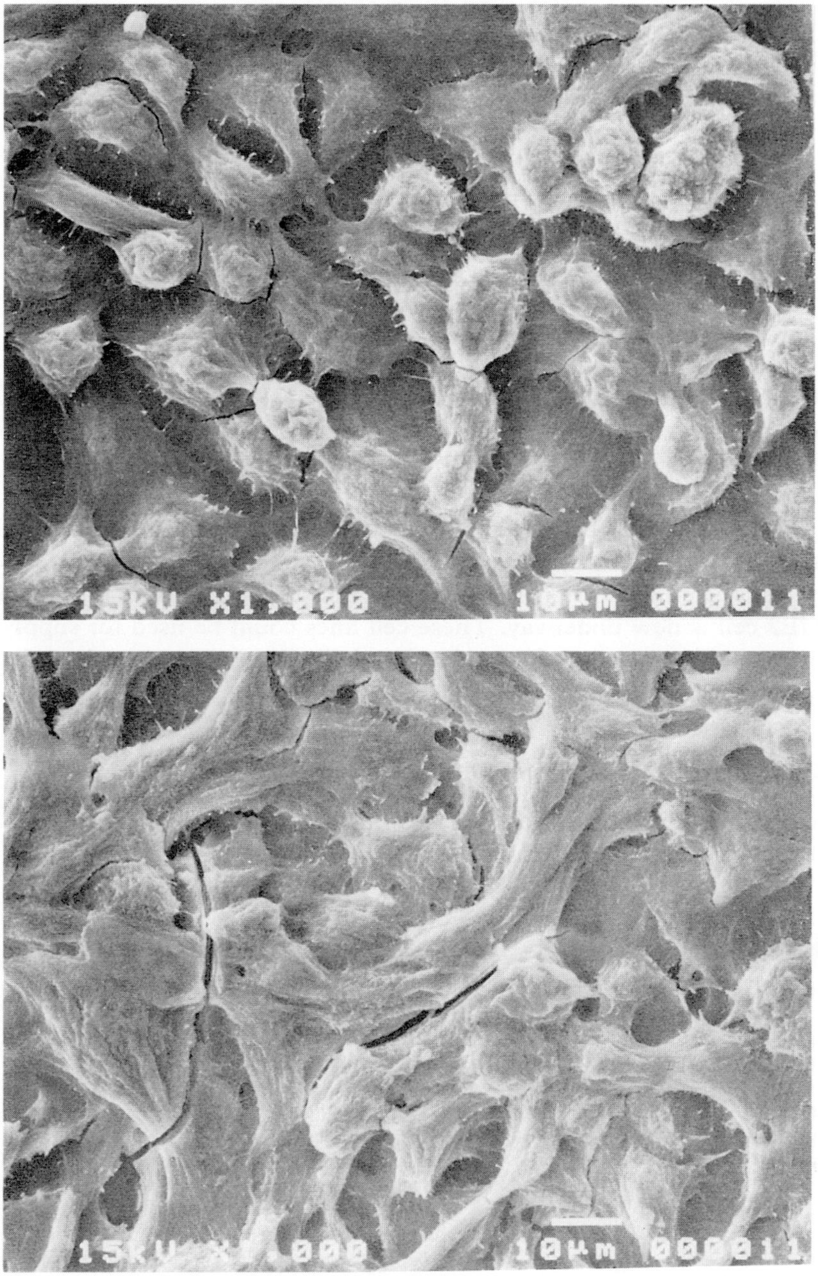

Fig. 6.6 Morphological changes of mp41 transformants revealed by scanning electron microscopy. Upper panel: vector-transfected t-HUE2 cells. Lower panel: mp41 cDNA transfected t-HUE2 cells, clone 2.5-11. mp41 is overexpressed in the latter clone, which showed more retractive morphology than the vector-transfected clone.

Table 6.2 Prepro ET-1 cDNA transcript and products in transfected human cells. prepro ET-1 mRNA level was determined by Western blot analysis and concentration of mature ET-1 in culture medium was measured by radioimmunoassay. Big ET was separated by HPLC and determined by radioimmunoassay. Note that Raji-1 cells expressed preproET-1 mRNA but did not produce mature ET-1. *Symbols:* [a] converting efficiency = mature ET/(mature ET + big ET), [b] mature ET = ET (1-21).

Cell type	Converting efficiency[a]	mRNA	Mature ET[b] mRNA
HUE	0.21	1.0	1.0
t-HUE2-1	0.75	2.9	11.8
Raji-1	—	0.5	—

HUE 2 transfectant is able to produce mature ET, presumably by cleaving precursor protein with a unique converting enzyme. In contrast, the Raji transfectant seemed to have some inhibitory activity for translation of prepro ET-1 mRNA.

The properties of the mp41 transfectant of t-HUE2 also suggest that the function of the endothelial cell line can be altered by gene transfection. The establishment of an immortal but nontumorgenic cell line from t-HUE2 cell is now underway. These cell lines could be used for supplying hormone-like substances by implanting the cells into the vascular tube or any other tissue.

ACKNOWLEDGMENTS

We wish to thank Renu Wadhwa for critically reading this manuscript and Ms. Chiiko Sakai for assistance in its preparation.

REFERENCES

Gorman C M, Moftat K F, Howard B H 1982 Recombinant genomes which express chloramphenicol acetyltransferase in mammalian cells. Mol Cell Biol 2: 1044-1051

Hasegawa N, Yamamoto M, Imamura T et al 1988 Evaluation of long-term cultured endothelial cells as a model system for studying vascular ageing. Mech Ageing Dev 46: 111-123

Imamura T, Mitsui Y 1987 Heparan sulfate and heparin as a potentiator or a suppressor of growth of normal and transformed vascular endothelial cells. Exp Cell Res 172: 92-100

Imamura T, Tokita Y, Mitsui Y 1991 Contact wtih basement membrane heparan sulfate enhances the growth of transformed vascular endothelial cells, but suppresses normal cells. Cell Struct Funct 16: 225-230

Ingber D E, Folkman J 1989 Mechanical switching between growth and differentiation during fibroblast growth factor-stimulated angiogenesis *in vitro*: role of extracellular matirx. J Cell Biol 109: 317-330

Inoue A, Yanagisawa M, Takuwa Y et al 1989 The human preproendothelin-1 gene: complete nucleotide sequence and regulation of expression. J Biol Chem 264: 14954-14959

Ishida N, Matsui M, Nishimatsu S et al 1994 Molecular cloning of a gene under control of the circadian clock and light in the rodent SCN. Mol Brain Res 26: 197-206

Ishida N, Noji S, Ono K et al 1991 Diurnal regulation of *per* repeat mRNA in the suprachiasmatic nucleus in rat brain. Neurosci Lett 122: 113-116

Ishida N, Tsujioka K, Tomoi M et al 1989 Differential activities of two distinct endothelin family peptides on ileum and coronary artery. FEBS Lett 247: 337-340

Ito Y, Yanagisawa M, Ohkubo S et al 1988 Cloning and sequence analysis of cDNA encoding the precursor of a human endothelium-derived vasoconstrictor peptide, endothelin: identity of human and porcine endothelin. FEBS Lett 231: 440-444

Kitayama J, Juji T, Atomi Y et al 1993 Transendothelial migration activity of lymphokine-activated killer (LAK) cells. J Immunol 151: 1663-1672

Kobayashi M, Kondo M, Mitsui Y 1991 Establishment of human endothelial cell lines in a serum-free culture and its application for expression of transfected prepro endothelin gene. Hum Cell 4: 296-304

Kondo M, Ishida N, Kobayashi M et al 1991 Establishment of a human cell line highly expressing endothelin in serum-free medium. J Cardiovasc Pharmacol 17: S52-S54

Kondo M, Ishida N, Kobayashi M et al 1992 Secretion of endothelin-1 in human endothelial cell line but not in B cell line by transfection of preproendothelin-1 cDNA. Biochim Biophys Acta 1134: 242-246

Kumazaki T, Fujii T, Kobayashi M et al 1994 Aging- and growth-dependent modulation of endothelin-1 gene expression in human vascular endothelial cells. Exp Cell Res 211: 6-11

Kumazaki T, Kobayashi M, Mitsui Y 1993 Enhanced expression of fibronectin during *in vivo* cellular aging of human vascular endothelial cells and skin fibroblasts. Exp Cell Res 205: 396-402

Matsui M, Mitsui Y, Ishida N 1993 Circadian regulation of *per* repeat mRNA in the SCN of rat brain. Neurosci Lett 163: 189-192

Mitsui Y, Hirokawa K 1984 Mechanisms of cellular aging. Cell Struct Funct 9: 127-133

Mitsui Y, Saida K 1991 Vasoactive intestinal contractor (VIC); its genetic analysis and biological activities. Now and Future 6: 5-8

Mitsui Y, Yamamoto M, Yamamoto K 1984 A new cell line of porcine diploid endothelial cells for the study of vascular function. In: Courtice F C et al (eds) Progress in Microcirculation Research, vol. II. University of New South Wales, Australia, pp 37-44

Mulligan R C, Berg P 1981 Selection for animal cells that express the *Escherichia coli* gene coding for xanthine-guanine phosphoribosyl transferase. Proc Natl Acad Sci USA 78: 2072-2076

Neichi T, Chang W, Mitsui Y, Murota S 1982 Comparison of prostaglandin biosynthetic activity between porcine aortic endothelial and smooth muscle cells in culture. Artery 11: 47-63

Okada T, Okuno H, Mitsui Y 1994 (in press) A novel *in vitro* assay system for transendothelial tumor cell invasion: significance of E-selectin and α3 integrin in the transendothelial invasion by HT1080 fibrosarcoma cells. Clin Exp Metastasis

Saida K, Mitsui Y 1991 cDNA cloning, sequence analysis and tissue distribution of a precursor for vasoactive intestinal contractor (VIC). Biochim Biophys Acta 1089: 404-406

Saida K, Mitsui Y, Ishida N 1989 A novel peptide, vasoactive intestinal contractor, of a new (endothelin) peptide family, molecular cloning, expression and biological activity. J Biol Chem 264: 14613-14616

Sawamura T, Kimura S, Shinmi O et al 1990 Characterization of endothelin converting enzyme activities in soluble fraction of bovine cultured endothelial cells. Biochem Biophys Res Comm 169: 1138-1144

Schneider E L, Mitsui Y 1976 The relationship between *in vitro* cellular aging and *in vivo* human age. Proc Natl Acad Sci USA 73: 3584-3588

Shin H S, Bargiello T A, Clark B T et al 1985 An unusual coding sequence from *Drosophila* clock gene is conserved in vertebrates. Nature 317: 445-448

Tokunaga O, Fan J, Watanabe T et al 1992 Endothelin: immunohistological localization in aorta and biosynthesis by cultured human aortic endothelial cells. Lab Invest 67: 210-217

Wadhwa R, Kaul S C, Sugimoto Y et al 1993 Induction of cellular senescence by transfection of cytosolic mortalin cDNA in NIH 3T3 cells. J Biol Chem 268: 22239-22242

Yanagisawa M, Kurihara H, Kimura S et al 1988 A novel potent vasoconstrictor peptide produced by vascular endothelial cells. Nature 332: 411-415

SECTION 3

Dysregulation of Vasomotor Tone

7

Endothelium-dependent and -independent vasodilator action of insulin: implications for the role of insulin in vasomotor tone regulation

Y. Ouchi, S.-Z. Han, H. Orimo

INTRODUCTION

Hyperinsulinaemia or insulin resistance has been receiving increasing attention as a pathogenetic factor for hypertension (Ferrannini et al 1987, Modan et al 1985). Insulin has been demonstrated to be involved in various biological actions, including glucose metabolism, lipid metabolism, electrolyte metabolism, cell proliferation and the modification of the sympathetic nervous system (Ferrari & Weidmann 1990). The common association of hypertension, dyslipoproteinaemia, obesity and impaired glucose tolerance has been well documented as a state of accumulated risk factors for atherosclerosis. This has been referred to as the insulin resistance syndrome (DeFronzo 1992) or syndrome X (Reaven 1988). However, some studies investigating the effect of insulin have shown that insulin acts as a vasodilator, by inhibiting vasoconstriction induced by certain vasoconstricting substances (Alexander & Oake 1977; Nudel et al 1977; Standley et al 1991; Yagi et al 1988; Zemel et al 1989). Moreover, insulin infusion in animals does not always increase blood pressure (Anderson & Mark 1993). To explain the controversy concerning the association of hypertension with hyperinsulinaemia, and the possible role of insulin resistance, it is necessary to investigate the possibility of deficient insulin action in the pathogenesis of hypertension. A deficiency in the vasodilator action of insulin may result in hypertension (Standley et al 1991; Zemel et al 1989).

Various studies have revealed that the mechanism of insulin's vasodilator action may be mediated via β-receptor stimulation (Creager et al 1985), hyperpolarisation of muscle cells (Zierler & Rogus 1981), stimulation of Ca^{2+} efflux from vascular smooth muscle cells (Zemel et al 1989)] and/or inhibition of Ca^{2+}influx into the cells (Standley et al 1991). However, the precise mechanism of insulin's vasodilator action has not been clarified.

The present study was therefore performed to investigate the effect of insulin on vascular tone, and also to investigate the endothelium-independent and -dependent mechanisms with special reference to intracellular free calcium concentration ($[Ca^{2+}]i$) in rat aortic preparations.

ENDOTHELIUM-INDEPENDENT VASODILATOR ACTION OF INSULIN

The endothelium-independent vasodilator action of insulin (porcine insulin crystal; Sigma Chemical Co., St. Louis, USA) was investigated by examining its effect on the tension of rat aortic ring preparations without endothelium, derived from male Wistar rats, precontracted with norepinephrine (noradrenaline). In another series of experiments, the effects of insulin on $[Ca^{2+}]i$ concentrations and tension were measured in smooth muscle cells of aortic strip spiral preparations without endothelium.

EFFECT OF POST-ADDITION OF INSULIN ON $[Ca^{2+}]i$ AND NOREPINEPHRINE-INCREASED TENSION

We first determined the effect of insulin post-addition on the tension of rat aortic ring preparations precontracted with norepinephrine. Thoracic aortas were isolated under ether anaesthesia from 5- to 6-week old male Wistar rats (Nippon Bio-Supply Center, Tokyo, Japan). The adventitia was carefully removed and the endothelium rubbed off by finger. The aortic spiral preparation (2 mm in width and 10 mm in length) was placed in a balanced salt solution (BSS), which consisted of NaCl 12 mmol/l, KCl 5 mmol/l, $CaCl_2$ 1.5 mmol/l, $MgCl_2$ 1 mmol/l, $NaHCO_3$ 23.8 mmol/l, EDTA 0.01 mmol/l and glucose 5.5 mmol/l. The solution was saturated with 95% O_2 and 5% CO_2 gas mixture and maintained at 37 °C and pH 7.4 during the experiment. The aortic ring preparations, to which an initial

Fig. 7.1 Effect of cumulative application of insulin (1-120 U/l) on the tension of rat aortic ring preparations without endothelium precontracted with norepinephrine (●; n = 10). Control study was performed using the same amounts of vehicle (○; n = 10). Data are expressed as percentage decrease in tension compared with the contraction induced by KCl 65 mmol/l as 100%. Values are given as means ± SEM. *Statistical significance:* *p <0.05, **p <0.01 versus vehicle.

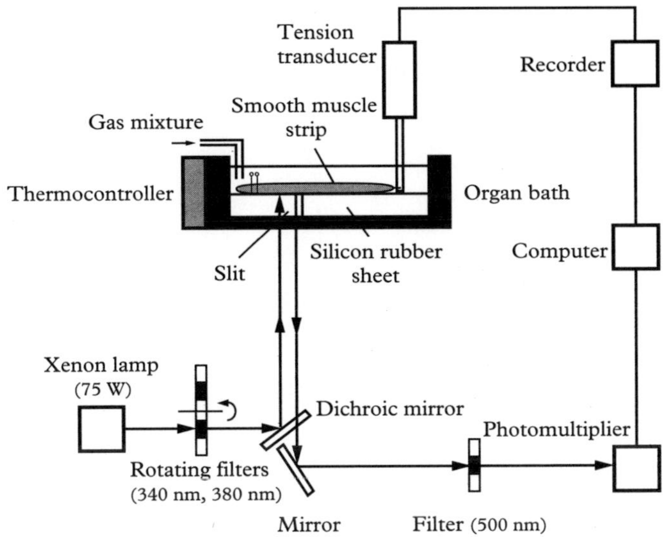

Fig. 7.2 Schematic diagram for the simultaneous measurement of intracellular free calcium concentration and tension of rat aortic spiral preparations.

tension of 0.5 g was applied, were precontracted with norepinephrine 0.1 μmol/l. Insulin (1-120 U/l), dissolved in BSS containing HCl 10 mmol/l, was then cumulatively added to the incubation bath. Vehicle alone (BSS containing HCl 10 mmol/l) was used as control. The tension increased by KCl 65 mmol/l was taken as 100%, and the percentage decrease in the tension was calculated. The absence of endothelium was confirmed by the elimination of any vasodilatation induced by acetylcholine 1 μmol/l of the norepinephrine-precontracted aortic preparations. As shown in figure 7.1, vehicle alone did not affect the tension of the aortic preparation, whereas insulin decreased tension in a dose-dependent manner.

Next, the effect of post-addition of insulin on $[Ca^{2+}]i$ and tension of the aortic preparation was investigated. Endothelium-free aortic spiral strips were prepared as described in the preceding section. $[Ca^{2+}]i$ was measured with fura-2, a fluorescent Ca^{2+} indicator. The aortic strip preparations were treated with fura-2 acetoxymethyl ester 7 μmol/l (fura-2/AM; Dojindo Laboratories, Kumamoto, Japan) for 3-5 h at room temperature. Fura-2/AM was dissolved in a noncytotoxic detergent, 0.02% cremophor EL (Nacalai Tesque Inc., Kyoto, Japan), and the solution was treated with an ultrasonic cell disrupter (Yamato Scientific Co., Ltd., Tokyo, Japan) to increase solubility. Experiments were performed with a fluorimeter designed to measure the fluorescence of living tissues (CAF-100, Japan Spectroscopic, Tokyo, Japan) as described previously (Ozaki et al 1981). A schematic diagram of the measurement is shown in figure 7.2. The fura-

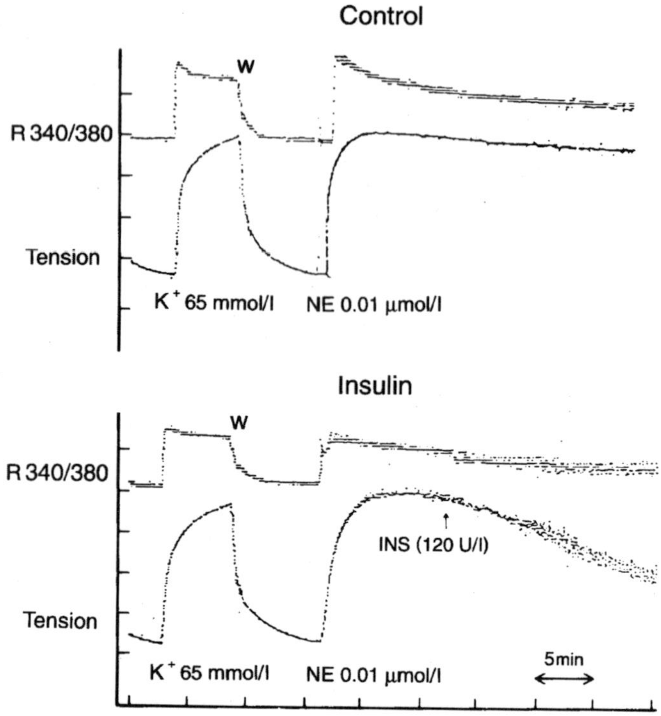

Fig. 7.3 Effect of insulin (INS; 120 U/l) on the intracellular free calcium concentration in smooth muscle as indicated by R340/380 ratio and the tension of rat aortic spiral preparations without endothelium precontracted with norepinephrine (NE). Control study was performed using the same amount of vehicle. *Abbreviation:* W = washing.

2/AM-loaded strip preparation was held horizontally on a silicon rubber sheet in a 5-ml organ bath maintained at 37 °C. One end of the strip was pinned to the silicon rubber sheet and the other end was connected to an isometric force transducer (Orientec, Tokyo, Japan). A part of the strip preparation was excited by light emitted from a xenon high-pressure lamp (75 W) equipped with a rotating filter wheel (48 Hz) having 340-nm and 380-nm (± 5.5 nm) interference filters. The light emitted from the strip preparation was collected into photomultiplier through a 500-nm (± 10.0 nm) filter. The fluorescence emitted from the aortic preparation excited at 340 nm (F340) and at 380 nm (F380) was serially measured with the fluorimeter, and the ratio (R340/380) was considered to be an index of $[Ca^{2+}]i$ in the aortic smooth muscle. The time constant of the optical channels was 1.0 sec. The resting tension of the strip preparation was adjusted to 0.8 g. Isometric tension and $[Ca^{2+}]i$ were then measured simultaneously. The aortic strip preparations were contracted with KCl 65 mmol/l, which was then washed out. After a subsequent equilibration period, the aortic preparation was contracted with norepinephrine 0.01 μmol/l. Then, either vehicle or insulin (120 U/l) was applied to the aortic preparation. As shown in figure 7.3, insulin decreased both $[Ca^{2+}]i$ and tension of the norepinephrine-precontracted aortic preparations. These effects were dose dependent (data not shown).

EFFECT OF INSULIN PRETREATMENT ON $[Ca^{2+}]i$ AND NOREPINEPHRINE-INCREASED TENSION

$[Ca^{2+}]i$ and tension of the aortic spiral strip preparations were measured as described earlier. The aortic preparations were contracted by KCl 65 mmol/l, which was then washed out. After a subsequent equilibration period, the preparations were incubated with either vehicle or insulin (12 and 120 U/l) for 30 min. The preparations were then contracted by the addition of norepinephrine, and the increases in R340/380 and tension were compared with those of the control experiment.

As shown in figure 7.4, pretreatment with insulin inhibited the increases in tension and in $[Ca^{2+}]i$ induced by norepinephrine in a dose-dependent manner. The $[Ca^{2+}]i$-tension relationship was not changed by preincubatation with insulin 12 U/l, but was significantly shifted the curve to the right with insulin 120 U/l. This indicates that the higher dose of insulin alters the sensitivity of contractile proteins to Ca^{2+} in aortic smooth muscle. Another series of experiments (data not shown) investigated the effect of incubation time (15-45 min) with insulin (30 U/l) on the tension development of the norepinephrine-contracted aortic preparations. The inhibition of tension development was found to be dependent on the incubation time.

These studies indicate that insulin relaxes norepinephrine-precontracted aortic preparations without endothelium in a dose-dependent manner. This endothelium-independent vasodilator action of insulin results from a direct action on vascular smooth muscle to inhibit norepinephrine-induced vasoconstriction. Other investigators have reported that insulin inhibits vasoconstriction via an endothelium-independent mechanism. For example, insulin attenuated the contractile response to norepinephrine in vascular smooth muscle (Alexander & Oake 1977; Nudel et al 1977), attenuated vasconstrictive responses to norepinephrine and angiotensin II in the rabbit femoral artery (Yagi et al 1988), and dilated canine carotid artery (D'Orleans-Juste et al 1985).

In order to investigate the underlying mechanism of the vasodilator action of insulin, we simultaneously measured $[Ca^{2+}]i$ and tension of the rat aortic spiral preparations. Insulin preincubation inhibited both the norepinephrine-induced increase in tension and smooth muscle $[Ca^{2+}]i$. This indicates that the antagonistic effect of insulin against norepinephrine-induced vasoconstriction may be caused by the inhibition of the increase in smooth muscle $[Ca^{2+}]i$ provoked by norepinephrine.

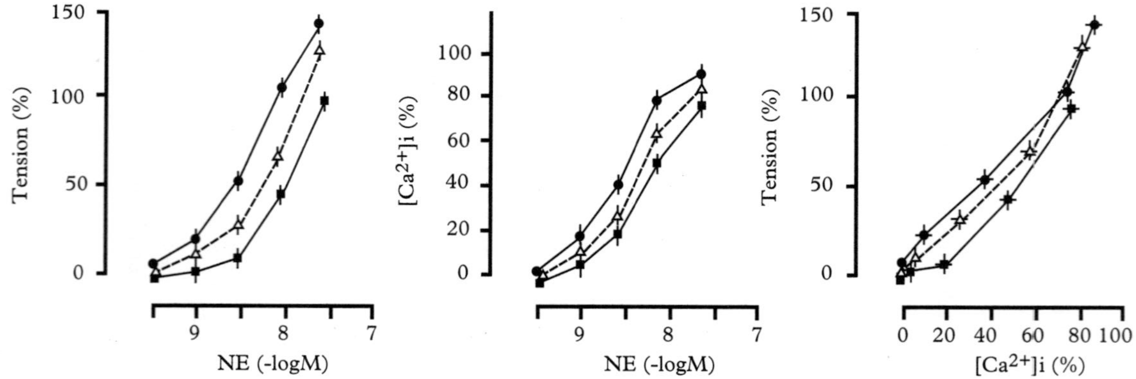

Fig. 7.4 Effect of preincubation with insulin 12 U/l (△) and 120 U/l (■)compared with vehicle alone (●) of rat aortic spiral preparations without endothelium precontracted with various concentrations of norepinephrine (NE) on the tension (left panel) and the intracellular free calcium concentration ($[Ca^{2+}]$i) in smooth muscle (middle panel). The $[Ca^{2+}]$i-tension relationship is shown in the right panel. Data are expressed as percentage decrease in tension compared with the contraction induced by KCl 65 mmol/l as 100%. Values are given as means ± SEM.

Two possible mechanisms should be considered with respect to the inhibitory effect of insulin on smooth muscle $[Ca^{2+}]i$. Firstly, insulin might inhibit Ca^{2+} influx via receptor-operated Ca^{2+} channels into the smooth muscle cell. Insulin has been previously reported to reduce Ca^{2+} influx into rat vascular smooth muscle cells via both receptor-operated and voltage-dependent Ca^{2+} channels (Standley et al 1991). Secondly, the stimulation of Ca^{2+} efflux from smooth muscle cells by insulin should be considered. Indeed, insulin has been shown to stimulate Ca^{2+} efflux by stimulating of Ca^{2+}-ATPase activity in rat aortic strip preparations (Ambrozy et al 1991).

In the present study, we also found that the preincubation of the rat aortic preparations with insulin 120 U/l shifted the $[Ca^{2+}]i$-tension relationship to the right. This indicates that a greater increase in $[Ca^{2+}]i$ is necessary to generate a similar level of tension, suggesting that a higher concentration of insulin decreases Ca^{2+} sensitivity of contractile protein in rat aortic smooth muscle cells. The modification of contractile protein Ca^{2+} sensitivity might be another mechanism underlying the vasodilator action of insulin in higher concentrations.

ENDOTHELIUM-DEPENDENT VASODILATOR ACTION OF INSULIN

The endothelium-dependent vasodilator action of insulin was investigated in a series of experiments similar to those described above, but in which the endothelium was not removed from the aortic preparations. The

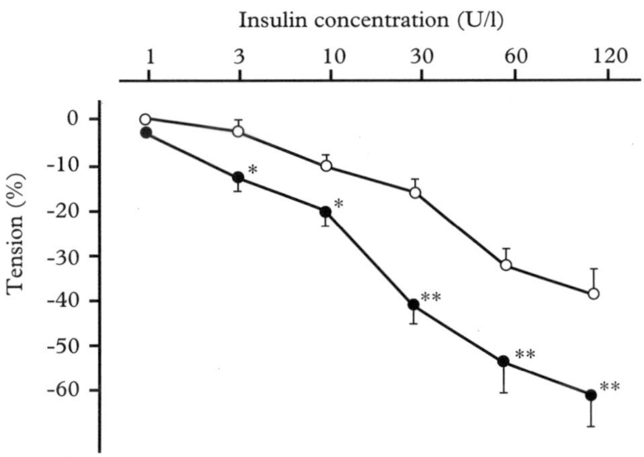

Fig. 7.5 Effect of cumulative application of insulin (1-120 U/l) on the tension of rat aortic ring preparations with (●; n = 10) or without endothelium (○; n = 10). Data are expressed as percentage decrease in tension compared with the contraction induced by KCl 65 mmol/l as 100%. Values are given as means ± SEM. *Statistical significance:* *$p < 0.05$, **$p < 0.01$ versus without endothelium.

preservation of endothelium in the aortic preparations was confirmed by demonstrating that acetylcholine (1 μmol/l) relaxed aortic preparations contracted by norepinephrine (0.1 μmol/l). The magnitude of vasodilator effect of insulin on the aortic preparation with endothelium was compared with that without endothelium. As shown in figure 7.5, the vasodilator effect of insulin was significantly greater in preparations with endothelium than in those without endothelium.

To investigate the mechanism underlying the endothelium-dependent vasodilator action of insulin, the effect of pretreatment with indomethacin was investigated. The aortic ring preparation was incubated with indomethacin (10 μmol/l) dissolved in DMSO or with vehicle for 15 min, and norepinephrine 0.05 μmol/l was then applied to the preparation. Insulin (1-120 U/l) was then cumulatively applied to the preparation. As shown in figure 7.6, the indomethacin preincubation did not affect the vasodilator action of insulin in the aortic preparations with endothelium.

Next, the effect of L-N^G-monomethylarginine monoacetate (L-NMMA; Calbiochem), a nitric oxide (NO) synthase inhibitor, on the vasodilator action of insulin was investigated. After the norepinephrine-induced increase in tension became stable, insulin (60 U/l) was applied to the aortic preparation. When the vasodilator action of insulin became maximal, L-NMMA (10 μmol/l) dissolved in distilled water was added. As shown in figure 7.7, L-NMMA reversed the vasodilator action of insulin.

The response of $[Ca^{2+}]i$ in the aortic endothelial cells to insulin was also investigated by examining the fluorescence from the endothelial surface of the aortic preparation without any precontraction according to the method

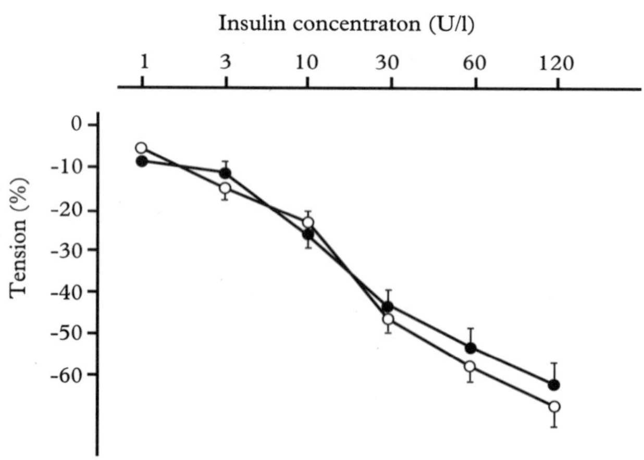

Fig. 7.6 Effect of pretreatment with indomethacin 10 μmol/l (●; n = 6) compared with vehicle alone (○; n =6) on the tension of rat aortic ring preparations with endothelium. Data are expressed as percentage decrease in tension compared with the contraction induced by KCl 65 mmol/l as 100%. Values are given as means ± SEM.

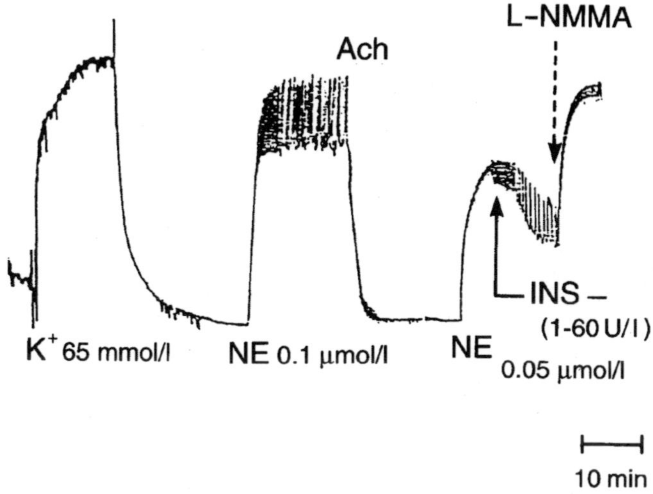

Fig. 7.7 Effect of L-N^G-monomethylarginine monoacetate (L-NMMA) on the cumulative application of insulin (INS; 1-60 U/l) to rat aortic ring preparations with endothelium contracted with norepinephrine (NE). The preservation of endothelium is confirmed by showing that acetylcholine (Ach) decreases tension of the aortic preparations precontracted by NE.

described by Sato et al (1990). As shown in figure 7.8, acetylcholine (1 µmol/l) increased endothelial $[Ca^{2+}]i$ and slightly decreased tension. After washing with BSS, insulin (200 U/l) was added and there was an increase in endothelial $[Ca^{2+}]i$ and a small decrease in the tension. These effects of insulin were essentially same as those induced by acetylcholine. The increase in $[Ca^{2+}]i$ induced by insulin was considered to be endothelial in origin because both insulin (200 U/l) and acetylcholine (1 µmol/l) did not affect $[Ca^{2+}]i$ and tension in the aortic preparations without endothelium.

In the present studies, we have found that the vasodilator action of insulin is greater in aortic preparations with endothelium than that in those without endothelium. This finding indicates that insulin exerts an endothelium-dependent vasodilator action. This endothelium-dependent vasodilator action of insulin was not affected by the presence of indomethacin, indicating that the production of vasodilator prostanoids, such as prostacyclin and prostaglandin E_2, is not involved. The vasodilator action of insulin was completely reversed by L-NMMA, suggesting that the endothelium-dependent vasodilator action of insulin is associated with NO production in the endothelium. The reversal was found to exceed the maximal level of contraction induced by norepinephrine. This might be explained by the fact that NO is also produced by norepinephrine, which would also be inhibited by L-NMMA.

Insulin increased $[Ca^{2+}]i$ in the aortic endothelium. The synthesis and release of NO has been reported to be regulated by $[Ca^{2+}]i$ in vascular

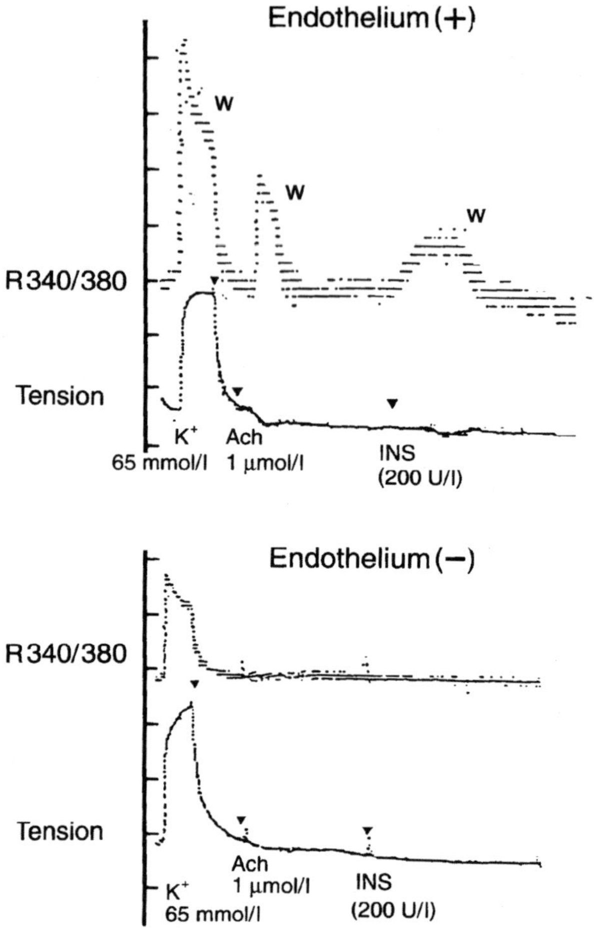

Fig. 7.8 Effect of insulin (INS; 200 U/l) on the intracellular free calcium concentration of the endothelial cells (as indicated by R340/380) and tension of rat aortic spiral preparation with endothelium (upper panel). Insulin increases the intracellular free calcium concentration and decreases the tension slightly. These changes are not observed in the aortic preparations without endothelium (lower panel), indicating these signals originated from the endothelium. Acetylcholine (Ach) exerts similar effects in the aortic preparation with endothelium (upper panel) and these effects are diminished in the aortic preparation without endothelium (lower panel). *Abbreviation:* W = washing.

endothelial cells: the increase in $[Ca^{2+}]i$ caused by either Ca^{2+} influx from the extracellular space or Ca^{2+} release form the intracellular store was essential for the synthesis and release of NO (Peach et al 1987). Moreover, NO-induced cGMP production and the resulting vasorelaxation are inhibited by elimination of Ca^{2+} from the extracellular space (Hughes et al 1986). Based on these findings, it is likely that the endothelium-dependent vasodilator action of insulin is mediated by a release of NO from the endothelial cells.

IMPLICATION FOR THE ROLE OF INSULIN IN VASOMOTOR TONE REGULATION

We have shown in the present studies that insulin exhibits both endothelium-independent and -dependent vasodilator activity in rat aortic preparation. If the present findings were also found in small resistance vessels, insulin resistance might negate the vasodilator action of insulin, leading to increased vascular resistance and hypertension. In Zucker rats with insulin resistance, Zemel et al (1989, 1990) have shown that raised blood pressure was associated with an increased vascular contractile response to phenylephrine, serotonin and KCl. Shehin et al (1989) found that Ca^{2+} efflux was diminished in vascular smooth muscle of Zucker rat. Furthermore, Kappagoda et al (1989) have shown that endothelium-dependent relaxation is attenuated in streptozotocin-induced diabetic rats and diabetic BB rats.

The association between insulin and hypertension has received considerable attention since Ferrannini and colleagues (1987) documented that hyperinsulinaemia and insulin resistance are present in hypertensive patients. Insulin stimulates sympathetic nervous system activity and increases plasma catecholamine levels, even when hypoglycaemia does not develop (Anderson et al 1991; Rowe et al 1981). Insulin has been reported to increase sodium resorption in the proximal tubules of the kidney (Ferrari & Weidmann 1990; Gesek & Schoolwerth 1991). Furthermore, insulin exerts a growth factor-like action via stimulation of Na^+/H^+ antiport in the cell membrane, leading to the medial hypertrophy of blood vessels (Ferrari & Weidmann 1990). Based on these reports, some investigators have insisted that hyperinsulinaemia is responsible for the development of hypertension. However, at least from the viewpoint of vascular function, insulin resistance may be more important in the development of hypertension rather that hyperinsulinemia *per se*.

CONCLUSION

In conclusion, we have shown that insulin dilates rat aortic preparations through both endothelium-independent and -dependent mechanisms. The endothelium-independent vasodilatation is associated with the decrease in $[Ca^{2+}]i$ in vascular smooth muscle cells. The decreased Ca^{2+} sensitivity of contractile proteins in vascular smooth muscle is also involved in the endothelium-independent vasodilator action of insulin at high concentrations. Endothelium-dependent vasodilatation is related to NO release from endothelial cells, which in turn is associated with the $[Ca^{2+}]i$ increase in endothelial cells. The diminished vasodilator action of insulin may contribute to hypertension in the syndrome of insulin resistance.

ACKNOWLEDGMENTS

We thank Prof. H. Karaki, Department of Veterinary Medicine, Faculty of Agricultural Sciences, University of Tokyo for his helpful discussions and criticism. This study was supported by a Grant-in-Aid from the Ministry of Education, Science and Culture of Japan (No. 05670597) and a grant from the Japan Milk Association. This study was presented at the 14th Scientific Meeting of the International Society of Hypertension, Madrid, Spain, June 1992.

REFERENCES

Alexander W D, Oake R J 1977 The effect of insulin on vascular reactivity to norepinephrine. Diabetes 26: 611-614

Ambrozy S A, Sowers J R, Zemel M B 1991 Insulin stimulation of vascular smooth muscle Ca^{++} pump activity. FASEB J 5: A1106

Anderson E A, Hoffman R P, Balon T W et al 1991 Hyperinsulinemia produces both sympathetic neural activation and vasodilation in normal humans. J Clin Invest 87: 2246-2252

Anderson E A, Mark A L 1993 The vasodilator action of insulin. Implications for the insulin hypothesis of hypertension. Hypertension 21: 129-135

Creager M A, Liang C S, Coffman J D 1985 Beta-adrenergic mediated vasodilator response to insulin in the human forearm. J Pharmacol Exp Ther 235: 709-714

D'Orleans-Juste P, Dion S, Mizrahi J et al 1985 Effects of peptides and non-peptides on isolated arterial smooth muscles. Eur J Pharmacol 114: 9-21

DeFronzo R A 1992 Insulin resistance, hyperinsulinemia, and coronary artery disease; a complex metabolic web. J Cardiovasc Pharmacol 20 (suppl 11): S1-15

Ferrannini E G, Buzzigoli R, Bondonna M A et al 1987 Insulin resistance in essential hypertension. N Engl J Med 317: 350-357

Ferrari P, Weidmann P 1990 Insulin, insulin sensitivity and hypertension. J Hypertens 8: 491-500

Gesek F A, Schoolwerth A C 1991 Insulin increases Na^{+}-H^{+} exchange activity in proximal tubules from normotensive and hypertensive rat. Am J Physiol 260: F695-703

Hughes A, Thom S, Martin G et al 1986 Endothelial dependent relaxation of human arteries by peptide hormones. Clin Sci 70: 88P

Kappagoda T, Jayakody L, Rajotte R et al 1989 Endothelium-dependent relaxation to acetylcholine in the aorta of streptozocin-induced diabetic rat and the BB-diabetic rat. Clin Invest Med 12: 187-193

Modan M, Halkin H, Almog S et al 1985 Hyperinsulinemia. A link between hypertension obesity and glucose intolerance. J Clin Invest 75: 809-817

Nudel D B, Lee J C, Downing S E 1977 Reciprocal inhibition of cardiac responses to norepinephrine and insulin. Am J Physiol 23: H665-669

Ozaki H Sato K, Satoh T et al 1981 Simultaneous recordings of calcium signals and mechanical activity using fluorescent dye fura 2 in isolated strips of vascular smooth muscle. Jpn J Pharmacol 45: 429-433

Peach M J, Singer H A, Izzo N J et al 1987 Role of calcium in endothelium-dependent relaxation of arterial smooth muscle. Am J Cardiol 59: 35-43A

Reaven G M 1988 Role of insulin resistance in human disease. Diabetes 37: 1495-1607

Rowe J W, Young J B, Miaker K L et al 1981 Effect of insulin and glucose infusions on sympathetic nervous system activity in normal man. Diabetes 30: 219-225

Sato K, Ozaki H, Karaki H 1990 Differential effects of carbachol on cytosolic calcium levels in vascular endothelium and smooth muscle. J Pharmacol Exp Ther 225: 114-119

Shehin S E, Reddy S, Chiou C 1989 Hypertension in the Zucker obese rat: role of altered calcium kinetics in vascular smooth muscle. FASEB J 3: A233

Standley P R, Zhang F, Ram L J et al 1991 Insulin attenuates vasopressin-induced calcium transients and a voltage-dependent calcium response in rat vascular smooth muscle cells. J Clin Invest 88: 1230-1236

Yagi S, Takata S, Kiyokawa H et al 1988 Effects of insulin on vasoconstrictive responses to norepinephrine and angiotensin II in rabbit femoral artery and vein. Diabetes 37: 1064-1067

Zemel M B, Reddy S, Shehin S et al 1989 Vascular reactivity in Zucker obese rats: role of insulin resistance. Hypertension 14: 358

Zemel M B, Sowers J R, Shehin S et al 1990 Impaired calcium metabolism associated with hypertension in Zucker obese rats. Metabolism 39: 704-708

Zierler K, Rogus E 1981 Rapid hyperpolarization of rat skeletal muscle induced by insulin. Biochim Biophys Acta 640: 687-692

8

Endothelium-derived nitric oxide and atherosclerosis

K. Hirata, S. Kawashima, M. Yokoyama

INTRODUCTION

In 1980, Furchgott and Zawadzki reported that acetylcholine-induced endothelium-dependent relaxation in isolated arteries depends on the release of a labile and diffusible substance from vascular endothelial cells, which was named endothelium-derived relaxing factor (EDRF) [Furchgott 1983; Furchgott & Zawadzki 1980]. Vascular endothelium, which produces EDRF, prostacyclin (PGI_2) and endothelin (Yanagisawa et al 1988) in response to physical and neurohumoral stimuli, plays a key role in the regulation of not only vascular tone but also smooth muscle growth and blood coagulability (Moncada et al 1991). EDRF was recently identified as nitric oxide (NO) or its related compounds (Myers et al 1990; Palmer et al 1987). NO is generated from terminal guanidino nitrogen of L-arginine by the action of NO synthase (Nathan 1992; Palmer et al 1988). NO represents an endogenous nitrosovasodilator, which produces cyclic GMP via the activation of soluble guanylate cyclase in vascular smooth muscle, and in turn causes dephosphorylation of myosin light chain leading to vasorelaxation. Endothelium-dependent relaxation is reduced in atherosclerotic arteries obtained from experimental animals and humans (Bossaller et al 1987; Cohen et al 1988; Freiman et al 1986; Hirata et al 1992; Shimokawa & Vanhoutte 1989). This endothelial dysfunction in hyperlipidaemia and atherosclerosis may predispose the blood vessel to vasospasm or to a further progression of the disease process (Maseri et al 1990).

The observation that the presence of an intact endothelium over atherosclerotic lesion areas of an artery suggests the possibility that the endothelial cells may actively participate in the atherogenic process. One of the earliest events in atherosclerosis is the enhanced adherence of leucocytes to the endothelium (Cybulski & Gimbrone 1991). NO has been shown to decrease adhesion of leucocytes to the endothelium (Kubes et al 1991). In this article, we review the impairment of endothelium-dependent relaxation in atherosclerotic vessels and the effects of oxidatively-modified low-density lipoprotein (LDL) and lysolipids on the responsiveness of isolated arteries to vasodilators. Recent reports on possible relationships between reduced EDRF production and atherosclerotic progression are also summarized.

IMPAIRMENT OF ENDOTHELIUM-DEPENDENT RELAXATION IN ATHEROSCLEROTIC VESSELS

EDRF, which is identified as NO or its related compounds (Myers et al 1990; Palmer et al 1987), plays an important role in the regulation of vascular tone and blood vessel function. EDRF induces vascular relaxation (Furchgott & Zawadzki 1980), inhibits smooth muscle proliferation (Garg & Hassid 1990), platelet aggregation (Radomski et al 1987) and leucocyte adhesion to vascular endothelium (Kubes et al 1991), and modulates endothelial permeability (Kurose et al 1993). Previous studies have demonstrated that the impairment in endothelial dilatory activity which occurs in atherosclerotic or hypercholesterolaemic blood vessels reflects an impairment in the ability of the endothelial cells to respond to specific stimuli (Bossaller et al 1987; Freiman et al 1986; Shimokawa & Vanhoutte 1989). We and other groups have demonstrated that endothelium-dependent relaxation progressively decreased as the severity of atherosclerotic lesion increased in Watanabe heritable hyperlipidaemic (WHHL) rabbits (Hirata et al 1992; Kolodgie et al 1990) [Fig. 8.1]. Impaired endothelium-dependent relaxation was accompanied by decreased cyclic GMP production in smooth muscle cells. The impairment of endothelium-dependent relaxation was not associated with impairment of endothelium-independent relaxation to nitrosovasodilators such as nitroglycerin (glyceryl trinitrate) and sodium nitroprusside, which may be considered as exogenous mimics of EDRF/NO, and activate soluble guanylate cyclase in smooth muscle cells, resulting in arterial relaxation. Therefore, these results may suggest that the endothelial dysfunction does not result from an inability of the smooth muscle cells to respond to EDRF/NO, but reflects an impaired production and/or release of the mediator from the endothelial cells or increased NO degradation.

A selective impairment of responsiveness to endothelium-dependent vasodilator agents has been demonstrated in a variety of animal models of atherosclerosis induced by high cholesterol diet and in atherosclerotic human vessels (Bossaller et al 1987; Freiman et al 1986; Shimokawa & Vanhoutte 1989). Several reports have demonstrated a selective dysfunction in receptor-dependent relaxation without an alteration in response to the receptor-independent calcium ionophore, A23187. Bossaller et al (1987) have observed that endothelium-dependent relaxation induced by A23187 is unchanged in coronary artery and aorta obtained from cholesterol-fed rabbits but that responses to acetylcholine were significantly reduced. Similar findings have been reported in atherosclerotic vessels obtained from cholesterol-fed pigs, cynomolgus

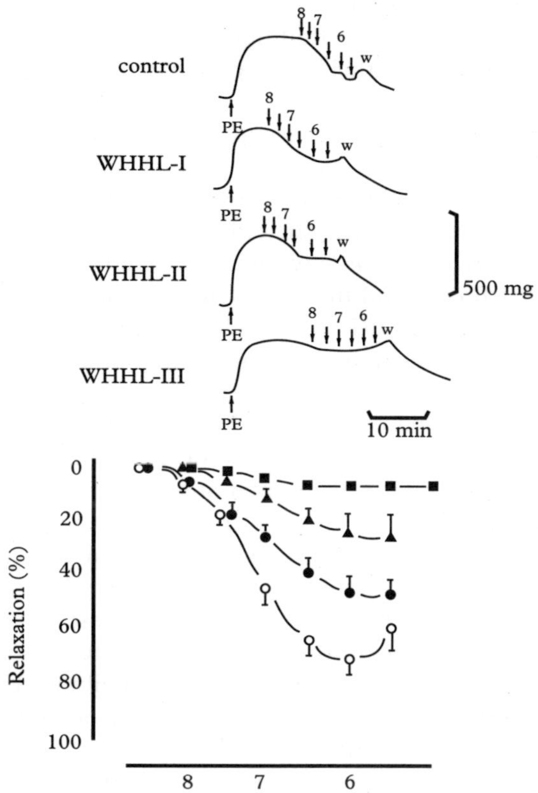

Fig. 8.1 Endothelium-dependent relaxation induced by acetylcholine in control (○ = 15) and Watanabe heritable hyperlipidaemic (WHHL) rabbits. Concentrations of acetylcholine are expressed as negative logarithm. The endothelium-dependent relaxation evoked by acetylcholine was progressively reduced in proportion to the degree of atherosclerosis. WHHL-I, 5-9 months (●, n = 8); WHHL-II, 10-22 months (▲, n = 11); and WHHL-III, 23-28 months (■, n = 6). Values in the graph are given as means ± SEM. *Abbreviations:* PE = phenylephrine (0.3 μmol/l); w = wash.

monkeys and humans with atherosclerotic coronary arteries. From these data, it is speculated that there are selective alterations of muscarinic receptors in atherosclerotic vessels and that other features of endothelium-dependent relaxation, including NO synthase activity, are preserved.

Several mechanisms have been proposed as being involved in the impairment of endothelium-dependent relaxation in atherosclerotic vessels. Verbeuren et al (1986) used a bioassay technique measuring intraluminal EDRF release to address the question of whether EDRF production is reduced in atherosclerotic vessels or not. These studies showed that intraluminal EDRF production is similar in the abdominal aorta of atherosclerotic and normal rabbits but is reduced in the thoracic aorta of atherosclerotic animals. These findings suggest that several factors may contribute to reduced endothelium-dependent relaxation in the aorta of cholesterol-fed rabbits.

Another mechanism of impaired endothelium-dependent relaxation is that the atherosclerotic lesion including intimal thickening plays a barrier to EDRF diffusion (Keitoku et al 1986). The intima of atherosclerotic vessels is markedly thickened, particularly in human and diet-induced primate atherosclerosis. It is conceivable that the increased distance between endothelial cells and the underlying vascular smooth muscle cells is so great that most of EDRF is degraded or inactivated before reaching its site of action, since EDRF is very labile compound. It has been reported that the half-life of EDRF is from several seconds to 30 seconds under physiological experimental conditions. Some insight into the possible role of intimal thickening as a barrier may be gained from studies of the regression of atherosclerosis (Harrison et al 1987). Following regression of atherosclerosis produced by dietary treatment, there is resorption at intimal lipids and inflammatory cells, but intimal thickening remains. These studies have demonstrated that endothelium-dependent relaxation returned to normal with the regression of atherosclerosis. This might suggest that intimal thickening does not provide a barrier to EDRF diffusion. However, it does not exclude the possibility that the intimal thickening of atherosclerotic vessels provides a functional barrier to EDRF by increasing degradation or inactivation.

Alternatively, EDRF might be inactivated by oxygen free radicals produced by inflammatory cells in the intima of atherosclerotic vessels. In fact, polyethylene glycolated superoxide dismutase can partially restore impaired endothelium-dependent relaxation of atherosclerotic vessels (Mügge et al 1991). Ohara et al (1993) demonstrated that there is an excess superoxide anion generation within hypercholesterolaemic vessels, and that the source of superoxide anions is not the smooth muscle cell layer but the endothelial cell itself or perhaps monocytes or macrophages closely associated with the endothelium. This increased superoxide anion release might result in accelerated degradation of either NO or a related component to an inactive form.

Shimokawa et al (1991) have proposed that hyperlipidaemia might influence the Gi protein-mediated signal transduction system in vascular endothelial cells. In porcine coronary arteries, endothelium-dependent relaxation was depressed during hypercholesterolaemia. Although the endothelium-dependent relaxation induced by bradykinin, which was coupled to Gq protein, or A23187 were similar in coronary arteries from control and hypercholesterolaemic pigs, endothelium-dependent relaxation evoked by agonists that activated the pertussis toxin-sensitive G protein were all reduced in blood vessels from hypercholesterolaemic animals.

Because of the similarity in inhibitory effects of pertussis toxin and hypercholesterolaemia, the authors suggested that hypercholesterolaemia might act by inhibiting the Gi protein-dependent intracellular signal transduction pathway in endothelial cells.

Minor et al (1990) have reported a paradoxical increase in the amount of NO released from atherosclerotic vessels measured by chemi-luminescence despite the decreased vasodilatory response. It was therefore proposed that EDRF is a more potent vasodilator than NO, indicating that EDRF is not NO but rather NO-containing compounds such as nitrosothiol (Myers et al 1990). This suggested that decreased endothelium-dependent relaxation in hypercholesterolaemic rabbits is due to an impairment of NO incorporation into parent substances acting as EDRF.

Recently, NO synthase has been purified and molecularly cloned from cerebellum (Bredt & Snyder 1990; Bredt et al 1991), endothelial cells (Janssens et al 1992; Lamas et al 1992; Marsden et al 1992; Nishida et al 1992; Pollock et al 1991; Sessa et al 1992), smooth muscle cells (Nunokawa et al 1993) and macrophages (Lyons et al 1992; Xie et al 1992; Yui et al 1991). Endothelial NO synthase was regulated by Ca^{2+}/calmodulin and modulated by phosphorylating enzymes including protein kinase C (Michel et al 1993). However, it is possible that an inducible type of NO synthase might be expressed in atherosclerotic vessels, resulting in a loss of receptor-mediated endothelium-dependent relaxation but increased NO basal release. In preliminary experiments, endothelial NO synthase mRNA or immunoreactivity was not decreased in atherosclerotic arteries obtained from rabbits or humans, indicating that the impaired endothelium-dependent relaxation in atherosclerotic arteries may not be derived from decreased NO synthase mRNA expression or protein content (Sundell et al 1992). The enzyme activity and gene expression of NO synthase in atherosclerotic arteries will be further characterized in future studies.

INHIBITORY EFFECT OF OXIDIZED-LDL AND LYSOPHOSPHATIDYLCHOLINE ON ENDOTHELIUM-DEPENDENT RELAXATION

Oxidized-LDL (ox-LDL) has been implicated as an important cause of atherosclerosis (Steinberg et al 1989). The hypothesis that modified forms of LDL, especially ox-LDL, play an important role in the atherogenic process has been strengthened by the recent *in vivo* observation that ox-LDL exists in human and rabbit atherosclerotic lesions (Rosenfeld et al 1990; Ylä-Herttuala et al 1989), and that long-term administration of antioxidants, including probucol, inhibits atherosclerotic lesion formation in Watanabe heritable hyperlipidaemic and cholesterol-fed rabbits (Carew et al 1987; Kita et al 1987). The presence of ox-LDL may have additional effects on the behaviour of cells resident within the artery. Over the past few years the focus of research on ox-LDL has broadened to include more generalized effects of ox-LDL on cellular metabolism, cytotoxity, vascular tone and coagulation. Furthermore, it is reported that lysophosphatidylcholine (LPC), which is a major lipid component of ox-LDL, plays an important role in the atherosclerotic process. In atherosclerotic aorta, several-fold increases of LPC were demonstrated in nutritionally-induced atherosclerosis (Portman et al 1970). Atherosclerotic human arteries have been also reported to exhibit 4- to 5-fold increases in LPC concentration compared with nonatherosclerotic arteries (Ylä-Herttuala et al 1987).

Our own and other groups (Kugiyama et al 1990; Yokoyama et al 1990) have clearly demonstrated that LPC in ox-LDL inhibits endothelium-dependent relaxation, indicating that ox-LDL may contribute to impaired endothelium-dependent relaxation in atherosclerotic arteries (Fig. 8.2). Ox-LDL (10-500 μg protein/ml) but not native LDL (<2 mg protein/ml) inhibits endothelium-dependent relaxation. Oxidative modification of LDL was achieved by treatment with Cu^{2+} or incubation with cultured endothelial cells. The impairment of endothelium-dependent relaxation was completely recovered by washing with Krebs buffer containing defatted albumin, indicating the functional integrity of endothelium was preserved after exposure to modified LDL. On the other hand, ox-LDL did not inhibit the relaxation induced by nitroglycerin, an endothelium-independent vasodilator. The inhibitory ability of ox-LDL on endothelium-dependent relaxation is heat stable and is associated with the lipid fraction of the molecule. Although lipid extracts from native LDL had no effect on endothelium-dependent relaxation, lipids from ox-LDL inhibited endothelium-dependent relaxation. One of characteristics of ox-LDL is its increased LPC content. During oxidative modification of LDL, as much as 40% of phosphatidylcholine (PC) is converted to LPC, causing LPC to be present at high concentrations in ox-LDL but not in native LDL.

In our experiments, fractionation of individual lipids revealed that LPC derived from ox-LDL inhibited endothelium-dependent relaxation in rabbit aorta, whereas the remaining lipids, including oxidized free fatty acids, sphingomyelin, cholesterol and other phospholipids, had no effect. Moreover, the effect of ox-LDL could be mimicked by using synthetic LPC (1-palmitoyl), whereas other phospholipids (e.g. phosphatidylethanolamine [PE] and PC) or lysolipid (e.g. lysophosphatidylethanolamine [LPE]) were ineffective. Furthermore, modified LDL treated with phospholipase A_2 (phospholipase A_2-treated LDL) markedly inhibited endothelium-dependent relaxation in rabbit aorta. After incubation with phospholipase A_2, PC in LDL was almost completely converted to LPC without producing oxidative lipid products. This strengthened our conclusion that LPC plays an important role in the endothelial dysfunction induced by modified LDL. From these results, we concluded that the

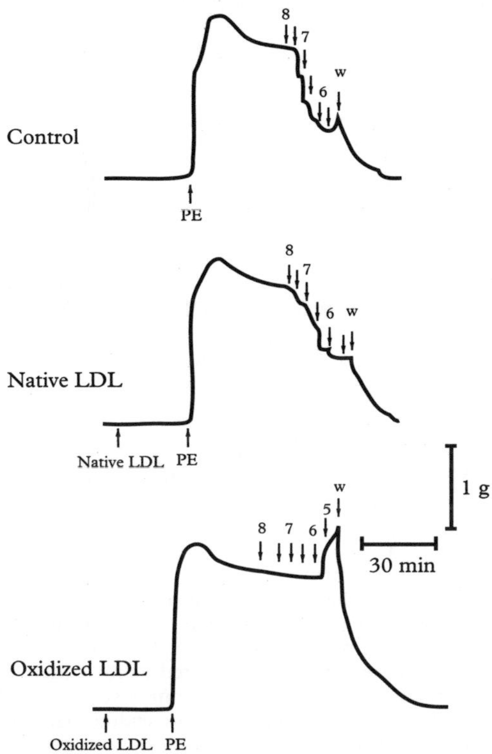

Fig. 8.2 Traces of typical response to acetylcholine by rabbit aorta in the absence or presence of native LDL (1 mg protein/ml) or oxidized-LDL (0.5 mg protein/ml). Oxidized LDL but not native LDL inhibits endothelium-dependent relaxation to acetylcholine. *Abbreviation:* PE = phenylephrine (0.3 μmol/l); w = wash.

inhibitory effects of ox-LDL on endothelium-dependent relaxation were to a large extent related to a transfer of amphiphilic lipids (LPC) from modified lipoproteins to endothelial cell membranes. Margin et al (1993) demonstrated that ox-LDL lost its inhibitory activity on endothelium-dependent relaxation after it was treated with defatted albumin or lysophospholipase (phospholipase B), both of which reduce LPC content. LPC in ox-LDL generated during oxidative modification was therefore the main inhibitory factor in the impairment of endothelium-dependent relaxation.

Tanner et al (1991) have demonstrated that, in porcine coronary arteries treated with ox-LDL, endothelium-dependent relaxation induced by serotonin is impaired but can be improved if the vessels are pretreated with L-arginine. These results suggest that the inhibitory effects of ox-LDL are

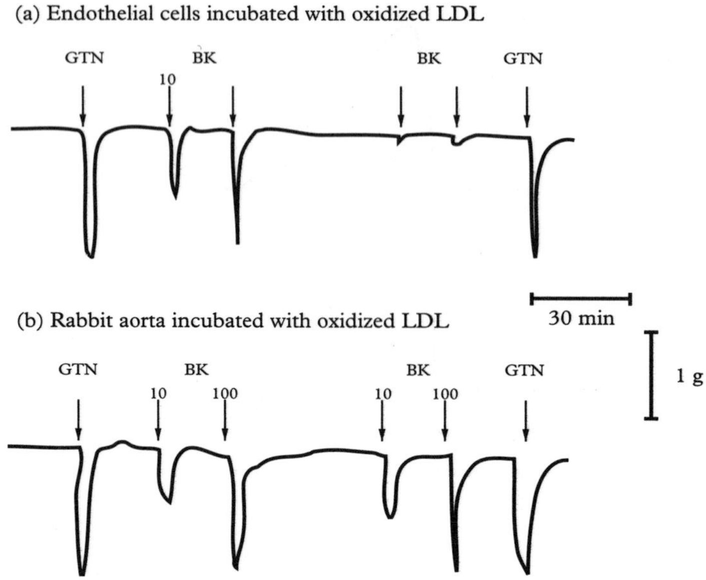

Fig. 8.3 Traces of relaxation of rabbit aorta helical strips without endothelium induced by endothelium-derived relaxing factor (EDRF) released by bradykinin (BK) at concentrations of 10 and 100 nmol/l. A column packed with 3-5 x 10^7 bovine aortic endothelial cells cultured on microcarriers was perfused with oxygenated Krebs buffer. The sensitivity of the bioassay tissues was standardized by administration of nitroglycerin (GTN) 100 nmol/l before and after each experiment. Pretreatment of bovine aortic endothelial cells with oxidized LDL (0.5 mg protein/ml) almost abolished the relaxations induced by EDRF (panel a). Pretreatment of the bioassay tissues with oxidized LDL (0.5 mg protein/ml) did not alter the relaxations induced by EDRF (panel b).

derived from impaired intracellular availability of L-arginine and/or by interference with receptor-operated amino acid synthesis. In contrast to our experiments, they also suggest that the inhibitory effects of ox-LDL are not mimicked by the addition of LPC to porcine coronary arteries. It is unclear what accounts for the differences in these experimental results.

Many studies have focused on the effects of ox-LDL on cellular function, including the EDRF synthesis in endothelial cells. However, some of these experiments show different effects of ox-LDL on endothelium-dependent relaxation. When LDL is oxidized in the presence of certain metal ions or by cells *in vitro*, a myriad of oxidation products are formed from both the peroxidation of the lipid component of LDL and oxidative degradation of apoprotein B. Variability of ox-LDL may be depend on the cell type or the exact metal ion concentration used, incubation time, presence of endogenous antioxidants, and LDL size or density. The variability of ox-LDL and experimental conditions may contribute to some of the differences in the effects of ox-LDL on endothelium-dependent relaxation.

Ox-LDL can cause foam cell formation via the scavenger receptors in macrophages. Poly G, a scavenger receptor antagonist, did not affect the inhibitory activity of ox-LDL, indicating that modified LDL inhibits the production of EDRF without mediation by the scavenger receptor (Hirata et al 1990). The mechanism underlying the inhibitory effect of ox-LDL may involve the impairment of production and/or release of EDRF, or the promotion of inactivation of EDRF after it is released. We have used a bioassay system to evaluate the site of action of ox-LDL on the impaired endothelium-dependent relaxation (Hirata et al 1990). EDRF was released from bovine aortic endothelial cells cultured on microcarrier beads in response to bradykinin and was detected by bioassay on helical strips of rabbit aorta. Treatment of these cells with ox-LDL or LPC for 30 min abolished relaxation of detector arteries by EDRF (Fig. 8.3). On the other hand, after the detector arteries were treated with ox-LDL or LPC, EDRF-induced relaxation was not altered. These results indicate that ox-LDL inhibits the release of EDRF from cultured bovine aortic endothelial cells but does not promote the degradation or inactivation of NO.

NATIVE LDL AND EDRF

According to some investigators, native LDL appears to be able to inhibit endothelium-dependent relaxation by a rapid and reversible mechanism that may result from a direct interaction between LDL and EDRF/NO. In 1987, Andrews et al (1987) reported that incubation of isolated rabbit aorta with human LDL preparations (500-2000 μg/ml) for 30 min impaired acetylcholine-induced relaxation. Galle et al (1991) demonstrated that native LDL and ox-LDL could inactivate EDRF/NO. These authors proposed that EDRF/NO might be sequestered and inactivated within the hydrophobic core of the lipoprotein molecule. They indicated that the vasoactive effects of LDL depend on the binding at native LDL to endothelial LDL receptors and that chemically-modified LDL was inactive. Conversely, several studies have failed to demonstrate any effect of native LDL on endothelium-dependent relaxation. Simon et al (1990) demonstrated that oxidative incubation of porcine coronary arteries with native LDL in the absence of antioxidants evoked slow increases in vascular tone. The inhibitory effect of native LDL may result from the conversion of LDL to ox-LDL by the highly oxygenated environment used in these physiological studies. Jacobs et al (1990) demonstrated that an inhibitory effect of LDL could only be observed if the arterial rings were precontracted by norepinephrine (noradrenaline) or serotonin, but not by phenylephrine. Tomita et al (1990) examined the effects of lipoprotein fractions from porcine serum on the endothelium-dependent relaxation of isolated porcine coronary arteries. Heat- or acid-treated LDL lost its inhibitory effect. From these observations, an inhibitory effect of native LDL remains controversial, since it is difficult to prevent oxidative modification of LDL in the experimental environment. Further and more precise experiments will be needed to clarify this problem.

CELLULAR MECHANISM OF ACTION BY OX-LDL AND LPC IN CULTURED BOVINE AORTIC ENDOTHELIAL CELLS

It has been proposed that the EDRF synthesis is regulated by an intracellular Ca^{2+} signal through a receptor-mediated phospholipase C-coupled transduction system that hydrolyzes phosphatidylinositol-4,5-diphosphate to produce diacylglycerol, the specific activator of protein kinase C, and inositol-1,4,5-trisphosphate (IP_3), a compound which mobilizes Ca^{2+} from intracellular Ca^{2+} stores. To clarify the underlying mechanism of reduced EDRF synthesis in endothelial cells elicited by ox-LDL or LPC, we examined the effects of ox-LDL and LPC on the receptor-mediated signal transduction system in cultured bovine aortic endothelial cells. Bradykinin (0.1 nmol/l -1 μmol/l) elicited rapid generation of inositol phosphates (IP_1, IP_2, IP_3), whereas ox-LDL or LPC alone did not induce IP_3 formation. Accumulation of IP_3 stimulated by bradykinin was markedly inhibited by ox-LDL (100-500 μg protein/ml) or LPC (1-40 μmol/l) [Hirata et al 1991; Inoue et al 1992]. Furthermore, at higher concentrations, LPC (20-40 μmol/l) inhibited IP_3 accumulation induced by AlF_4, which is a direct stimulator for G protein. However, PC (1-20 μg/ml) had no effect on bradykinin-induced IP_3 accumulation.

To investigate the effects of ox-LDL and LPC on the intracellular signalling pathway, intracellular calcium concentration ($[Ca^{2+}]i$) was monitored. LPC (10-20 μmol/l) itself induced a biphasic increase in $[Ca^{2+}]i$, which consisted of a rapid increase followed by a sustained increase. The initial component was a result of mobilization from intracellular calcium stores without a detectable increase of IP_3 (Inoue et al 1992). Ox-LDL and LPC inhibited the increase in $[Ca^{2+}]i$ induced by bradykinin and ATPγS, an endothelium-dependent vasodilator, in cultured bovine aortic endothelial cells. These findings allow us to speculate that ox-LDL and LPC inhibit the intracellular signal transduction which links receptor stimulation to biosynthesis of a secondary messenger in endothelial cells, leading to an endothelial defect in the generation of appropriate intracellular calcium signals necessary for activation of Ca^{2+}/calmodulin-dependent NO synthase, and impaired EDRF production and/or release (Fig. 8.4). Reduced IP_3 production caused by uncoupling between receptor and G protein may be involved in the inhibition of Ca^{2+} release from intracellular Ca^{2+} stores.

However, the mechanism of the inhibitory effect of LPC on bradykinin-stimulated Ca^{2+} influx is unknown, because the precise mechanism of the Ca^{2+} influx stimulated by agonists in endothelial cells is not fully

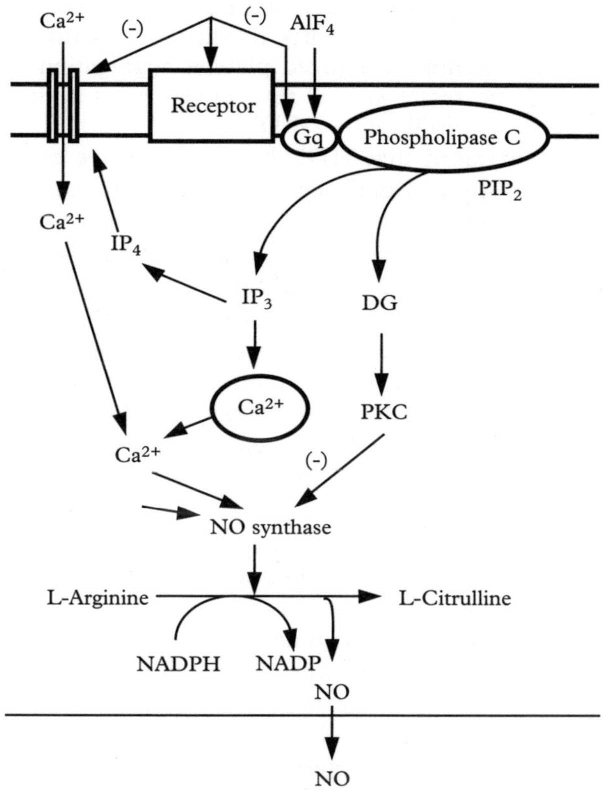

Fig. 8.4 Effect of oxidized LDL and lysophosphatidylcholine on the intracellular signal transduction system in cultured bovine aortic endothelial cells. *Abbreviations:* AlF_4 = alminium fluoride; DG = diacylglycerol; IP_3 = inositol-1,4,5-trisphosphate; IP_4 = inositol-1,3,4,5-tetrakisphosphate; LPC = lysophosphatidylcholine; PIP_2 = phosphatidylinositol-4,5-diphosphate; PKC = protein kinase C.

established. The inhibitory effect of LPC is probably due to the direct interaction with the plasma membrane of endothelial cells (Inoue et al 1992). Alterations of plasma membrane properties by LPC may cause the inhibitory effects of LPC on phospholipase C-mediated phosphoinositide hydrolysis, the generation of secondary messengers, and Ca^{2+} influx across the plasma membrane in endothelial cells.

EFFECT OF HIGH-DENSITY LIPOPROTEIN ON EDRF INHIBITION BY OX-LDL AND LPC

High-density lipoprotein (HDL) is known to exert its antiatherogenic effect through the promotion of reverse cholesterol transport. In addition,

HDL attenuates the cytotoxic effect of LDL on vascular smooth muscle and endothelial cells, and prevents oxidative modification of LDL. Furthermore, HDL inhibits enhanced platelet aggregation evoked by ox-LDL. Thus, HDL possesses several protective effects against a variety of unfavourable actions of LDL and ox-LDL.

We have demonstrated that HDL has a preventive effect on the ox-LDL-induced inhibition of endothelium-dependent relaxation in rabbit aorta strips (Matsuda et al 1993). In the presence of HDL (1 mg protein/ml), the inhibitory effect of ox-LDL (0.5 mg protein/ml) on the endothelium-dependent relaxation induced by acetylcholine was markedly reduced. HDL by itself had no effect on the resting tension, phenylephrine-induced contraction or endothelium-dependent relaxation. We examined whether HDL had any effect on the inhibitory action of LPC and ox-LDL on endothelium-dependent relaxation. Endothelium-dependent relaxation induced by acetylcholine disappeared completely after incubation with LPC 10 mmol/l, but was almost completely prevented by concurrent addition of HDL (1 mg protein/ml). We then looked at the effect of HDL on the incorporation of radiolabelled LPC into cultured bovine aortic endothelial cells and the removal of LPC from these cells by HDL. After culture of the cells for 30 min in Dulbecco's minimal essential medium (DMEM) containing [^{14}C]-LPC (10 mmol/l), 11.7% of the LPC added to the medium was incorporated into the cells. In the presence of HDL (1 mg protein/ml) in the medium, however, the incorporation of LPC into cells was decreased to 0.6%. After another 30-min incubation of [^{14}C]-LPC-incorporated cells with fresh DMEM, only 4.7% of the initially incorporated LPC was released into the medium and 95.3% remained in the cells. On the other hand, another 30-min incubation of LPC-incorporated cells with fresh DMEM containing HDL (1 mg protein/ml) promoted the release of the initially incorporated LPC into the medium up to 53.7% and reduced the LPC remaining in the cells to 46.3%. The results obtained from these LPC transfer experiments with HDL are in accordance with those of the previously mentioned vasorelaxation experiments. We concluded that HDL markedly reduced the incorporation of LPC into cultured bovine aortic endothelial cells and promoted the release of cell-incorporated LPC into the medium, resulting in a reduction of the LPC remaining in the cells. After incubation of ox-LDL with HDL, LPC in ox-LDL was transferred into HDL particle.

These results indicate that HDL reverses the ox-LDL-induced impairment of endothelium-dependent relaxation by removing LPC from ox-LDL and preventing LPC from acting on the endothelium. Recently, Kuhn et al (1991) reported that there is a positive correlation between HDL-cholesterol and normal acetylcholine-induced coronary vasoreactivity in patients undergoing coronary arteriography, implying the relevance of our findings. Thus, HDL may have a salutary effect against the impairment of endothelium-mediated vasodilatation in atherosclerotic arteries.

ENDOTHELIAL NO SYNTHASE ACTIVITY BY LYSOLIPIDS

Recently, several types of NO synthase have been purified and cloned not only from endothelium but also from cerebellum, macrophage, smooth muscle and hepatocyte. NO synthase exists as at least two discrete families or isoforms: one form is constitutively expressed, which is present in endothelium and cerebellum, and the other is inducible. Activity of endothelial constitutive NO synthase is mainly regulated by Ca^{2+}/calmodulin in the presence of (6R)-5,6,7,8-tetrahydrobiopterin, NADPH and FAD as cofactors. We have investigated the effects of lipids, especially LPC on particulate NO synthase purified from cultured bovine aortic endothelial cells using an assay of L-arginine to L-citrulline conversion (Ohashi et al 1993). NO synthase activity was enhanced up to about 3 fold by PC, LPC and PE in the presence of Ca^{2+} and calmodulin. Arachidonic acid (100-1000 μmol/l) tended to decrease NO synthase activity. Other lipids, e.g. LPE, phosphatidylinositol, lysophosphatidylinositol, phosphatidylserine, phosphatidic acid, palmitic acid and oleic acid, did not have any effect on NO synthase activity. From these results, the impaired NO production by LPC would not appear to be related to NO synthase activity.

CONCLUSION - CLINICAL RELEVANCE OF IMPAIRMENT OF ENDOTHELIUM-DEPENDENT RELAXATION

Patients with atherosclerosis are prone to develop vascular spasm, particularly spasm of coronary arteries (MacAlpin 1983). Attenuation of the basal release of EDRF may substantially augment vascular tone in response to vasoactive agents. Furthermore, serotonin, a potential mediator of vascular spasm, produces augmented vascular responses when the endothelium is removed. Thus, an alteration in the production and/or release of EDRF in atherosclerosis would predispose to vascular spasm. This altered endothelial modulation of vascular tone may be responsible for a variety of clinical manifestations of atherosclerotic vascular disorders.

There is accumulating evidence that diminished NO production may accelerate coronary artery disease by promoting interaction between platelets and the vessel wall through loss of NO-mediated platelet inhibition. In diseased vessels, products of activated platelets, such as serotonin and platelet-derived growth factor, may lead to vasoconstriction and the proliferation of vascular smooth muscle, processes that tend to accelerate the progression of coronary artery disease. Infusion of L-arginine or long-term treatment with L-arginine markedly restores decreased endothelium-dependent relaxation in hypercholesterolaemia or atherosclerosis. Moreover, Cooke et al (1992) tested the effect of L-arginine on the formation of atherosclerotic lesions in cholesterol-fed animals. They found a 3-fold decrease in lesion area in cholesterol-fed rabbits when the rabbits were simultaneously fed with L-arginine, but not with D-arginine. From these results, L-arginine could serve as a therapeutic tool to prevent atherosclerotic progression.

To determine whether an abnormal NO synthase gene may play a role in the aetiology of atherosclerosis, the structure of NO synthase genes and their expression in blood vessels of patients with atherosclerosis will need to be studied. Advances in molecular biology may also permit new therapeutic approaches, such as the direct insertion of cDNA for endothelial NO synthase into the vessel walls of coronary and peripheral arteries, to prevent atherosclerotic progression and restenosis after percutaneous transluminal coronary angioplasty.

REFERENCES

Andrews H E, Bruckdorfer K R, Dunn R C et al 1987 Low-density lipoproteins inhibit endothelium-dependent relaxation in rabbit aorta. Nature 327: 237-239

Bossaller C, Habib G B, Yamamoto H et al 1987 Impaired muscarinic endothelium-dependent relaxation and cyclic guanosine 5-monophosphate formation in atherosclerotic human coronary artery and rabbit aorta. J Clin Invest 79: 170-174

Bredt D S, Hwang P, Glatt C E et al 1991 Cloned and expressed nitric oxide synthase structurally resembles cytochrome P-450 reductase. Nature 351: 714-719

Bredt D S, Snyder S H 1990 Isolation of nitric oxide synthase, a calmodulin-requiring enzyme. Proc Natl Acad Sci USA 87: 682-685

Carew T E, Schwenke D C, Steinberg D 1987 Antiatherogenic effect of probucol unrelated to its hypocholesterolemic effect: evidence that antioxidants *in vivo* inhibit low density lipoprotein degradation in macrophage-rich fatty streaks and slow the progression of atherosclerosis in the Watanabe heritable hyperlipidemic rabbits. Proc Natl Acad Sci USA 84: 7725-7729

Cohen R A, Zitnay K M, Haudenschild C C et al 1988 Loss of selective endothelial cell vasoactive functions caused by hypercholesterolemia in pig coronary arteries. Circ Res 64: 903-910

Cooke J P, Singer A H, Tsao P et al 1992 Antiatherogenic effects of L-arginine in the hypercholesterolemic rabbit. J Clin Invest 90: 1168-1172

Cybulski M I, Gimbrone Jr M A 1991 Endothelial expression of a mononuclear leukocyte adhesion molecule during atherogenesis. Science 251: 788-791

Freiman P C, Mitchell G G, Heistad D D et al 1986 Atherosclerosis impairs endothelium-dependent vascular relaxation to acetylcholine and thrombin in primates. Circ Res 58: 783-789

Furchgott R F, Zawadzki J M 1980 The obligatory role of endothelial cells in the relaxation of arterial smooth muscle by acetylcholine. Nature 288: 373-376

Furchgott R F 1983 Role of endothelium in responses of vascular smooth muscle. Circ Res 53: 557-573

Galle J, Mulsch A, Busse R et al 1991 Effects of native and oxidized low density lipoproteins on formation and inactivation of endothelium-derived relaxing factor. Arterioscler Thromb 11: 198-203

Garg U C, Hassid A 1990 Nitric oxide generating vasodilators and 8-bromo-cyclic GMP inhibit mitogenesis and proliferation of cultured rat vascular smooth muscle cells. J Clin Invest 83: 1774-1777

Harrison D G, Armstrong M L, Freiman P C et al 1987 Restoration of endothelium-dependent relaxation by dietary treatment of atherosclerosis. J Clin Invest 80: 1808-1811

Hirata K, Akita H, Yokoyama M et al 1992 Impaired vasodilatory response to atrial natriuretic peptide during atherosclerosis progression. Arterioscler Thromb 12: 99-105

Hirata K, Akita H, Yokoyama M 1991 Oxidized low density lipoprotein inhibits bradykinin-induced phosphoinositide hydrolysis in cultured bovine endothelial cells. FEBS Lett 287: 181-184

Hirata K, Yokoyama M, Matsuda, Y et al 1990 Lysophosphatidylcholine in modified low density lipoprotein inhibits production of endothelium-derived relaxing factor in endothelial cells. Circulation 82 (suppl 3): 111-171

Inoue N, Hirata K, Yamada M et al 1992 Lysophosphatidylcholine inhibits bradykinin-induced phosphoinositide hydrolysis and calcium transient in cultured bovine aortic endothelial cells. Circ Res 71: 1410-1421

Jacobs M, Plane F, Bruckdorfer K R 1990 Native and oxidized low density lipoproteins have different inhibitory effects on endothelium-derived relaxing factor in the rabbit aorta. Br J Pharmacol 100: 21-26

Janssens S P, Shimouchi A, Quertermous T et al 1992 Cloning and expression of a cDNA encoding human endothelium-derived relaxing factor/nitric oxide synthase. J Biol Chem 267: 14519-14522

Keitoku M, Maruyama T, Takishima T 1986 Unfavorable effect of intimal thickening on endothelium-dependent relaxation in human coronary artery. Circulation 74 (suppl 2): 498

Kita T, Nagano Y, Yokode M et al 1987 Probucol prevents the progression of atherosclerosis in Watanabe heritable hyperlipidemic rabbit an animal model for familial hypercholesterolemia. Proc Natl Acad Sci USA 84: 5298-5931

Kolodgie F D, Virmani R, Rice H E et al 1990 Vascular reactivity during the progression of atherosclerotic plaque. A study in Watanabe heritable hyperlipidemic rabbits. Circ Res 66: 1112-1126.

Kubes P, Suzuki M, Granger D N 1991 Nitric oxide: an endogenous modulator of leukocyte adhesion. Proc Natl Acad Sci USA 88: 4651-4655

Kugiyama K, Kerns S A, Morrisett J D et al 1990 Impairment of endothelium-dependent relaxation by lysolecithin in modified low-density lipoproteins. Nature 344: 160-162

Kuhn F E, Mohler E R, Satler L F et al 1991 Effects of high-density lipoprotein on acetylcholine-induced coronary vasoreactivity. Am J Cardiol 68: 1425-1430

Kurose I, Kubes P, Wolf R et al 1993 Inhibitrion of nitric oxide production: mechanisms of vascular albumin leakage. Circ Res 17: 164-171

Lamas S, Marsden P A, Li G K et al 1992 Endothelial nitric oxide synthase: molecular cloning and characterization of a distinct constitutive enzyme isoform. Proc Natl Acad Sci USA 89: 6348-6352

Lyons C R, Orloff G J, Cunningham J M 1992 Molecular cloning and functional expression of an inducible nitric oxide synthase from a murine macrophage cell line. J Biol Chem 267: 6370-6374

MacAlpin R 1983 Relation of coronary arterial spasm to sites of organic stenosis. Am J Cardiol 46: 143-153

Margin Jr E L, Kugiyama K, Nguy J H et al 1993 Effects of lysolipids and oxidatively modified low density lipoprotein on endothelium-dependent relaxation of rabbit aorta. Circ Res 72: 161-166

Marsden P A, Schappert K T, Chen H S et al 1992 Molecular cloning and characterization of human nitric oxide synthase. FEBS Lett 307: 287-293

Maseri A, Davies G, Hackett D et al 1990 Coronary artery spasm and vasoconstriction. The case for a distinction. Circulation 81: 1983-1991

Matsuda Y, Hirata K, Inoue N et al 1993 High density lipoprotein reverses inhibitory effect of oxidized low density lipoprotein on endothelium-dependent relaxation. Circ Res 72: 1103-1109

Michel T, Li G K, Busconi L 1993 Phosphorylation and subcellular translocation of endothelial nitric oxide synthase. Proc Natl Acad Sci USA 90: 6252-6256

Minor R L, Myers P R, Guerra R et al 1990 Diet-induced atherosclerosis increases the release of nitrogen oxides from rabbit aorta. J Clin Invest 86: 2109-2116

Moncada S, Palmer R M J, Higgs E A 1991 Nitric Oxide: Physiology, pathophysiology, and pharmacology. Pharmacol Rev 43: 109-142

Mügge A, Elwell J H, Peterson T G et al 1991 Chronic treatment with polyethylene-glycolated superoxide dismutase partially restores endothelium-dependent vascular relaxations in cholesterol-fed rabbits. Circ Res 69: 1293-1300

Myers P R, Minor R L, Guerra R et al 1990 Vasorelaxant properties of the endothelium-derived relaxing factor more closely resemble S-nitrosocysteine than nitric oxide. Nature 345: 161-163

Nathan C 1992 Nitric oxide as a secretory product of mammalian cells. FASEB J 6: 3051-3064

Nishida K, Harrison D G, Navas J P et al 1992 Molecular cloning and characterization of constitutive bovine aortic endothelial cell nitric oxide synthase. J Clin Invest 90: 2092-2096
Nunokawa Y, Ishida N, Tanaka S 1993 Cloning of inducible nitric oxide synthase in rat vascular smooth muscle cells. Biochem Biophys Res Commun 191: 89-94
Ohara Y, Peterson T M, Harrison D G 1993 Hypercholesterolemia increases endothelial superoxide anion production. J Clin Invest 91: 2546-2551
Ohashi Y, Katayama M, Hirata K et al 1993 Activation of nitric oxide synthase from cultured aortic endothelial cells by phospholipids. Biochem Biophys Res Commun 195: 1314-1320
Palmer R M J, Ashton D S, Moncada S 1988 Vascular endothelial cells synthesize nitric oxide from L-arginine. Nature 333: 664-666
Palmer R M J, Ferrige A G, Moncada S 1987 Nitric oxide release accounts for the biological activity of endothelium-derived relaxing factor. Nature 327: 524-526
Pollock J S, Förstermann U, Mitchell J A et al 1991 Purification and characterization of particulate endothelium-derived relaxing factor synthase from cultured and native bovine aortic endothelial cells. Proc Natl Acad Sci USA 88: 10480-10484
Portman Q W, Soltys P, Alexander M et al 1970 Metabolism of lysolecithin *in vivo*: effects of hyperlipidemia and atherosclerosis in squirrel monkeys. J Lipid Res 11: 596-604
Radomski N W, Palmer R M J, Moncada S 1987 Endogenous nitric oxide inhibits human platelet adhesion to vascular endothelium. Lancet 338;2: 1057-1058
Rosenfeld M E, Palinski W, Ylä-Herttuala S et al 1990 Distribution of oxidation specific lipid-protein adducts and apolipoprotein B in atherosclerotic lesions of varying severity from WHHL rabbits. Arteriosclerosis 10: 336-349
Sessa W C, Harrison J K, Barber C M et al 1992 Molecular cloning and expression of a cDNA encoding endothelial cell nitric oxide synthase. J Biol Chem 267: 15274-15276
Shimokawa H, Flavahan N A, Vanhoutte P M 1991 Loss of endothelial pertussis toxin-sensitive G-protein function in atherosclerotic porcine coronary arteries. Circulation 83: 652-660
Shimokawa H, Vanhoutte P M 1989 Impaired endothelium-dependent relaxation to aggregating platelets and related vasoactive substances in porcine coronary arteries in hypercholesterolemia and atherosclerosis. Circ Res 64: 900-914
Simon B C, Cunningham L D, Cohen R A 1990 Oxidized low density lipoproteins cause contraction and inhibit endothelium-dependent relaxation in the pig coronary artery. J Clin Invest 86: 75-79
Steinberg G, Parthasarathy S, Carew T E et al 1989 Beyond cholesterol: modifications of low density lipoprotein that increases its atherogenicity. N Engl J Med 320: 915-924
Sundell C L, Marsden P A, Subramanian R R et al 1992 Nitric oxide synthase is expressed by endothelial cells overlying human atherosclerotic plaques. Circulation 86 (suppl 1): 472
Tanner F C, Noll G, Boulanger C M et al 1991 Oxidized low density lipoproteins inhibit relaxations of porcine coronary arteries. role of scavenger receptor and endothelium-derived nitric oxide. Circulation 83: 2012-2020
Tomita T, Ezaki M, Miwa M et al 1990 Rapid and reversible inhibition by low density lipoprotein of the endothelium-dependent relaxation to hemostatic substances in porcine coronary arteries. Circ Res 66:18-27
Verbeuren T J, Jordaens F H, Zonnekeyn L L et al 1986 Effect of hypercholesterolemia on vascular reactivity in the rabbit. I. Endothelium-dependent and endothelium-independent contractions and relaxations in isolated arteries of control and hypercholesterolemic rabbits. Circ Res 58: 552-564.
Xie Q W, Cho H J, Calaycay J et al 1992 Cloning and characterization of inducible nitric oxide synthase from mouse macrophage. Science 256: 225-228
Yanagisawa M, Kurihara H, Kimura S et al 1988 A novel potent vasoconstrictor peptide produced by vascular endothelial cells. Nature 332: 411-415
Ylä-Herttuala S, Palinski W, Rosenfeld M E et al 1989 Evidence for the presence of oxidatively modified low density lipoprotein in atherosclerotic lesions of rabbit and man. J Clin Invest 84: 1086-1095
Ylä-Herttuala S, Sumuvuori H, Karkola K et al 1987 Atherosclerosis and biochemical composition of coronary arteries in Finnish men. Atherosclerosis 65: 109-115
Yokoyama M, Hirata K, Miyake R et al 1990 Lysophosphatidylcholine: essential role in the inhibition of endothelium-dependent vasorelaxation by oxidized low-density lipoprotein. Biochem Biophys Res Commun 168: 301-308
Yui Y, Hattori K, Kosuga K et al 1991 Purification of nitric oxide synthase from macrophage. J Biol Chem 266: 12544-12547

9

Endothelial dysfunction in diabetes: role of endothelium-derived relaxing factor

T. Taminato, S. Sen, H. Kato, G. Sarwar

INTRODUCTION

Prevention and treatment of the chronic vascular complications is the central therapeutic problem in diabetes mellitus. Prolonged exposure to hyperglycaemia is the primary factor associated with the development of diabetes-specific microvascular disease, and the relationship between deranged glucose metabolism and arterial disease is complicated by many other factors that influence atherogenesis in nondiabetics. Hypertension and other vascular diseases are more prevalent in diabetic patients than in the general population.

Damage of vascular endothelium and disturbance of endothelium-dependent responses have been shown to be early events of diabetic micro- and macroangiopathy. Increased blood flow and vascular leakage of proteins preferentially affect tissues that are sites of diabetic complications in humans and animals. Recently, interest has focused on a factor, endothelium-derived relaxing factor (EDRF), which has been investigated for its role in the physiology or pathogenesis of vascular diseases. The synthesis and release of EDRF from vascular endothelial cells, which regulates the calibre of resistance blood vessels, may play a part in controlling vascular perfusion within individual organs (Archer 1993; Nathan 1992).

ENDOTHELIAL DYSFUNCTION IN DIABETES

Endothelial-dependent vascular relaxation has been investigated in many studies using aortae from diabetic rats. In brief, when acetylcholine was used as an agonist, most laboratories have shown impaired relaxation (Durante et al 1988; Kamata et al 1989; Meraji et al 1987; Oyama et al 1986; Pieper & Gross 1988), whereas other laboratories have reported no change (Fortes et al 1983; Harris & MacLeod 1988; Head et al 1987; Wakabayashi et al 1987). Reports which showed impairment of endothelium-dependent vascular relaxation induced by acetylcholine have also presented evidence of impairment of relaxation induced by other endothelial-dependent vasodilators such as histamine (Meraji et al 1987; Oyama et al 1986) and the calcium ionophore A23187 (Durante et al

1988; Oyama et al 1986). In other species, EDRF-mediated relaxation of cerebral arterioles *in vivo* and aorta *in vitro* is suppressed in diabetic rabbits (Tesfamariam et al 1989). Similarly, penile arterial relaxation to EDRF is imparied in diabetic men (De Tajada et al 1989).

It is noteworthy that the impairment of endothelium-dependent responses has been shown only when hyperglycaemia has developed whatever the diabetes model used, although the WBN/Kob diabetic rat model is an exception (Durante et al 1988; Kamata et al 1989). Furthermore, in aortae from diabetic rabbits or in those from normal rabbits exposed to elevated glucose for 6 h, acetylcholine-induced relaxation is impaired (Tesfamariam et al 1989, 1990). These observations indicate that suppression of vascular dilatation to EDRF occurs early in diabetic state.

ROLE OF EDRF IN VASCULAR FUNCTION

Interest has now been focused on nitric oxide (NO), since the recent discovery that EDRF is in fact NO or a closely related compound. NO is a small, gaseous, paramagnetic radical with a high affinity for interaction with ferrous haemoproteins such as soluble guanylate cyclase and haemoglobin. In addition to being a potent endogenous vasodilator and inhibitor of platelet aggregation, NO has a role in inflammation, thrombosis, immunity and neurotransmission. NO's effects on such diverse pathophysiological processes might be related to its ability to oxidise numerous important compounds (thiols, haem groups, and iron-sulphur centres) [Archer 1993].

NO is synthesized from the guanidino nitrogen of L-arginine and molecular oxygen, a process hat can be inhibited by N^G-substituted L-arginine analogues such as N^G-monomethyl L-arginine (NMMA) [Nathan 1992], NO is produced in macrophages, endothelial cells, neutrophils and cerebellum by dioxygenases, known as nitric oxide synthetase (NOS) [Nathan 1992]. There are two basic types of NOS, a constitutive form that accounts for the rapid, transient, Ca^{2+}-dependent production of EDRF/NO by the endothelium, and an inducible form, which causes the slow onset of Ca^{2+}-independent NO synthesis in inflammatory cells (after stimulation with cytokines or lipopolysaccharide). It now appears that the constitutive form of NOS binds calmodulin loosely and produces NO when transient elevations of cytosolic Ca^{2+} induce close association of calmodulin with NOS. Inducible forms of NOS have such a close coupling with calmodulin under normal conditions that enzyme activity is not susceptible to modulation by Ca^{2+} transients (Nathan 1992). NADPH is a cosubstrate for NOS, and flavin adenine dinucleotide, flavin mononucleotide, haem and tetrahydrobiopterin are cofactors (Nathan 1992). NOS produces L-citrulline as a coproduct of L-arginine metabolism.

The vasodilator effect of acetylcholine in preconstricted rings or bands of isolated arteries and on resistance blood vessels of perfused organs is mediated by EDRF (Furchgott & Zsawadzki 1989). Conversely, impaired production of EDRF may contribute to the vasospasm of coronary arteries associated with angina pectoris and with the increased peripheral resistance in hypertension. Reduced biosynthesis of EDRF has been shown in the aorta of diabetic rats (Bhardwaj & Moore 1988; Oyama et al 1986; Pieper & Gross 1991).

POSSIBLE MECHANISMS FOR DETERIORATED VASCULAR RESPONSES IN DIABETES

A decrease in the release of EDRF/NO has recently been proposed as occurring in diabetes (Bhardwaj & Moore 1988; Oyama et al 1986; Pieper & Gross 1991). Several hypotheses, especially related to the impaired production of EDRF and/or quenching of EDRF, have been put forward to explain the vascular dysfunction in diabetic or high glucose conditions.

INCREASED GENERATION OF OXYGEN RADICALS

In the intestinal microvasculature of insulin-dependent diabetic rats, Lash and Bohlen (1991) demonstrated that arteriolar dilatation in response to acetylcholine is severely depressed within 1 week of the onset of hyperglycaemia, and that this depression is maintained for at least 7 to 8 weeks during hyperglycaemia. However, vasodilatation in response to sodium nitroprusside was completely normal in these diabetic rats. Relaxation of vascular smooth muscle induced by sodium nitroprusside and EDRF is accomplished through a common intracellular guanosine 3', 5'-cyclic monophosphate (cGMP) mechanism (Moncada 1990). Mayhan et al (1991) found a similar situation for cerebral arterioles in insulin-dependent diabetic rats. These results indicate that diabetes is associated with a deficiency in EDRF function which develops rapidly, possibly related to decreased production or increased destruction of EDRF.

Kontos et al (1989) have shown that arachidonic acid metabolism is associated with the generation of oxygen radicals that interfere with, or destroy, EDRF. This observation raises the question of whether hyperglycaemia, or lack of insulin action, could cause increased eicosanoid synthesis, which could in turn interfere with EDRF production or action. Tesfamariam and Cohen (1992) has shown that *in vitro* exposure of the aorta to D-glucose 44 mmol/l (~800 mg/dl) for 6 h results in increased prostanoid synthesis. These events occur simultaneously with a suppression of EDRF-mediated vasodilatation, which can be substantially prevented by addition of oxygen radical scavengers or blockade of eicosanoid synthesis. A potential source for increased arachidonic acid metabolism during hyperglycaemia may be the increased production of diacylglycerol, a precursor of arachidonic acid (Lee et al 1989b). Both Mayhan et al (1991) and Tesfamariam et al (1989, 1990) have shown that suppression of eicosanoid production and action effectively restores EDRF function during long-term hyperglycaemia in diabetic animals.

Bohlen et al (1993) have demonstrated that pretreatment with superoxide dismutase, catalase, indomethacin or meclofenamic acid preserved EDRF-mediated vasodilatation during exposure to a D-glucose concentration of 500 mg/dl. Their results indicate that oxygen radicals, formed in part by increased eicosanoid synthesis during exposure to D-glucose hyperglycaemia, interfere with the EDRF mechanism before its action on the microvascular smooth muscle.

GLYCATED HAEMOGLOBIN AND ADVANCED GLYCOSYLATION END-PRODUCTS

Long-term hyperglycaemia produces glycated proteins, and protein glycosylation has been proposed as a pathogenic mechanism producing long-term diabetic effects. Moreover, recent articles (Bucala et al 1991; Tooke et al 1991; Sandman et al 1992) have connected the percentage of glycosylated haemoglobin with the generation of advanced glycosylation end-products (AGEs) formed spontaneously from a post-Amadori modification of haemoglobin as well as with increased capillary pressure in diabetic patients. Oxyhaemoglobin is one of the best known modulators of these endothelium-dependent responses. Rodriguez-Manas (1993) postulated that high levels of plasma glycosylated haemoglobin, a frequent profile in diabetic patients, may be the cause of the disturbance in endothelium-dependent relaxation and/or contraction. Their results demonstrated that glycosylated human haemoglobin impairs endothelial-mediated vasoactive responses. Furthermore, in animals treated with insulin, this impairment of endothelium-dependent vasodilatation is restored, suggesting that a hyperglycaemia-linked event plays a role in determining all these impaired responses (Rodriguez-Manas et al 1993). Interestingly, this impairment in animal models of diabetes appears to be time dependent (Bucala et al 1991; Mulhern et al 1989). It becomes present between 21 and 30 days after the development of hyperglycaemia, but not at earlier stages, and reaches a plateau at 2 to 3 months. This time dependency is coincident with the time taken to reach steady-state glycosylated haemoglobin concentrations in plasma, 6-13 weeks.

The mechanism mediating the effect of glycosylated haemoglobin on endothelium-dependent, NO-mediated vasorelaxant responses has not yet been elucidated, but generation of AGEs may be involved. Bucala et al (1991) suggest these effects are linked to advanced glycosylation of vessel wall proteins, especially collagen modification, but haemoglobin glycosylation may also be involved in producing impairment of endothelium-dependent vasodilatation. AGEs may exacerbate this process by quenching nitric oxide.

Corbett et al (1992) reported that aminoguanidine, an inhibitor of AGE formation, prevented glucose-induced vascular changes in nondiabetic rats. Furthermore, they tested the potency of aminoguanidine in inhibiting interleukin-1β-induced nitrite formation (an oxidation product of NO) and cGMP accumulation using a rat β-cell insulinoma cell line RINm5F. They found that aminoguanidine was equipotent to the strong NOS inhibitor, NMMA, in inhibiting the above mentioned parameters as well as the formation of iron-nitrosyl complexes by islets of Langerhans. In contrast, NMMA is 40 times more potent than aminoguanidine in elevating blood pressure in nondiabetic rats. These results demonstrate that aminoguanidine inhibits NO production and suggest a role for NO in the pathogenesis of diabetic vascular complications.

ACTIVATION OF PROTEIN KINASE C

A basic and common mechanism underlying vascular dysfunction in the hyperglycaemic diabetic state is increased protein kinase C (PKC) activity. Hyperglycaemia increases the *de novo* synthesis of diacylglycerol in cultured endothelial cells and in microvessels (Lee et al 1989a; Wolf et al 1991) and activates PKC in cultured endothelial cells (O'Donnell 1989). Increased PKC activity inhibits the synthesis and release of EDRF/NO and secondarily diminishes Na^+,K^+-ATPase activity in vascular smooth muscle. Moreover, PKC activation increases the release of vasoconstrictor prostanoids.

Decreased Na^+, K^+-ATPase activity

A reversible hyperglycaemia-associated consequence of decreased Na^+, K^+-ATPase activity is impaired endothelial-dependent arterial relaxation (Tesfamariam et al 1991). It has been suggested that hyperglycaemia might exert such effects by inhibiting Na^+,K^+-ATPase activity. Decreased Na^+,K^+-ATPase activity appears to decrease the release of the EDRF/NO or a closely-related molecule (Gupta et al 1992).

N^+,K^+-ATPase maintains the cellular ionic milieu and influences functions such as growth, differentiation and contraction of vascular smooth muscle. Simmons and Winegrad (1991) have recently suggested that hyperglycaemia specifically inhibits an adenosine-regulated Na^+,K^+-ATPase. PKC activation in arteries induced by direct-acting phorbol esters and by vasoconstrictive agents is associated with an increase in Na^+,K^+-ATPase activity in the smooth muscle (Gupta et al 1991; Navran et al 1988). Direct activation of PKC by phorbol esters has been shown to inhibit the release of EDRF/NO from cultured porcine aortic endothelial cells (Smith & Lang 1990) and from isolated canine femoral arteries (Rubanyi et al 1989). Thus, PKC has been proposed as playing a role in the synthesis and release of EDRF/NO. The impairment of endothelial-dependent relaxation by hyperglycaemia appears to be mimicked by pretreatment with a phorbol ester and it is prevented by an inhibitor of PKC in rabbit aorta (Tesfamariam et al 1991). A postulated consequence is that hyperglycaemia, by increasing PKC activity in endothelial cells, inhibits the synthesis and release of EDRF/NO and this secondarily diminishes Na^+,K^+-ATPase activity in vascular smooth muscle. Gupta et al (1992) suggest that the decrease in vascular Na^+,K^+-ATPase activity induced by hyperglycaemia is related, at least in part, to a decrease in the basal release of EDRF/NO. They also suggest that alterations in basal EDRF/NO release and possibly Na^+,K^+-ATPase activity contribute to the impairment in vascular relaxation caused by hyperglycaemia and diabetes.

Increased release of vasoconstrictor prostanoids

Another important event that might explain the impaired receptor-mediated endothelium-dependent relaxation in diabetes mellitus is an increased release of vasoconstrictor prostanoids. Impaired vascular relaxation in diabetic animals is found after weeks of sustained hyperglycaemia or 6-h exposure to hyperglycaemia, and in both cases, EDRF-dependent vasodilatation could be substantially improved by blockade of prostaglandin synthesis or thromboxane A_2 receptor blockade (Tesfamariam et al 1989; Mayhan et al 1991).

Acetylcholine, a stimulator of EDRF release, also elicits release of vasoconstrictor prostanoids, including thromboxane A_2 from aortic segments with intact endothelium, but not without endothelium, in both diabetic and elevated glucose conditions (Tesfamariam et al 1989, 1990). This is consistent with a role for vasoconstrictor prostanoids in causing abnormal vascular relaxation. Agonists like acetylcholine initiate their endothelial cell response by muscarinic receptor-mediated activation of phospholipase C, which causes phosphatidylinositol breakdown and subsequent inositol trisphosphate formation. This in turn causes the release of intracellular Ca^{2+} and diacylglycerol which activates PKC. Exposure to high glucose concentrations has been reported to stimulate *de novo* diacylglycerol production in various cells, including endothelial cells, by providing a substrate for phosphatidic synthesis, and this is associated with PKC activation (Wolf et al 1991). In so far as the response to acetylcholine is modulated by diacylglycerol-activated PKC, one might expect that acetylcholine-induced vascular relaxation would be altered in arteries exposed to elevated glucose conditions. As mentioned earlier, Tesfamariam et al (1991) found that 4-phorbol, 12-myristate, 13-acetate (PMA) caused a significant increase in basal and acetylcholine-stimulated release of vasoconstrictor prostanoids, including thromboxane A_2 from aortic segments with intact endothelium, but not in those without endothelium. PKC inhibitors, H-7 or sphingosine, restored acetylcholine-induced relaxation to normal and also suppressed the abnormal release of prostanoids in aortae exposed to elevated glucose conditions. These findings suggest that the dysfunction of receptor-mediated endothelium-dependent relaxation associated with exposure to elevated glucose conditions is due to increased production of vasoconstrictor prostanoids by the endothelium as a consequence of PKC activation.

CONCLUSION

Exposure to reversible hyperglycaemia for a short time results in decreased Na^+,K^+-ATPase activity and a consequent impairment of EDRF release. Hyperglycaemia also causes a quenching of EDRF via an increase in arachidonic acid metabolism and via the augmented generation of oxygen radicals, which interfere with or destroy EDRF. Long-term hyperglycaemia causes glycosylation of functional proteins, such as haemoglobin, and the generation of AGEs. Glycosylated haemoglobin may be the cause of the disturbance in endothelium-dependent vascular relaxation. Attempts at restoration EDRF release and EDRF action with an aldose reductase inhibitor, aminoguanidine or superoxide dismutase will help to raise new insights into the pathophysiology of diabetes and other vascular diseases.

REFERENCES

Archer S 1993 Measurement of nitric oxide in biological models. FASEB J 7: 349-360

Bhardwaj R, Moore P K 1988 Increased vasodilator response to acetylcholine of renal blood vessels from diabetic rats. J Pharm Pharmacol 40: 739-742.

Bohlen H G, Lash J M 1993 Topical hyperglycemia rapidly suppresses EDRF-mediated vasodilation of normal rat arterioles. Am J Physiol 265: H219-225

Bucala R, Tracey H I, Calami A 1991 Advanced glycosylation products quench nitric oxide and mediate defective endothelial-dependent vasodilation in experimental diabetes. J Clin Invest 87: 432-438

Corbett J A, Tilton R G, Chang K et al 1992 Aminoguanidine, a novel inhibitor of nitric oxide formation, prevents diabetic vascular dysfunction. Diabetes 421: 552-556

De Tajada I, Goldstein S I Azadzoi K et al 1989 Impaired neurogenic and endothelial-relaxation of penile smooth muscle form diabetic men with impotence. N Engl J Med 320: 1025-1030

Durante W, Sen A K, Sunahara F A 1988 Impairment of endothelium-dependent relaxation in aortae from spontaneously diabetic rats. Br J Pharmacol 94: 463-468

Fortes Z B, Leme J G, Scivoletto R 1983 Vascular reactivity in diabetes mellitus: role of the endothelial cell. Br J Pharmacol 79: 771-781

Furchgott R F, Zsawadzki J V 1980 The obligatory role of the endothelial cells in the relaxation of arterial smooth muscle by acetylcholine. Nature 288: 373-376

Gupta S, Ruderman N B, Cragoe Jr E J et al 1991 Endothelin stimulates Na^+-K^+ ATPase activity by a protein kinase C dependent pathway in rabbit aorta. Am J Physiol 261: H38-45

Gupta S, Sussman I, McArthur C S et al 1992 Endothelial-dependent inhibition of Na^+-K^+ ATPase activity in rabbit aorta by hyperglycemia. Possible role of endothelial-derived nitric oxide. J Clin Invest 90: 727-732

Harris H H, MacLeod K M 1988 Influence of the endothelium on contractile responses of arteries from diabetic rats. Eur J Pharmacol 153: 55-64

Head R H, Longhurst P A, Panek R L et al 1987 A contrasting effect of the diabetic state upon the contractile responses of aortic preparations from the rabbit. Br J Pharmacol 91: 275-286

Kamata K, Miyata N, Kasuya Y 1989 Impairment of endothelium dependent relaxation and changes in levels of cyclic GMP in aorta from streptozotocin-induced diabetic rats. Br J Pharmacol 97: 614-618

Kontos H A, Wei E P, Povlishock R C T et al 1989 Inhibition by arachidonate of cerebral arteriolar dilation from acetylcholine. Am J Physiol 256: H665-671

Lash J M, Bohlen H G 1991 Structural and functional origins of suppressed acetylcholine vasodilation in diabetic rat intestinal arterioles. Circ Res 69: 1259-1268

Lee T S, MacGregor L C, Fluharty S J et al 1989a Differential regulation of protein kinase C and (Na, K)-adenosine triphosphatase activities by elevated glucose levels in retinal capillary endothelial cells. J Clin Invest 83: 90-94

Lee T S, Saltsman K A, Ohashi H et al 1989b Activation of protein kinase C by elevation of glucose concentration: proposal for a mechanism in the development of diabetic vascular complications. Proc Nat Acad Sci USA 86: 5141-5145

Mayhan W G, Simmons L K, Sharpe G M 1991 Mechanism of impaired responses of cerebral arterial during diabetes mellitus. Am J Physiol 260: H219-326

Meraji S, Jayakody L, Senaratne M P J et al 1987 Endothelium-dependent relaxation in aorta of BB rat. Diabetes 36: 978-981

Moncada S, Palmer R M J, Hoggs E A 1991 Nitric oxide: physiology, pathophysiology and pharmacology. Pharm Rev 43: 109-142

Mulhern M, Docherty J R 1989 Effects of experimental diabetes on the responsiveness of rat aorta. Br J Pharmacol 97: 1007-1012

Nathan C 1992 Nitric oxide as a secretory product of mammalian cells. FASEB J 6: 3051-3054

Navran S S, Adair S E, Jemelka S K et al 1988 Sodium pump stimulation by activation of two alpha adrenergic receptor subtypes in canine blood vessels. J Pharmacol Exp Ther 245: 608-613

O'Donnell M E 1989 Regulation of Na-K-Cl cotransport in endothelial cells by atrial natriuretic factor. Am J Physiol 257: C36-44

Oyama Y, Kawasaki H, Hattori Y et al 1986 Attenuation of endothelium-dependent relaxation in aorta from diabetic rats. Eur J Pharmacol 131: 75-78

Pieper G M, Gross G J 1988 Oxygen free radicals abolish endothelium-dependent relaxation in diabetic rat aorta. Am J Physiol 255: H825-832

Pieper G M, Gross G J 1991 Endothelial dysfunction in diabetes. In: Rubanyi G M (ed) Cardiovascular Significance of Endothelium-derived Vasoactive Factors. Futura Publishing Co., Inc., Mount Kisco, New York, pp 223-249

Rodriguez-Manas L, Arribas S, Giron C et al 1993 Interference of glycosylated human hemoglobin with endothelial-dependent responses. Circulation: 88: 2111-2116

Rubanyi G M, Desiderio D, Luisi A et al 1989 Phorbol dibutyrate inhibits release and action of endothelium-derived relaxing factor(s) in canine blood vessels. J Pharmacol Exp Ther 249: 858-863

Sandeman I D, Shore A C, Awoke M E 1992 Relation of skin capillary pressure in patients with insulin-dependent diabetes mellitus to complications and metabolic control. N Eng J Med 327: 760-764

Simmons D A, Winegrad A I 1991 Elevated extracellular glucose inhibits an adenosine-(Na^+-K^+)-ATPase regulatory system in rabbit aortic wall. Diabetologia 34: 157-163

Smith J A, Lang D 1990 Release of endothelium-derived relaxing factor from pig cultured endothelial cells, as assessed by changes in endothelial cell cyclic GMP content, is inhibited by a phorbol ester. Br J Pharmacol 99: 565-571

Tesfamariam B, Brown M L, Cohen R A 1991 Elevated glucose impairs endothelium-dependent relaxation by activated protein kinase C. J Clin Invest 87: 1643-1648

Tesfamariam B, Brown M L, Keykin D et al 1990 Elevated glucose promotes generation of endothelium-derived vasoconstrictor prostanoids in rabbit aorta. J Clin Invest 85: 929-932

Tesfamariam B, Cohen R A 1992 Free radicals mediate endothelial cell dysfunction caused by elevated glucose. Am J Physiol 263: H321-326

Tesfamariam B, Jakubowski J A, Cohen R A 1989 Contraction of diabetic rabbit aorta caused by endothelium-derived PGH_2-TXA_2. Am J Physiol 257: H1327-1333

Tooke M E, Sandeman M E, Shore A C 1991 Microvascular hemodynamics in hypertension and diabetes. J Cardiovasc Pharmacol 16 (suppl 2): S51-S53

Wakabayashi I, Hatake K, Kimura N et al 1987 Modulation of vascular tonus by the endothelium in experimental diabetes. Life Sci 40: 643-648

Wolf B A, Williamson J R, Jason R A et al 1991 Diacylglycerol accumulation and microvascular abnormalities induced by elevated glucose levels. J Clin Invest 87: 31-38

SECTION 4

Accelerated Atherogenesis

10

A possible mechanism for vascular endothelial cell injury elicited by activated leucocytes: a significant involvement of adhesion molecules, CD11/CD18 and ICAM-1

H. Fujita, I. Morita, S. Murota

INTRODUCTION

Diabetes mellitus induces vasculopathy as a result of various metabolic abnormalities. Diabetic vasculopathy occurs in both major and minor vessels. In macroangiopathy, major vessels such as aorta and its first branches undergo atherosclerotic change. The result of such macroangiopathic atherosclerotic changes in diabetes can lead to various complications such as arteriosclerosis obliterans and myocardial infarction. On the other hand, arteriosclerosis in some organs is characterized by microangiopathy, e.g. nephropathy, neuropathy. It is well known that leucocytes play an important role in the process of the atherosclerosis (Munro & Contran 1988). Because of their anatomical location, vascular endothelial cells are the only kind of cells, other than blood cells themselves, which are directly exposed to various forms of oxidative stress by the bloodstream. Endothelial cell injury elicited by activated leucocytes is known to be the initial stage of various vascular disorders, such as diabetic vasculopathy, and is mainly due to active oxygen species released from activated leucocytes, e.g. superoxide anions, hydrogen peroxide, hydroxyl radicals (Varani et al 1985; Weiss et al 1981). Recently, the phenomenon of monocyte adhesion to the endothelium was recognized as an important process whereby monocytes cause endothelial cell injury (Peri et al 1990). Adhesion of leucocytes to the endothelium is mediated by various kinds of adhesion molecules (Bevilacqua et al 1989; Diamond et al 1991; Elices et al 1990; Foxall et al 1992; Johnson et al 1989; Lasky et al 1992; Marlin & Springer 1987; Miyake et al 1990; Phillips et al 1990). In a previous paper (Fujita et al 1991), we reported that endothelial cell injury induced by phorbol myristate acetate (PMA)-activated neutrophils was due to the adhesion of the leucocytes to the endothelium via the binding of CD11/CD18 (except CD11c) and ICAM-1.

In the present report using an interactive laser cytometer with Adherent Cell Analysis and Sorting-570 (ACAS 570), we detected newly synthesized peroxides in endothelial cells as well as the influx of peroxides from leucocytes to endothelial cells. We show: 1) an increased level of the intracellular peroxides in endothelial cells exposed to PMA-stimulated leucocytes, and that the increase was due to hydrogen peroxide derived from both leucocytes and endothelial cells themselves; 2) monoclonal antibodies against CD11a, CD11b, CD18 and ICAM-1 inhibited the increase of peroxides in the endothelial cells elicited by PMA-stimulated leucocytes; and 3) the increased level of peroxides was well correlated with endothelial cell injury. These data suggest that binding of CD11/CD18 to ICAM-1 may regulate the influx of hydrogen peroxide from leucocytes into endothelium or may stimulate the production of peroxides by endothelial cells themselves.

METHODS

All the procedures have been previously described in detail (Fujita et al 1991, 1994). These include: isolation of endothelial cells from freshly excised bovine carotid arteries; isolation of human polymorphonuclear leucocytes (PMNLs) from normal healthy donors; measurement of intracellular peroxides; cytotoxicity assay; and hydrogen peroxide assay.

Anti-CD11a (clone 25.3.1), anti-CD11b (clone BEAR1), anti-CD11c (clone BU15) and anti-CD18 (clone BL5) antibodies were purchased from Cosmo Bio Co. Ltd (Tokyo, Japan). Anti-ICAM-1 antibody (clone 84H10) was obtained from Immunotech S. A. (Marseilles, France). Catalase, superoxide dismutase, deferoxamine mesylate, allopurinol and PMA were from Sigma Chemical Co. (St Louis, Missouri, USA). 2,7-Dichlorofluorescein diacetate (DCFDA), hydrogen peroxide and mouse IgG were obtained from Wako Pure Chemical Industries Ltd (Osaka, Japan).

All results are expressed as means ± SEM. The Student's t test was used for statistical analysis and p values <0.05 were considered as significant.

RESULTS

EFFECTS OF OXYGEN-RELATING ENZYMES AND DRUGS ON ENDOTHELIAL CELL INJURY INDUCED BY PHORBOL-STIMULATED LEUCOCYTES

As demonstrated in our previous paper (Fujita et al 1991), PMA-stimulated leucocytes caused severe injury to cultured vascular endothelial cells. When catalase (700 U/ml), a hydrogen peroxide-decomposing enzyme, was added to this system, the injury was only partly suppressed (42.2 ± 3.2% inhibition). However, it was almost completely inhibited (inhibition 95.6 ± 1.2%) by the addition of deferoxamine mesylate (1 mmol/l), an iron-chelating agent. The addition of superoxide dismutase

(SOD), a superoxide anion-decomposing enzyme, to the assay system had little effect on the endothelial cell injury induced by PMA-stimulated leucocytes (0.7 ± 0.2% inhibition).

To elucidate the contribution of hydrogen peroxide released from leucocytes in the assay system of the endothelial cell injury, we firstly measured the amount of hydrogen peroxide produced by PMA-activated leucocytes alone. The concentration of hydrogen peroxide produced by 10^6 leucocytes activated by PMA (10 ng/ml) was 12.7 ± 1.5 mmol/l, which is almost the same concentration as previously reported (Nathan et al 1989). However, when 50 mmol/l of hydrogen peroxide was added to the culture medium, it did not induce endothelial cell injury at all (specific ^{51}Cr release 1.9 ± 0.2%). The number of leucocytes was equivalent to that used in our previous experiments.

INCREASE IN PEROXIDE LEVEL IN ENDOTHELIAL CELLS EXPOSED TO PMA-STIMULATED LEUCOCYTES

To elucidate the mechanism by which PMA-stimulated leucocytes caused endothelial cell injury, we next measured the change in intracellular peroxide level in cultured endothelial cells. Endothelial cells prelabelled with DCFDA, which is a fluorescent marker for peroxide level, were exposed to PMA-stimulated leucocytes. Fluorescence intensity in the

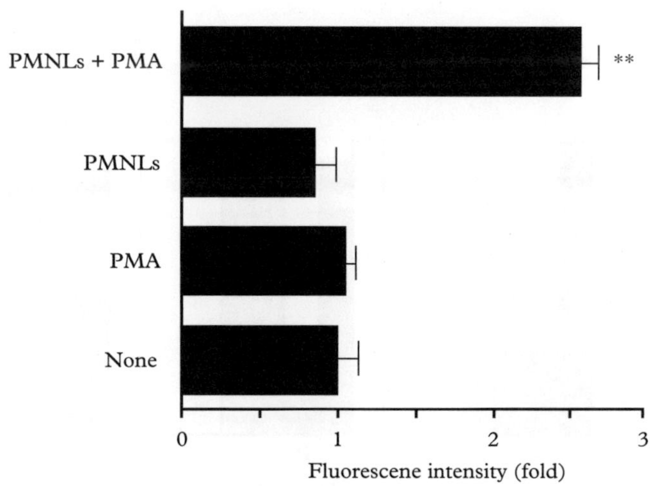

Fig. 10.1 Increase of the intracellular peroxide level of endothelial cells exposed to phorbol (PMA)-stimulated leucocytes. PMA, leucocytes (PMNLs) and PMA plus PMNLs were added to confluent monolayers of cultured endothelial cells prelabelled with 2,7-dichlorofluorescein diacetate. Intensity of fluorescence was measured after 15 min. Values are given as means ± SEM of 20 cells. *Statistical significance:* **p <0.01.

endothelial cells was measured from the image obtained using a laser cytometer with Adherant Cell Analysis and Sorting (ACAS 570). Untreated endothelial cells exhibited a low fluorescence intensity (purple colour), while endothelial cells exposed to PMA-stimulated leucocytes exhibited higher intensity (blue-green-yellow-red-white colour, depending on the conditions). The cells exhibited little variation in response. Intracellular fluorescence increased significantly within 5 min after the addition of leucocytes and PMA, but the time to maximal fluorescence intensity varied in each experiment (5-20 min). As shown in figure 10.1, the addition of PMA alone or unstimulated leucocytes alone to endothelial cell monolayers did not cause any increase in the intracellular fluorescence level at all.

RELATIONSHIP BETWEEN INTRACELLULAR PEROXIDE LEVELS AND ENDOTHELIAL CELL INJURY

We have found that endothelial cell injury induced by PMA-stimulated leucocytes was completely inhibited by 1-mm separation of the leucocytes and the endothelial cell monolayer using a special Intercell culture dish. Specific ^{51}Cr release was 20.3 ± 2.9% without Intercell and 0.8 ± 0.1% with Intercell. This suggests that the leucocyte adhesion to endothelial cells may be very important for the leucocytes to induce cytotoxicity. In a

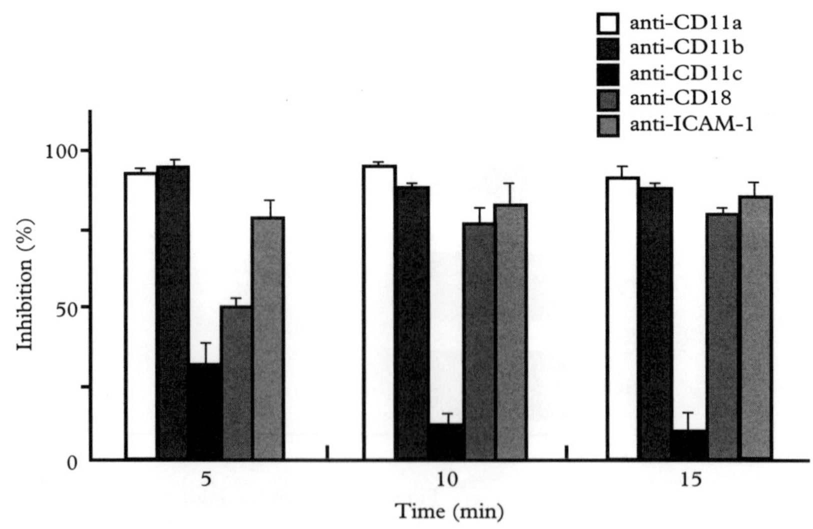

Fig. 10.2 Inhibitory effect of anti-adhesion molecule monoclonal antibodies on the increase in fluorescence of endothelial cells prelabelled with 2,7-dichlorofluorescein diacetate exposed to phorbol-stimulated leucocytes. Values are given as means ± SEM of 20 cells.

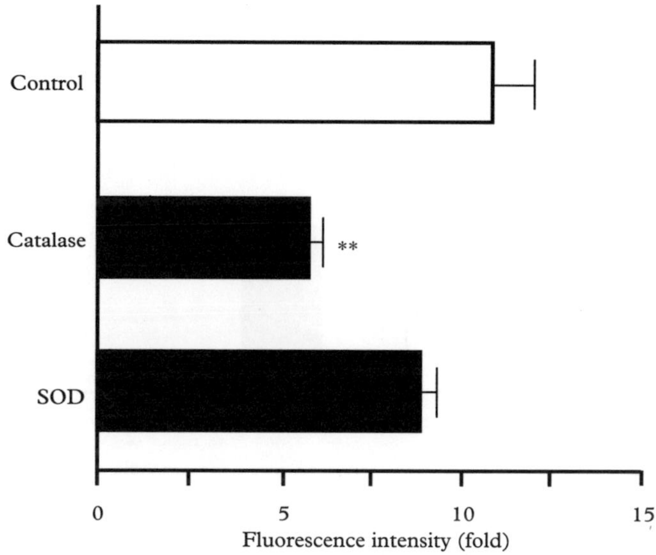

Fig.10.3 Effect of superoxide dismutase (SOD) [1000 U/ml] and catalase (700 U/ml) on the increase in fluorescence of endothelial cells prelabelled with 2,7-dichlorofluorescein diacetate exposed to phorbol-stimulated leucocytes. Values are given as means ± SEM of 20 cells. *Statistical significance:* **$p < 0.01$.

previous report (Fujita et al 1991), we demonstrated that antibodies against CD11a, CD11b, CD18 and ICAM-1 also abolished endothelial cell injury induced by PMA-activated leucocytes. The possibility that the antibodies against these adhesion molecules might therefore affect the intracellular peroxide level of endothelial cells was examined. The addition of antibodies against CD11a, CD11b, CD18 and ICAM-1 to the assay system abolished the increase in the fluorescence in endothelial cells after exposure to PMA-stimulated leucocytes, the only exception being the anti-CD11c antibody (Fig. 10.2). The time course and inhibition value in each experiment varied dependent on the conditions of the endothelial cells and isolated leucocytes. This peroxide inhibitory pattern of the antibodies was the same as that previously reported for endothelial cell injury (Fujita et al 1994). Mouse IgG (10 μg/ml) had no inhibitory effect on endothelial cell injury (91.0 ± 3.0% versus control) or peroxide production (7.5 ± 4.8% inhibition) elicited by PMA-stimulated leucocytes (Fujita et al 1994). These data strongly suggest that the early increase in the intracellular peroxide level is closely related to the late endothelial cell injury induced by PMA-stimulated leucocytes.

Next, we investigated the origin of the peroxide (hydrogen peroxide), the direct precursor of hydroxyl radicals in endothelial cells. We first examined the effects of SOD and catalase on the increase in the intracellular

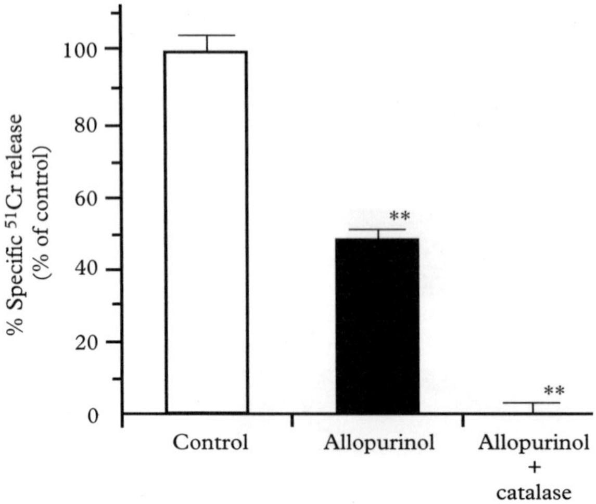

Fig. 10.4 Effect of catalase (700 U/ml) and allopurinol (1 mmol/l) on endothelial cell injury measured as specific ^{51}Cr release elicited by phorbol-stimulated leucocytes. Values are given as means ± SEM of 3 dishes. *Statistical significance:* **p <0.01.

peroxide levels in endothelial cells exposed to PMA-stimulated leucocytes. As shown in figure 10.3, catalase reduced intracellular fluorescence intensity by 50% at 15 min. However, SOD had no significant effect on fluorescence, despite a tendency towards a reduction in fluorescence intensity. We have previously demonstrated (Fujita et al 1994) that catalase had a suppressive effect on endothelial cell injury by PMA-stimulated leucocytes similar to that now reported on the peroxide level. SOD, however, had no inhibitory action on the endothelial cell injury despite the slight inhibition of the intracellular peroxide level.

To examine the possibility that endothelial cells generate peroxides by themselves via the xanthine-xanthine oxidase system, allopurinol, an inhibitor of xanthine oxidase, was added to the assay system. Allopurinol pretreatment (1 mmol/l for 18 h) significantly inhibited the endothelial cell injury by PMA-activated leucocytes (58.5 ± 4.5% inhibition), but it was not completely abolished. The concomitant addition of catalase to the assay system for the allopurinol-pretreated endothelial cells caused a complete abolition of the endothelial cell injury induced by PMA-activated leucocytes (Fig. 10.4). Allopurinol also inhibited the increase in the intracellular peroxide level of endothelial cells induced by PMA-stimulated leucocytes. As shown in figure 10.5, the production of intracellular peroxide in allopurinol-pretreated endothelial cells was almost completely inhibited at least up to 5 min, but increased thereafter gradually.

DISCUSSION

It has been recognized that endothelial cell injury induced by activated leucocytes is primarily caused by the release of various leucocyte-produced factors, such as active oxygen species, proteases, cytokines and metabolites of arachidonic acid. Among these substances, it has been accepted that active oxygen species have the most injurious effect on endothelial cells. Active oxygen species other than hydrogen peroxide are very unstable, and their diffusible distance is too limited for them to reach the endothelial cell membrane and to cause cellular injury. Hydrogen peroxide is therefore the most probable candidate among these mediators as the main cause of endothelial cell injury. This is supported by data showing that catalase inhibited endothelial cell injury induced by activated leucocytes (Weiss et al 1981) and that deferoxamine mesylate, an iron-chelating agent, also inhibited endothelial cell injury (Varani et al 1985). This suggests that after penetration of hydrogen peroxide into the endothelial cells it is converted to the hydroxyl radical in the presence of Fe^{2+} within the cell, and that the newly produced hydroxyl radical causes the endothelial cell injury. It is noteworthy that the inhibitory effect of deferoxamine mesylate is almost

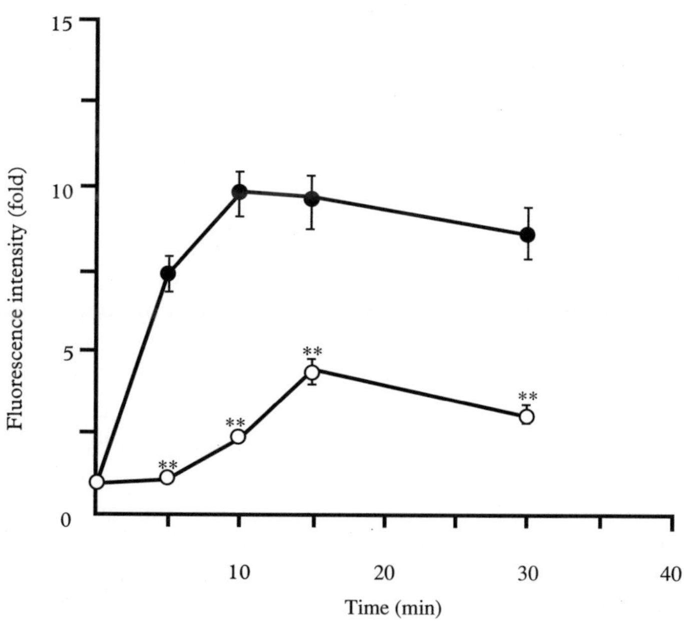

Fig. 10.5 Effect of pretreatment of endothelial cells with allopurinol (1 mmol/l for 18 h) on the increase in intracellular fluorescence intensity of endothelial cells prelabelled with 2,7-dichlorofluorescein diacetate exposed to phorbol-stimulated leucocytes. Values are given as means ± SEM of 20 cells. *Statistical significance:* $^{**}p < 0.01$.

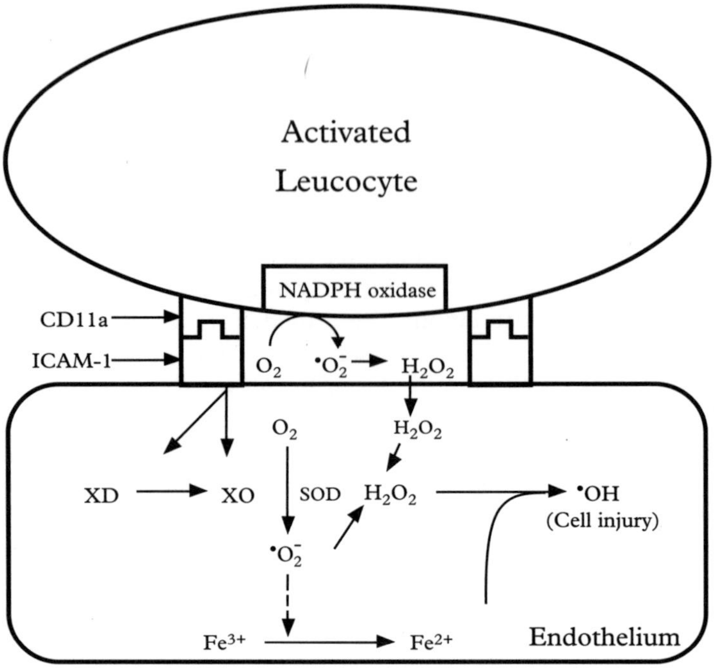

Fig. 10.6 Hypothetical scheme of the mechanism by which phorbol-activated leucocytes injured endothelial cell. We hypothesize that the binding of CD11/CD18 and ICAM-1 may stimulate the conversion of xanthine dehydrogenase (XD) to xanthine oxidase (XO) or activate xanthine oxidase activity, or may make the penetration of hydrogen peroxide into the endothelial cells easier. *Abbreviation:* SOD = superoxide disinutase.

complete and much more potent than that of catalase. In addition, when hydrogen peroxide 50 mmol/l was exogenously added to endothelial cell monolayers, no endothelial cell injury occurred. This concentration of hydrogen peroxide is about 4 times higher than that produced by PMA-activated leucocytes. This suggests that there must be some synergistic system within endothelial cells for leucocyte-induced cell injury. One possibility is that the conversion of hydrogen peroxide to hydroxyl radicals by the Harber-Weiss reaction is necessary for exogenous hydrogen peroxide to cause endothelial cell cytotoxicity and that the Harber-Weiss reaction must be accelerated by the specific binding of ICAM-1 and CD11/CD18 (except CD11c). This hypothetical scheme is shown in figure 10.6.

In the present study, we have demonstrated that endothelial cells have the capacity to produce peroxides and that the peroxides produced are closely related to endothelial cell injury on the basis of the following data: 1) peroxide production by endothelial cells exposed to PMA-stimulated leucocytes was partly inhibited by catalase; 2) peroxide production by endothelial cells exposed to PMA-stimulated leucocytes was inhibited by allopurinol, an inhibitor of xanthine oxidase; and 3) allopurinol inhibited endothelial cell injury induced by activated leucocytes. In addition, as shown in figure 10.5, allopurinol pretreatment caused the almost complete inhibition of the initial rise in the intracellular peroxide level for at least up to 5 min after the addition of PMA-stimulated leucocytes. On the other hand, we have shown in a previous paper that catalase could not block the initial rise as completely as allopurinol (Fujita et al 1994). These data suggest that the initial rise in the intracellular peroxide level must be dependent on some peroxide-generating system present in endothelial cells, and that after 10 min it must be due to hydrogen peroxide derived from activated leucocytes. Concomitant addition of catalase and allopurinol completely suppressed the endothelial cell injury as well as the peroxide increase in endothelial cells induced by PMA-stimulated leucocytes. The increase in the intracellular peroxides up to 15 min seems to be closely related to endothelial cell injury elicited by PMA-activated leucocytes after 5 h. In other words, endothelial cell injury induced by PMA-stimulated leucocytes resulted from the overproduction of hydrogen peroxide by leucocytes and endothelial cells.

Phan et al (1989) claimed that the superoxide anion generated by xanthine oxide could change Fe^{3+} to Fe^{2+} by reduction. In endothelial cells, the hydrogen peroxide produced by endothelial cells themselves, as well as that derived from leucocytes, must be converted to hydroxyl radicals through the action of Fe^{2+}, and the radicals can trigger and propagate lipid peroxidation, followed by endothelial cell injury. 2,7-Dichlorofluorescein diacetate is known to react with the lipid peroxides derived from hydroxyl radicals as well as hydrogen peroxide (Bass et al 1983; Cathcart et al 1983). In the present paper, we show that when allopurinol inhibited xanthine oxidase in endothelial cells, the peroxide level and the injury of endothelial cells elicited by PMA-activated leucocytes decreased by about 50% and 40%, respectively. These data suggest that the function of xanthine oxidase in endothelial cell injury is not only via the reduction of Fe^{3+} to Fe^{2+}, but also by the direct or indirect production of hydrogen peroxide. However, among the products released from leucocytes, proteases, platelet-activating factor and lipoxygenase products of arachidonic acid (e.g. leukotrienes and hydroperoxy-eicosatetraenoic acid) might participate in peroxide production in addition to the hydrogen peroxide derived directly from leucocytes and endothelial cells. More detailed studies for the origin of and the kind of peroxides in endothelial cells is in progress in our laboratory.

We recently obtained data supporting our hypothesis that the binding of CD11/CD18 and ICAM-1 could activate xanthine oxidase, thereby causing an increase the intracellular peroxide measured by fluorescence intensity. We found that even dead leucocytes were able to increase fluorescence intensity in endothelial cells. In this experiment, leucocytes were activated with PMA for 5 h so that their adhesion molecules were expressed on the surface of the cell membrane. The leucocytes were then fixed with ethanol to kill them. The fixed leucocytes were no longer able to release active oxygen radicals, but they exhibited some ability to bind to endothelial cells through their adhesion molecules. The endothelial cells to which the dead leucocytes adhered showed a significant increase in fluorescence intensity, suggesting that xanthine oxidase was activated by the binding of certain adhesion molecules.

We have also demonstrated that monoclonal antibodies against ICAM-1 and CD11/CD18, but not the anti-CD11c antibody, had a protective effect on endothelial cell injury elicited by PMA-stimulated leucocytes. The data suggest that the binding through these adhesion molecules plays an important role in the induction of endothelial cell injury. The mechanisms underlying the endothelial cell injury induced through the adhesion molecules may be as follows: 1) the production of hydrogen peroxide in activated leucocytes increases with the activation of CD11/CD18; 2) the penetration of hydrogen peroxide in endothelial cells increases through the specific adhesion; 3) the xanthine-xanthine oxidase system is activated by the specific adhesion through ICAM-1; and 4) the sensitivity to injurious substances increases with the endothelial cell. The first hypothesis is supported by Shappell et al (1990) who showed that antibodies against CD11b as well as CD18 inhibited the production of hydrogen peroxide released from fMLP (formyl-Met-Leu-Phe)-stimulated leucocytes, but they claimed that the antibody against CD11a did not. However, in the present study the chemiluminescence of PMA-stimulated leucocytes was not affected by any antibodies against these adhesion molecules under our experimental conditions. This is probably due to the difference in stimuli. The second and third possibilities are also examined in this paper. Monoclonal antibodies against CD11a, CD11b and CD18 almost completely prevented the increase in the intracellular peroxide level in endothelial cells, as well as endothelial cell injury. These data support the concept that binding between activated leucocytes and endothelial cells via the adhesion molecules, CD11/CD18 and ICAM-1, may be necessary for the intracellular peroxide level to increase in endothelial cells. Peri et al (1990) showed that the cytotoxicity of activated monocytes toward endothelial cells was not due to injurious agents such as active oxygen species or proteases released from the monocytes, but to adhesion between monocytes and endothelial cells, such as via CD11a/CD18. It has also been claimed that adhesion via CD18 might induce cytotoxicity by a means unrelated to suppression of the effect of the anti-CD18 antibody on the rate of adherence of monocytes to endothelial cells (Jonjic et al 1992).

The mechanism of intracellular signal transduction via these adhesion molecules is still unclear, but Tohma et al (1991) demonstrated that T cell-dependent B-cell activation occurred via CD11a and ICAM-1 adhesion molecules between T lymphocytes and B cells. Namely, the binding of CD11a/CD18 on T cells to ICAM-1 on B cells can cause B-cell activation. ICAM-1 may stimulate the signal transduction by B cells. Moreover, Huang et al (1993) have reported that endothelial cell calcium increased when neutrophils migrated through endothelial cell monolayers. The cytosolic calcium level of endothelial cells was therefore increased when neutrophils adhered to endothelium. Conversion of xanthine dehydrogenase to xanthine oxidase is known to be Ca^{2+}-dependent (Granger et al 1986). Therefore, we propose the hypothesis that ICAM-1 activation through binding to CD11/CD18 may stimulate xanthine oxidase activation via a Ca^{2+}-signal transduction. More precise definition of the mechanism of this intracellular signal transduction is in progress in our laboratory. Clarification of the mechanism of vascular endothelial cell damage induced by leucocytes may help in resolving the problem of diabetic vasculopathy.

CONCLUSION

To clarify the mechanism of vascular endothelial cell injury induced by activated leucocytes, we investigated intracellular peroxide levels in endothelial cells. The change in the intracellular peroxide level was measured using the fluorescence of 2,7-dichlorofluorescein diacetate. The fluorescence intensity of the endothelial cells exposed to PMA-stimulated leucocytes increased with time up to 15 min, although neither PMA alone nor unstimulated leucocytes alone showed any such increase. When catalase, which degrades hydrogen peroxide produced by leucocytes, was added to this system, the peroxide level in endothelial cells decreased significantly. Pretreatment of endothelial cells with allopurinol, a specific inhibitor of xanthine oxidase, also caused significant inhibition of the increase in peroxide levels in the endothelial cells. Monoclonal antibodies against CD11a, CD11b, CD18 and ICAM-1 showed almost complete inhibition of the increase in intracellular peroxide levels of the endothelial cells exposed to PMA-stimulated leucocytes, whereas the anti-CD11c antibody had no effect. Endothelial cell injury elicited by activated leucocytes was partially inhibited by catalase alone (about 40%) and allopurinol alone (about 60%), but it was completely inhibited by concomitant treatment with catalase and allopurinol. Specific antibodies against adhesion molecules such as ICAM-1 and CD11/CD18, but not CD11c/CD18, also significantly blocked endothelial cell injury. These data suggest that there is a good correlation between the early increase in intracellular peroxides and endothelial cell injury elicited by PMA-stimulated leucocytes, and that the adhesion of activated leucocytes to endothelial cells via CD11a/CD18 and ICAM-1 must be deeply involved in these phenomena.

ACKNOWLEDGMENTS

We thank Mr Y. Wakabayashi for his excellent assistance. This work was supported in part by a Grant-in-Aid for Scientific Research from the Ministry of Education and Culture of Japan and by a research grant from the Uehara Memorial Foundation.

REFERENCES

Bass D A, Parce J W, Dechatelet L R et al 1983 Flow cytometric studies of oxidative product formation by neutrophils. J Immunol 130: 1910-1917

Bevilacqua M P, Stengelin S, Gimbrone M A et al 1989 Endothelial leukocyte adhesion molecule-1: an inducible receptor for neutrophils related to complement regulatory proteins and lectins. Science 243: 1160-1165

Cathcart R, Schweisers E, Ames B N 1983 Detection of picomole levels of hydroperoxides using a fluorescent dichlorofluorescein assay. Anal Biochem 134: 111-116

Diamond M S, Staunton D E, Marlin et al 1991 Binding of the integrin Mac-1 (CD11b/CD18) to the third immunoglobulin-like domain of ICAM-1 (CD54) and its regulation by glycosylation. Cell 65: 961-971

Elices M J, Osborn L, Takada Y et al 1990 VCAM-1 on activated endothemium interacts with the leukocytes integrin VLA-4/fibronectin binding stie. Cell 60: 577-584

Foxall C, Watson S R, Dowbenko D et al 1992 The three members of the selectin receptor family recognize a common carbohydrate epitope, the sialyl Lewis(x) oligosaccharide. J Cell Biol 117: 895-902

Fujita H, Morita I, Murota S 1991 Involvement of adhesion molecules (CD11a-ICAM-1) in vascular endothelial cell injury elicited by PMA-stimulated neutrophils. Biochem Biophys Res Commun 177: 664-672

Fujita H, Morita I, Murota S 1994 A possible mechanism for vascular endothelial cell injury elicited by activated leukocytes: a significant involvement of adhesion molecules, CD11/CD18, and ICAM-1. Arch Biochem Biophys 309: 62-69

Granger D N, Hollwarth M E, Parks D A 1986 Ischemia-reprofusion injury: role of oxygen-derived free radicals. Acta Physiol Scand 548: 47-63

Huang A J, Manning J E, Bandak T M et al 1993 Endothelial cell cytosolic free calcium regulates neutrophil migration across monolayers of endothelial cells. J Cell Biol 120: 1371-1380

Johnson G I, Cook R G, McEver R P 1989 Cloning of GMP-140, a granule membrane protein of platelets and endothelium. Cell 56: 1033-1044

Jonjic N, Jilek P, Bernasconi S et al 1992 Molecules involved in the adhesion and cytotoxicity of activated monocytes on endothelial cells. J Immunol 148: 2080-2083

Lasky L A, Singer M S, Dowbenko D et al 1992 An endothelial ligand for L-selectin is a novel mucin-like molecule. Cell 69: 927-938

Marlin S D, Springer T A 1987 Purified intercellular adhesion molecule-1 (ICAM-1) is a ligand for lymphocyte function-associated antigen 1 (LFA-1). Cell 51: 813-819

Miyake K, Underhill C B, Lesley J et al 1990 Hyaluronate can fuction as a cell adhesion molecule and CD44 participates in hyaluronate recognition. J Exp Med 172: 69-72

Munro J M, Contran R S 1988 Biology of disease. Lab Invest 58: 249-261

Nathan C, Srimal S, Farber C et al 1989 Cytokine-induced respiratory burst of human neutrophils: dependence on extracellular matrix proteins and CD11/CD18 integrins. J Cell Biol 109: 1341-1349

Peri G, Chiaffarino F, Bernasconi S et al 1990 Cytotoxicity of activated monocytes on endothelial cells. J Immunol 144: 1444-1448

Phan S H, Gannon D F, Varani J et al 1989 Xanthine oxidase activity in rat pulmonary artery endothelial cells and its alteration by activated neutrophils. Am J Pathol 134: 1201-1211

Phillips M L, Nudelman E, Geata F C et al 1990 ELAM-1 mediates cell adhesion by recognition of a carbohydrate ligand, sialyl Lewis X. Science 250: 1130-1132

Shappell S B, Toman C, Anderson D C et al 1990 Mac-1 (CD11b/CD18) mediates

adherence dependent hydrogen peroxide production in bovine vascular endothelial cells. J Immunol 144: 2702-2711
Tohma S, Hirohata S, Lipsky P E 1991 The role of CD11a/CD18-CD54 interactions in human T cell dependent B cell activation. J Immunol 146: 492-499
Varani J, Fligiel S E G, Till G O et al 1985 Pulmonary endothelial cell killing by human neutrophils. Lab Invest 53: 656-663
Weiss S J, Young J, LoBunglio A F et al 1981 Role of hydrogen peroxide in neutrophil-mediated destruction of cultured endothelial cells. J Clin Invest 68: 714-721

11

Interaction between endothelial cells and smooth muscle cells through platelet-derived growth factor: direct effects and phenotypic modulation

N. Morisaki, Y. Saito

INTRODUCTION

Smooth muscle cells play an important role in the formation of intimal thickening in atherosclerosis (Ross 1993). However, smooth muscle cells do not usually exist in the intima but migrate there from the media and proliferate in response to paracrine/autocrine migration/growth factors. Preceding such migration and proliferation, smooth muscle cells are subjected to phenotypic change in response to paracrine/autocrine factors (Campbell et al 1989). In some conditions, phenotypic change may result in autocrine regulation of smooth muscle cell growth. As endothelial cells are intricately involved in paracrine function, they are particularly important in affecting smooth muscle cell function, especially when they are activated. There are two ways for endothelial cells to affect smooth muscle cells function through humoral paracrine factors: 1) a direct effect through humoral factors; and 2) a change of smooth muscle cell phenotype through humoral factors, which then affects smooth muscle cell function. In the latter case, autocrine factors may play a role. In this review we focus on the regulation of smooth muscle cell growth by endothelial cells via these two mechanisms.

ENDOTHELIAL CELL-DERIVED SMOOTH MUSCLE CELL GROWTH FACTORS

Numerous factors which affect smooth muscle cell growth have been isolated from plasma and cells composing atherosclerotic lesions. Table 11.1 shows growth factors and table 11.2 growth inhibitors which may affect smooth muscle cells, together with their sources. The importance of some of these factors in the formation of intimal thickening remains to be clarified in more detail. In the following sections, we will concentrate on the affects of platelet-derived growth factor (PDGF) and some of the other factors secreted from endothelial cells whose affects have been better studied.

Table 11.1 Growth factors for vascular smooth muscle cells.

Growth factor	Origin
Platelet-derived growth factor (PDGF)	Platelets, macrophages, endothelial cells, smooth muscle cells
Basic fibroblast growth factor (bFGF)	Endothelial cells, macrophages, smooth muscle cells
Interleukin-1 (IL-1)	Macrophages, endothelial cells, smooth muscle cells
Angiotensin II	Plasma
Smooth muscle cell-derived growth factor (SDGF)	Smooth muscle cells
Endothelial cell-derived growth factor (ECDGF)	Endothelial cells
Epidermal growth factor (EGF)	Platelets, plasma
Heparin-binding EGF-like growth factor	Macrophages, smooth muscle cells
Somatomedin C	Plasma, smooth muscle cells
Endothelin	Endothelial cells
Transforming growth factor-β (TGF-β)	Platelets, endothelial cells, macrophages, etc.
Others (insulin, laminin, low-density lipoprotein, fibrin, phosphatidic acid, thrombin, interleukin-6, interferon-γ)	

Table 11.2 Growth inhibitors for vascular smooth muscle cells

Inhibitor	Origin
Transforming growth factor-β (TGF-β)	Platelets, macrophages, endothelial cells, etc.
Prostaglandins I_2 and E_1	Endothelial cells, smooth muscle cells
Heparin sulphate	Endothelial cells
Interferon-γ (IFN-γ)	T-lymphocytes
Cyclic AMP	All cells
α_2-Macroglobulin	Plasma

PLATELET-DERIVED GROWTH FACTOR

PDGF (for reviews see Betsholtz et al 1986; DiCorleto & Fox 1988; Heldin & Westermark 1990) was so named as it was first found in platelets. However, over recent years it has been clarified that it is secreted not only from platelets but also from other cell types, such as tumour cells and cells composing atherosclerotic lesions (e.g. endothelial cells, macrophages and smooth muscle cells) [Ross 1993]. The secretion of PDGF depends on the phenotype or activation of cells. As for endothelial cells, they must be activated in order to express and secrete PDGF.

PDGF is a dimer with a molecular weight about 30 kDa. There are two types of monomeric components, the A and B chain, which yield three types of dimers, PDGF-AA, -AB and -BB. Cultured endothelial cells can express both PDGF-A and -B chain genes depending on the conditions. Serum or plasma factors are not required for PDGF expression and secretion. Both growing and static endothelial cells secrete almost the same amount of PDGF-like activity per cell (Di Corleto & Fox 1988). An increase in pH stimulates PDGF secretion (Di Corleto & Fox 1988), PDGF secretion or expression of PDGF-B chain mRNA is enhanced by endotoxin, phorbol ester, thrombin and factor Xa (Table 11.3), as well as by interleukin-l (IL-1), tumour necrosis factor-α (TNF-α) and transforming growth factor-β (TGF-β) (Ross 1993). The expression of PDGF is also affected by haemodynamic factors. For example, sheer stress stimulates expression of PDGF-A and-B chain mRNA through activation of protein kinase C (Hsieh et al 1992). Anoxia also stimulates expression of PDGF-B chain mRNA (Kourembanas et al 1990).

Inhibitory mechanisms of PDGF expression in endothelial cells have also been studied (Table 11.3). Endothelial cells in a three-dimensional structure express an inhibitory factor, which is not secreted by cells cultured *in vitro*. PDGF secretion is decreased by endothelial cells cultured on dishes covered with the mixture of type I and type III collagens. Acetylated low-density lipoprotein (LDL) decreases PDGF secretion from endothelial cells. This effect may be mediated through uptake of lipoproteins because acetylated LDL is not effective in certain endothelial cells which do not metabolize them. Oxidized LDL also inhibits secretion of PDGF by an unknown mechanism (see DiCorleto & Fox 1988 for review). Interferon-γ inhibits the expression of PDGF-B chain. In atheromatous lesions *in vivo*, PDGF-A chain mRNA is expressed in endothelial cells with angiogenesis (Wilcox et al 1988).

There are two types of PDGF-receptor genes, alpha and beta (Claesson-Welsh et al 1989; Yarden et al 1986). Receptors are also believed to work

Table 11.3 Expression of platelet-derived growth factor genes and their regulation. *Abbreviations:* DMPA = dimethylpropane-diamine; LDL = low-density lipoprotein; $PDGF_C$= platelet-derived growth factor secreted by cells; PMA = phorbol myristic acid. (Adapted from DiCorleto & Fox 1988)

Regulatory factor	Endothelial cell source	Parameter quantified	Expression level (%)
STIMULATORS			
Endotoxin	Bovine aorta	$PDGF_C$	200
Phorbol esters (cytotoxic doses)	Bovine aorta	$PDGF_C$	350
Heparin	Bovine aorta	Mitogenic activity	300-500
Factor Xa	Bovine aorta	$PDGF_C$	1000
Thrombin	Human kidney	c-*sis* mRNA; $PDGF_C$	300-500; 210
PMA	Human kidney	c-*sis* mRNA; $PDGF_C$	1500; 240
Endotoxin	Human umbilical vein	c-*sis* mRNA	230
INHIBITORS			
'Tube formation'	Human umbilical vein	c-*sis* mRNA	23
Acetyl-LDL, oxidized LDL, DMPA-LDL	Human umbilical vein bovine aorta, porcine aorta	$PDGF_C$	0-25
Collagen	Bovine aorta	$PDGF_C$	34

as dimers. Dimerization of receptors after ligand binding is therefore the initial step for subsequent signal transduction by PDGF. The relationship between affinity of ligands and receptors is as follows: AA to alpha/alpha, AB to alpha/beta or alpha/alpha and BB to alpha/alpha, alpha/beta and beta/beta (Raines et al 1990). It has been believed that endothelial cells do not express PDGF receptors. This is true for endothelial cells from large vessels, but endothelial cells from microvessels, such as rat brain capillaries (Smits et al 1989) and rabbit retinal capillaries (Koyama et al 1994), at least express PDGF-beta receptors *in vivo* or *in vitro* and can grow in response to PDGF-AB or -BB. It is speculated that PDGF-alpha receptors are not expressed in these endothelial cells because they do not respond to PDGF-AA stimulation. On the other hand, cultured smooth muscle cells do express PDGF-receptors (especially beta receptors) and respond to mitogenic or migratory stimuli by PDGF. Medial smooth muscle cells under normal conditions *in vivo* are mostly of the contractile form (described later) and do not express PDGF receptors. However, medial smooth muscle cells in diabetes (Kanzaki et al 1994; Kawano et al 1993) and hypertension (Sarzani et al 1992) express PDGF-beta receptors. Moreover, some of the intimal smooth muscle cells in atheromatous lesions are of the synthetic form (described later) and express PDGF-beta receptors (Ross 1993). These smooth muscle cells possibly respond to B-chain containing PDGF (-AB and -BB) derived from endothelial cells. As for alpha receptors, there is little evidence that smooth muscle cells express PDGF-alpha receptors at sufficient levels, because PDGF-AA has little or no mitogenic (Kawano et al 1993) or migratory (Koyama et al 1992) effect on rabbit aortic smooth muscle cells. However, PDGF-AA 1-10 ng/ml inhibits migration of rat smooth muscle cells stimulated by PDGF-AB, PDGF-BB and fibronectin (Koyama et al 1992), suggesting that PDGF-alpha receptors are also sufficiently expressed in rat smooth muscle cells. In addition, Schollmann et al (1992) reported that basic fibroblast growth factor (bFGF), which can be derived from endothelial cells, stimulates expression of PDGF-alpha receptors.

These data underline the importance of PDGF-AA and PDGF-alpha receptor mechanisms in the interaction between endothelial and smooth muscle cells. The regulatory mechanism of PDGF-A chain expression in endothelial cells and PDGF-alpha receptors expression in smooth muscle cells remain to be clarified, together with any functional differences between PDGF-alpha and -beta receptors.

OTHER ENDOTHELIAL CELL-DERIVED GROWTH FACTORS

DiCorleto and Fox (1988) estimated that more than half of the mitogenic activity for smooth muscle cells secreted from endothelial cells was due to nonPDGF molecule(s), which was termed endothelial cell-derived growth factor (ECDGF) and is different from bFGF, epidermal growth factor (EGF) and IL-1. Besides PDGF and ECDGF, possible paracrine growth factors derived from endothelial cells are bFGF, IL-1 and TNF-α. bFGF is usually expressed by most cultured endothelial cells, but its secretion mechanism has not yet been elucidated because its gene product has no signal peptide (Vlodavsky et al 1991). Therefore, bFGF derived from endothelial cells may be significant only when endothelial cells are killed by some form of injury. mRNA of IL-1β is expressed *in vitro* in response to various stimuli, including IL-1 itself, lipopolysaccharide, TNF-α, phorbol esters and factor Xa. The mitogenic effect of IL-1 on smooth muscle cells is weakened by its stimulation of synthesis of prostaglandin (PG) I_2 (Libby 1988), which is itself an intrinsic inhibitor (Morisaki et al 1988b). IL-1 is a potent growth factor in the presence of cyclooxygenase inhibitors *in vitro* (Libby 1988). The mechanism of the mitogenic effect of IL-1 on smooth muscle cells is speculated to be indirect, i.e. stimulation of autocrine secretion of PDGF from smooth muscle cells (Raines et al 1989). TNF-α is also expressed by endothelial cells following stimulation with IL-1 *in vitro*, but it is not mitogenic to rabbit and rat aortic smooth muscle cells, unlike fibroblasts (unpublished data).

The paracrine growth factors derived from endothelial cells usually act as atherogenic factors but PDGF-AA may be antiatherogenic because of its inhibitory effect on smooth muscle cells migration. Moreover, bFGF may sometimes act as antiatherogenic factor because of its stimulation of repair in balloon-injured endothelial cells (Bjornsson et al 1991).

ENDOTHELIAL CELL-DERIVED GROWTH INHIBITORS

Growth inhibitors for smooth muscle cells are listed in table 11.2. TGF-β both stimulates and inhibits growth of smooth muscle cells depending on cell density, culture conditions, species and interaction with other factors (Morisaki et al 1991; Roberts & Sporn 1990). TGF-β can be expressed in various types of cells, including endothelial cells. The *in vivo* role of TGF-β in the formation of atherosclerosis is not well known. Our data shows that injection of TGF-β1 for 14 days into a rabbit balloon-catheter model accelerated intimal thickening through stimulation of extracellular matrix synthesis (manuscript submitted). TGF-β was clearly atherogenic in this model, but its role is still unclear in other types of atherosclerosis and in long-term lesion development. Heparin or heparin sulphate derived from endothelial cells is a well known inhibitor of smooth muscle cell growth *in vitro* and is believed to be antiatherogenic *in vivo* (Clowes & Clowes 1986).

PGI_2 is secreted from both endothelial and smooth muscle cells, but the principal source of PGI_2 *in vivo* is believed to be endothelial cells. PGI_2 and its long-acting analogue inhibit growth of smooth muscle cells by blocking transition from G_1 to S phases in the cell cycle (Morisaki et al

1988b). PGI_2 is believed to be secreted into the luminal side of endothelial cells *in vivo* for inhibition of platelet aggregation. However, it is not known whether it is secreted into subendothelial spaces. If so, PGI_2 could be a significant factor in regulating accelerated growth of smooth muscle cells. The problem is, as described later, smooth muscle cells derived from the atherosclerotic intima (intima-derived smooth muscle cells) are resistant to growth inhibition by PGI_2 (Morisaki et al 1988c).

In conclusion, some endothelial cells-derived factors including heparin sulphate, PGI_2 and PDGF-AA can be antiatherogenic, while other factors, such as B-chain containing PDGFs, bFGF, IL-1, TGF-β can be atherogenic. Further studies are required to evaluate the role of these paracrine factors in the formation of intimal thickening.

PHENOTYPIC CHANGES OF SMOOTH MUSCLE CELLS INDUCED BY ENDOTHELIAL CELLS

Growth and migratory responses of smooth muscle cells to various paracrine/autocrine factors are dependent on smooth muscle cell phenotype (Campbell et al 1989). The classic phenotypes of smooth muscle cells are 'contractile' and 'synthetic'. The synthetic phenotype is more related to atherogenesis (Campbell et al 1989). More recently, we have discovered subphenotypes of the synthetic phenotype, which are closely related to atherosclerosis. In this section, the properties and regulation of these phenotypes, including endothelial-smooth muscle cell interaction will be discussed.

CONTRACTILE VERSUS SYNTHETIC

Smooth muscle cells in the normal media are of the contractile form and can contract but cannot migrate or grow in response to various stimuli. In the process of atherogenesis, the contractile form of smooth muscle cells is probably the first to change its phenotype, to the synthetic phenotype which can then respond to migratory and growth stimuli. Some of smooth muscle cells in the intima of atherosclerotic lesions *in vivo* are of this synthetic form. Factors which stimulate phenotypic change from the contractile to the synthetic form are serum (Campbell et al 1989), fibronectin (Thyberg et al 1990) and heparinase derived from macrophages (Campbell & Campbell 1991). On the other hand, some smooth muscle cells in the intima also express the contractile phenotype, suggesting that a phenotypic change from the synthetic to the contractile form also occurs *in vivo*. Factors which stimulate phenotypic change in this direction are heparin, elastin and laminin (Thyberg et al 1990), and PGE_1 (Pomeranz & Hajjay 1989). Most cultured smooth muscle cells are of the synthetic form, which is different to the situation *in vivo*. It is very difficult for the synthetic form to revert to the contractile form *in vitro*. The morphological and functional properties of contractile and synthetic

Table 11.4 Comparison of smooth muscle cell phenotypes: contractile versus synthetic.

	Contractile		Synthetic
Function			
-contraction	+		-
-growth	-		+
-migration	-		+
-synthesis of substances		<<	
-lipid accumulation	-		+
Localization	normal media		thickened intima in cultured cells
Morphology			
-filament		>>	
-α-actin	++++		+/-
-β-actin	++++		+/-
-γ-actin	++		++
-myosin	+++		+/-
-desmin	+++		+/-
-vimentin	+		+
-myosin heavy chain isoforms	SM1, SM2		SM1, SMemb
-mitochondria		<<	
-ribosomes		<<	
-rough endoplasmic reticulum		<<	

phenotypes are summarized in table 11.4 (for review see Campbell et al 1989). Among the factors affecting phenotype change which are derived from endothelial cells, heparin may be antiatherogenic together with its inhibitory effect on smooth muscle cells growth.

INTIMA- VERSUS MEDIA-DERIVED SMOOTH MUSCLE CELLS

Smooth muscle cells are usually cultured from normal media (media-derived smooth muscle cells) and they are of the synthetic form. However, we have cultured smooth muscle cells from the intima of atherosclerotic lesions in a cannulation-injury rabbit model (Inaba et al 1992; Saito et al 1988), a high-cholesterol rabbit model (Morisaki et al 1988c) and a rabbit balloon-catheter model (unpublished data) [intima-derived smooth muscle cells]. We compared the properties of intima-derived and media-derived smooth muscle cells. Both are of the synthetic form, but expressed different phenotypes (subphenotypes). The differences are summarized in table 11.5. First, growth rate was much higher in intima-derived than in media-derived smooth muscle cells (Saito et al 1988). Intima-derived smooth muscle cells did not show the so-called 'hills & valleys pattern', which is typically observed in media-derived smooth muscle cells. The characteristics of intima-derived smooth muscle cells are as follows: 1) they are resistant to autocrine growth inhibition induced by PGI_2 (Morisaki et al 1988c), whereas media-derived smooth muscle cells are sensitive (Morisaki et al 1988b); 2) an autocrine growth factor, smooth muscle cell-derived growth factor (SDGF) (Morisaki et al 1988a), which is different from PDGF, is secreted from intima-derived but not from media-derived

Table 11.5 Comparison of smooth muscle phenotypes: media-derived versus intima-derived. *Abbreviations:* c-fms = M-CSF receptor; LDL = low-density lipoprotein; M-CSF = macrophage colony-stimulating factor; PGI_2 = prostaglandin I_2; SDGF = smooth muscle cell-derived growth factor; SDMF = smooth muscle cell-derived migration factor.

	Media-derived		Intima-derived
Growth		<<	
Hills and valley pattern	+		+/-
Inhibition by PGI_2	+		-
Synthesis of PGI_2		<<	
Secretion of SDGF	-		+
Secretion of SDMF		<	
Scavenger pathway	-		+
Expression of c-fms	-		+
Response to M-CSF	-		+
Response to growth scavenger pathway	-		+
Resistance of LDL cytotoxicity		<<	

smooth muscle cells (Morisaki et al 1989); and 3) intima-derived but not media-derived smooth muscle cells express macrophage-colony stimulating factor (M-CSF) receptors, c-fms, and respond to the mitogenic stimulus of M-CSF (Inaba et al 1992). The rapid growth of intima-derived smooth muscle cells is consistent with the mechanism of intimal thickening by smooth muscle cells. We have recently discovered an autocrine migration factor, smooth muscle cell-derived migration factor (SDMF) [Koyama et al 1993] and this factor is secreted more by intima-derived than media-derived smooth muscle cells (unpublished data).

These two types of smooth muscle cells show not only the above-mentioned differences in growth and migration but also differences in lipid metabolism. Intima-derived but not media-derived smooth muscle cells express the so-called 'scavenger pathway' (Inaba et al 1992; Saito et al 1988), which metabolizes acetylated LDL and oxidized LDL (Kodama et al 1990). In addition, intima-derived smooth muscle cells express more scavenger receptors in response to M-CSF stimulation (Inaba et al 1992).

This projects a new insight into the mechanism of smooth muscle cell-derived foam cell formation. The properties of intima-derived smooth muscle cells susceptible to growth stimulation and foam cell formation may in part explain the pathological findings observed in smooth muscle cells in atheromatous lesions, i.e. growth and lipid accumulation.

MECHANISM OF PHENOTYPIC CHANGE FROM THE MEDIA-DERIVED TO THE INTIMA-DERIVED FORM OF SMOOTH MUSCLE CELLS

Intimal smooth muscle cells are derived from the media and a phenotypic change from the contractile to the synthetic form probably occurs before migration of medial smooth muscle cells to the intima (Campbell et al 1989). It is not clear when and where the above-mentioned phenotypic change from the media-derived to the intima-derived form occurs. Presumably, it occurs after smooth muscle cells become synthetic. The regulatory mechanism of the phenotypic change is not known well. However, we will outline our recent *in vitro* data on the phenotype change from the media-derived to the intima-derived form of smooth muscle cells.

When rabbit media-derived smooth muscle cells were incubated with endothelial cells without smooth muscle cell-endothelial cell attachment, the incubated smooth muscle cells grew faster than control smooth muscle cells coupled with autocrine secretion of SDGF, even after removal of endothelial cells from the culture (Saito et al 1989). This rapid growth of smooth muscle cells continued for at least two passages after removal of the endothelial cells from the culture. The factor(s) responsible for the phenotype change should be humoral, as the smooth muscle and

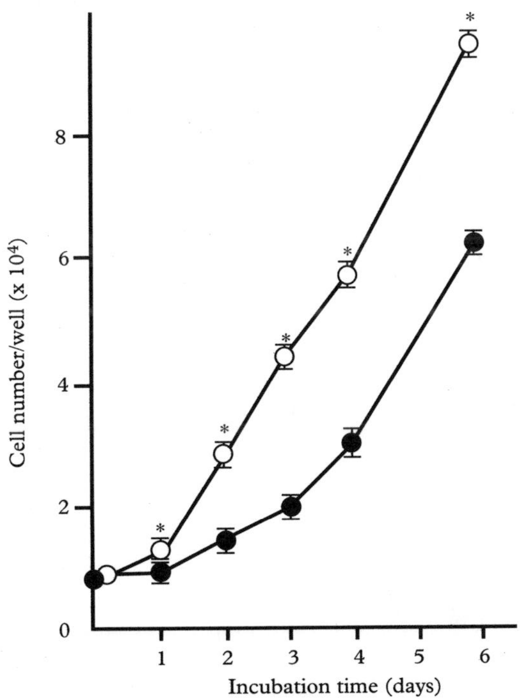

Fig. 11.1 Effects of preincubation with platelet-derived growth factor (PDGF)-AB on the growth phenotype of smooth muscle cells. Confluent smooth muscle cells at the second passage were seeded into 24-well plates at 3 x 10^4 cells/well and were cultured in 1 ml of culture medium in the presence (●) or absence (○) of PDGF 10 ng/ml for 3 days. After incubation, the cells were harvested and cell growth measured. Values are given as mean ± SD (n = 3). *Statistical significance:* *p <0.001 versus corresponding control values. (Reproduced and adapted from Morisaki et al 1992)

endothelial cells were separated from each other. It was later revealed that one of the factors was PDGF (Morisaki et al 1992). Rabbit media-derived smooth muscle cells were incubated with PDGF-AB for 3 days to confluency and PDGF was removed from the culture. The smooth muscle cells acquired the following properties, which intima-derived but not media-derived synthetic smooth muscle cells possessed: 1) they grew faster than control smooth muscle cells (Fig. 11.1), and this accelerated growth continued for at least two passages after removal of PDGF; 2) they secreted SDGF, which is different from PDGF; and 3) they expressed scavenger pathways. Incubation of media-derived smooth muscle cells with macrophages or macrophage-conditioned medium also resulted in rapid growth of these cells, even after removal of macrophages or macrophage-conditioned medium (Morisaki et al 1992). The phenotype-modifying activity in the macrophage-conditioned medium was completely neutralized by an anti-PDGF antibody, suggesting that the factor in macrophages responsible for the phenotypic change was also PDGF. Using these criteria as indicators of intima-derived smooth muscle cells, we tested whether various factors could regulate the phenotypic change, e.g. the three forms of PDGF, bFGF, TNF-α, IL-1β, and TGF-β. Among these, only PDGF-AB, PDGF-BB (Morisaki et al 1992) and TNF-α (Morisaki et al 1993) stimulated the phenotypic change from the media-derived to the

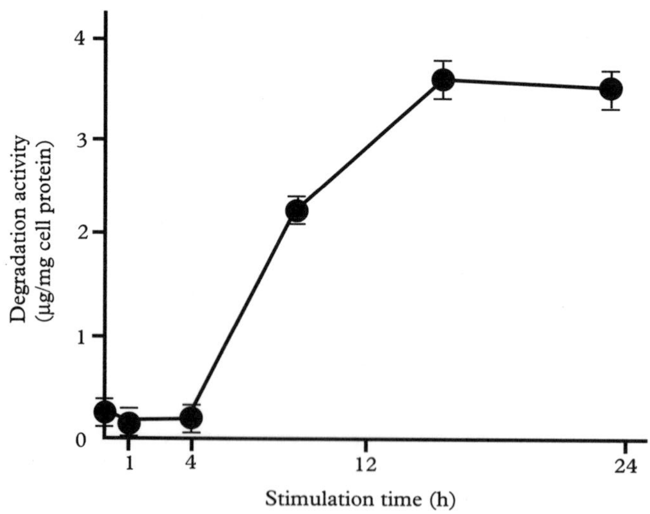

Fig. 11.2 Effect of stimulation time with 12-*O*-tetradecanoyl-phorbol-13-acetate (TPA) on degradation of ^{125}I-acetylated LDL by media-derived smooth muscle cells. Media-derived smooth muscle cells were incubated with TPA 10^{-8} mol/l for indicated times and then assayed for degradation activity 24 h after medium change with [^{125}I]-acetylated LDL 10 μg/ml. Values are given as means ± SD (n = 3).

intima-derived form. PDGF may affect the phenotypic change through PDGF-β receptor signalling pathway because PDGF-AA had no effect on the phenotype change (Morisaki et al 1992). Different from these data, a phorbol ester, 12-*O*-tetradecanoylphorbol-13-acetate stimulates expression of the scavenger pathway (Fig. 11.2) but did not induce rapid growth (unpublished data), suggesting that there may be more smooth muscle cell subphenotypes. From the above data, endothelial cells possibly affect growth and lipid metabolism of smooth muscle cells by modulating their phenotype from the media-derived to the intima-derived form through secretion of B-chain-containing PDGF and TNF-α.

CONCLUSION

Endothelial cells give positive or negative signals for growth, migration and lipid accumulation to smooth muscle cells through humoral factors either by direct action on smooth muscle cells or modulation of smooth muscle cell phenotype. These signals can lead to either atherogenic or antiatherogenic consequences. Current understanding of these paradoxical effects of endothelial cells may be summarized as follows: activated endothelial cells are atherogenic, whereas inactivated endothelial cells are antiatherogenic.

REFERENCES

Betsholtz C, Johnsson A, Heldin C-H et al 1986 cDNA sequence and chromosomal localization of human platelet-derived growth factor A-chain and its expression in tumour cell lines. Nature 320: 695-699

Bjornsson T D, Dryjski M, Tluczek J et al 1991 Acidic fibroblast growth factor promotes vascular repair. Proc Natl Acad Sci USA 88: 8651-8655

Campbell G R, Campbell J H, Manderson J A et al 1989 Arterial smooth muscle. A multifunctional mesenchymal cell. Arch Pathol Lab Med 112: 977-986

Campbell J H, Campbell G R 1991 The macrophage as an initiator of atherosclerosis. Clin Exp Pharmacol Physiol 18: 81-84

Claesson-Welsh L, Hammacher A, Westermark B et al 1989 cDNA cloning on the human A-type platelet- derived growth factor (PDGF) receptor establishes structural similarity to the B-type PDGF receptor. Proc Natl Acad Sci USA 86: 4917-1921

Clowes A W, Clowes M M 1986 Kinetics of cellular proliferation after arterial injury: IV. Heparin inhibits rat smooth muscle mitogenesis and migration. Circ Res 58: 839-845

DiCorleto P E, Fox P L 1988 Growth factor production by endothelial cells. In: Ryan U S (ed) Endothelial Cells. CRC Press, Boston, pp 51-61

Heldin C-H, Westermark B 1990 Platelet-derived growth factor: mechanism of action and possible *in vivo* function. Cell Regulation 1: 555-566

Hsieh H-J, Li N-Q, Frangos J A 1992 Shear-induced platelet-derived growth factor gene expression in human endothelial cells is mediated by protein kinase C. J Cell Physiol 150: 552-558

Inaba T, Yamada N, Gotoda T et al 1992 Expression of M-CSF receptor encoded by c-fms on smooth muscle cells derived from arteriosclerotic lesions. J Biol Chem 67: 5693-5699

Kanzaki T, Shinomiya M, Ueda S et al 1994 (in press) Enhanced arterial intimal thickening after balloon catheter injury in diabetic animals accompanied by PDGF beta-receptor expression of aortic media. Eur J Clin Invest

Kawano M, Koshikawa T, Kanzaki T et al 1993 Diabetes mellitus induces accelerated growth of aortic smooth muscle cells: association with overexpression of PDGF-beta-receptors. Eur J Clin Invest 23: 84-90

Kodama T, Freeman M, Rohrer L et al 1990 Type I macrophage scavenger receptor contains alpha-helical and collagen-like coiled coils. Nature 343: 531-535

Kourembanas S, Hannan R L, Faller D V 1990 Oxygen tension regulates the expression of the platelet-derived growth factor-B chain gene in human endothelial cells. J Clin Invest 86: 670-674

Koyama N, Harada K, Yamamoto A et al 1993 Purification and characterization of an autocrine migration factor for vascular smooth muscle cells (SMC), SMC-derived migration factor. J Biol Chem 268: 13301-13308

Koyama N, Morisaki N, Saito Y et al 1992 Regulatory effects of platelet-derived growth factor-AA homodimer on migration of vascular smooth muscle cells. J Biol Chem 267: 22806-22812

Koyama N, Tezuka M, Watanabe S et al 1994 Migratory and proliferative effect of platelet-derived growth factor (PDGF) in rabbit retinal endothelial cells: evidence of autocrine pathway of PDGF. J Cell Physiol 158: 1-6

Libby P 1988 Interleukin-1: a mitogen for human vascular smooth muscle cells that induce the release of growth-inhibitory prostanoids. J Clin Invest 81: 487-498

Morisaki N, Kanzaki T, Koshikawa T et al 1988a Secretion of a new growth factor, smooth muscle cell derived growth factor, distinct from platelet derived growth factor by cultured rabbit aortic smooth muscle cells. FEBS Lett 230: 186-190

Morisaki N, Kanzaki T, Motoyama N et al 1988b Cell cycle-dependent inhibition of DNA synthesis by prostaglandin I_2 in cultured rabbit aortic smooth muscle cells. Atherosclerosis 71: 165-171

Morisaki N, Kanzaki T, Saito Y et al 1988c Lack of inhibition of DNA synthesis by prostaglandin I_2 in cultured intimal smooth muscle cells from rabbits. Atherosclerosis 73: 67-69

Morisaki N, Kanzaki T, Saito Y et al 1989 Secretion of a new growth factor [smooth muscle cell derived growth factor (SDGF) distinct from platelet derived growth factor (PDGF)] by cultured rabbit smooth muscle cells from the aortic media and intima. Clinica Terapia Cardiovascolare 8: 257-260

Morisaki N, Kawano M, Koyama N et al 1991 Effects of transforming growth factor-beta 1 on growth of aortic smooth muscle ells. Atherosclerosis 88: 227-234

Morisaki N, Koyama N, Kawano M et al 1992 Human macrophages modulate the phenotype of cultured rabbit smooth muscle cells through secretion of platelet-derived growth factor. Eur J Clin Invest 22: 461-468

Morisaki N, Xu Q-P, Koshikawa T et al 1993 Tumor necrosis factor-alpha can modulate the phenotype of aortic smooth muscle cells. Scand J Clin Lab Invest 53: 347-352

Pomeranz K B, Hajjay D P 1989 Eicosanoids in regulation of arterial smooth muscle cell phenotype, proliferative capacity, and cholesterol metabolism. Arteriosclerosis 9: 413-429

Raines E W, Bowen-Pope D F, Ross R 1990 Platelet-derived growth factor. In: Sporn M B, Roberts A B (eds) Handbook of Experimental Pharmacology. Springer-Verlag, Berlin, pp 173-262

Raines E W, Dower S K, Ross R 1989 Interleukin-1 mitogenic activity for fibroblasts and smooth muscle cellsis due to PDGF-AA. Science 311: 669-671

Roberts A B, Sporn M B 1990 The transforming growth factor- betas. In: Sporn M B, Roberts A B (eds) Handbook of Experimental Pharmacology. Springer-Berlag, Berlin, pp 419-472

Ross R 1993 The pathogenesis of atherosclerosis: a perspective for the 1990s. Nature 362: 801-809

Saito Y, Bujo H, Morisaki N et al 1988 Proliferation and LDL binding of cultured intimal smooth muscle cells from rabbits. Atherosclerosis 69: 161-164

Saito Y, Kanzaki T, Morisaki N et al 1989 Modification of growth property of aortic smooth muscle cells by the endothelial cells. Clinica Terapia Cardiovascolare 8: 261-264

Sarzani R, Arnaldi G, Chobanian A V 1991 Hypertension-induced changes of platelet-derived growth factor receptor expression in rat aorta and heart. Hypertension 17: 888-895

Schollmann C, Grugel R, Tatje D et al 1992 Basic fibroblast growth factor modulates the mitogenic potency of the platelet-derived growth factor (PDGF) isoforms by specific upregulation of the PGF alpha factor in vascular smooth muscle cells. J Biol Chem 267: 18032-18039

Smits A, Hermansson M, Nister M et al 1989 Rat brain capillaries endothelial cells express functional PDGF B-type receptors. Growth Factors 2: 1-8

Thyberg J, Hedin U, Sjolund M et al 1990 Regulation of differentiated properties and proliferation of arterial smooth muscle cells. Arteriosclerosis 10: 966-990

Vlodavsky I, Bar-Shavit R, Ishai-Michaeli R et al 1991 Extracellular sequestration and release of fibroblast growth factor: a regulatory mechanism? Biochemistry in Israel 16: 268-271

Wilcox J N, Smith K M, Williams L T et al 1988 Platelet-derived growth factor mRNA detection in human atherosclerotic plaques by *in situ* hybridization. J Clin Invest 82: 1134-1143

Yarden Y, Escobedo J A, Kuang W J et al 1989 Structure of the receptor for platelet-derived growth factor helps define a family of closely related growth factor receptors. Nature 323: 4917-4921

12

Regulation of proteoglycans in endothelial cells: implication for atherogenesis and thrombogenesis

M. Nishinaga, M. Kobayashi, K. Shimada

INTRODUCTION

The endothelial surface plays an important role in the pathogenesis of atherosclerosis and the regulation of coagulation (Wall & Harker 1980). It has become increasingly clear that, while perturbed endothelial cells generate procoagulant activity (Nawroth & Stern 1985), under normal conditions they possess multiple antithrombotic and anticoagulant mechanisms, including generation of prostacyclin (Moncada & Vane 1979) and plasminogen activators (Lostkutoff & Edgington 1977), and synthesis of thrombomodulin as a cell surface cofactor for thrombin-catalyzed activation of protein C (Esmon 1983). In addition, anticoagulant-active heparan sulphate proteoglycans, including heparin-like molecules, are apparently present on the vascular surface (Wight 1980). However, information on factors influencing these properties and possible consequence of their alternation have been quite limited.

In this article, following a brief review on the structure and functions of proteoglycans including anticoagulant-active heparan sulphate, we discuss their modification by various atherothrombogenic stimuli including cytokines and homocysteine.

STRUCTURE AND FUNCTIONS OF HEPARAN SULPHATE PROTEOGLYCAN

Proteoglycans are macromolecules in which sulphated glycosaminoglycan chains are covalently linked to a protein core, e.g. heparan sulphate proteoglycan (Fig. 12.1) [Wight 1980, 1989]. Proteoglycans are a diverse group of proteins, grouped together solely because of their glycosaminoglycan content. Despite the diversity of the structure, function and expression of their core proteins, there is some justification for considering the various proteoglycans together because the glycosaminoglycan component gives them a certain uniformity. A glycosaminoglycan is a linear heteropolysaccharide possessing a characteristic disaccharide repeat sequence. One monosaccharide of the disaccharide repeat is an amino sugar with D-glucosamine or

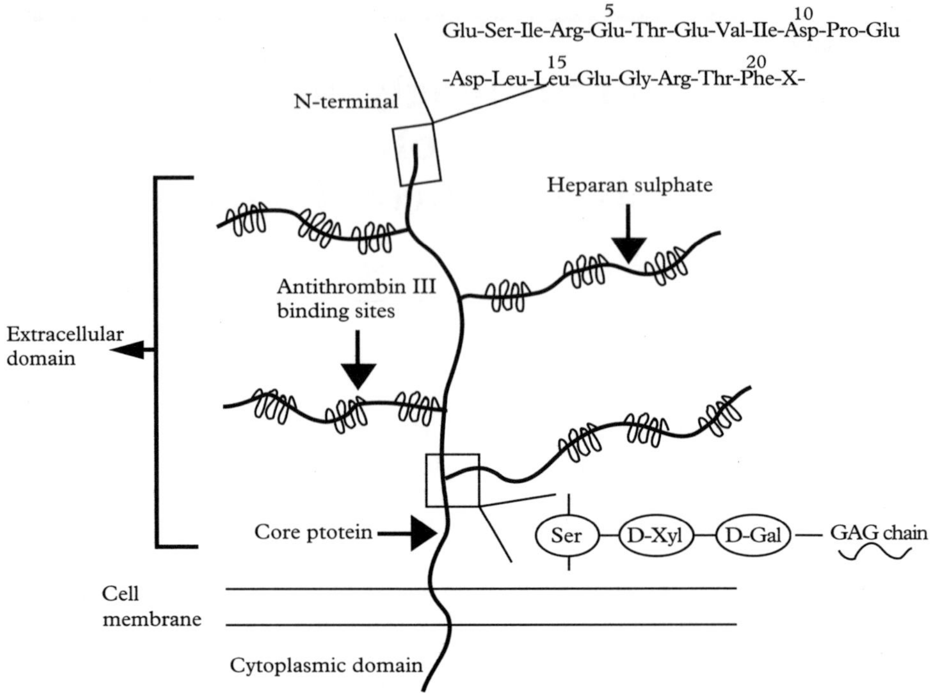

Fig. 12.1 Structures of heparin-like compounds on endothelial cell surface. *Abbreviation:* GAG = glycosaminoglycan.

galactosamine, and the other unit is typically, but not always, an uronic acid residue of either D-glucuronic acid or iduronic acid. Both units are variably *N*- and *O*-sulphated, which adds to the heterogeneity of these complex macromolecules. The most common glycosaminoglycan structure are chondroitin sulphate, dermatan sulphate, heparan sulphate, keratan sulphate, hyaluronic acid and heparin; representative structures for each disaccharide are shown in figure 12.2 (Jackson et al 1991). With the exceptions of heparin and hyaluronic acid, glycosaminoglycan chains are covalently attached at their reducing end through an *O*-glycosidic linkage to a serine residue or *N*-linked asparagine in a core protein; the resulting macromolecule is termed a proteoglycan.

Of these proteoglycans, heparan sulphate proteoglycan is involved in thrombogenesis and atherogenesis. This is because a certain class of heparan sulphate proteoglycans associated with the endothelial surface can bind antithrombin III in plasma and can accelerate thrombin inactivation by protease inhibitor (Rosenberg & Rosenberg 1984). The binding of heparan sulphate on cell surface to antithrombin III is responsible for an acceleration of complex formation between certain enzymes (such as thrombin and Xa) and their inhibitors (Damus et al 1973). Evidence

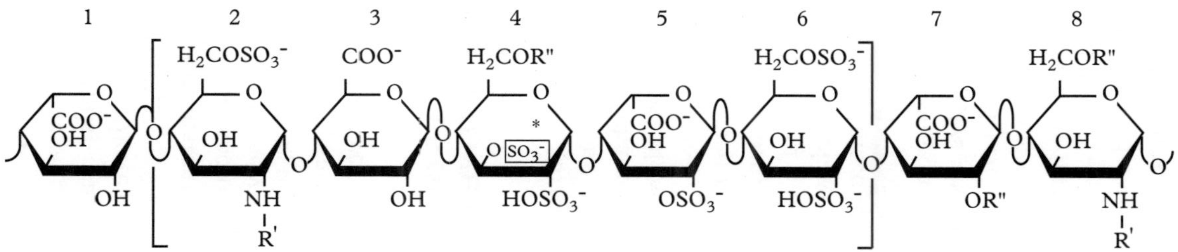

Fig. 12.2 Structure of the antithrombin III-binding octasaccharide. The 2,5-anhydro-D-mannose unit 8 corresponds to an N-sulphated D-glucosamine residue in the intact polysaccharide. The actual binding region is represented by the pentasaccharide sequence (units 2-6) within brackets. Structural variants are indicated by R' (-$COCH_3$ or -SO_3), R" (-H or -SO_3), and by the sugar residue (unit 7). The 3-*O*-sulphate group of unit 4 (marked by an asterisk) is unique to the antithrombin-binding region of the heparan sulphate molecule. In addition, each one of the sulphate groups indicated by an asterisk is essential to the high affinity binding of antithrombin III.

suggests that heparan sulphate proteoglycans synthesized by vascular endothelial cells also possess such anticoagulant properties. The anticoagulant activity of heparan sulphate (proteoglycan) is related to the presence of a pentasaccharide sequence (Fig. 12.2) [Pejler et al 1987], the distinguishing feature of which is a 3-*O*-sulphated glucosamine residue. Polysaccharide chains possessing this sequence bind with high affinity to antithrombin III and, thus, drastically increase the rate by which this proteinase inhibitor inactivates enzymes involved in the coagulation process (Pejler et al 1987).

Recent studies demonstrated that a specific heparan sulphate proteoglycan is not only located on cell surface but also along the abluminal side of the endothelium, namely the basement membrane or extracellular matrix produced by endothelial cells (de Agostini et al 1990b). However, the relative roles of the heparan sulphate proteoglycan on cell surface or basement membrane has not yet been completely clarified.

EFFECT OF CYTOKINES OR HOMOCYSTEINE ON ANTICOAGULANT-ACTIVE HEPARAN SULPHATE (PROTEOGLYCAN)

These proteoglycans have various biological functions and undergo changes in response to various stimuli, such as stress, inflammation and hormonal influences. The changes are generally governed by local cellular activity. Recent studies have shown that the cytokines, such as interleukin-1 and tumour necrosis factor-α, potent immunological and inflammatory mediators released by activated monocytes and macrophages, can induce a whole sequence of procoagulant reactions on the endothelial cell surface, starting with the expression of a tissue factor-like activity (Bevilacqua et al 1986a; Colucci et al 1983; Nawroth & Stern 1986; Rogers and Shuman 1983), and suppressing anticoagulant activity through decreased cell surface thrombomodulin (Esmon 1987; Moore et al 1989; Nawroth et al 1986) and heparin-like compounds on endothelial cells (Kobayashi et al 1990). These cytokines have also been shown to suppress anticoagulant activity through decreased cell surface thrombomodulin, thus inhibiting the anticoagulant effects of protein C and protein S. These mechanisms may contribute to thrombus formation and vasculopathy associated with inflammatory responses.

Homocysteinaemia caused by inborn error is usually associated with serious thromboembolic complications and premature atherosclerotic lesions in most large and medium-sized arteries at an early age (Boers et al 1985; Brattstrom et al 1984; Malinow et al 1989). In addition, some investigators reported that homocysteine damages cultured endothelial cells *in vitro* (Hayashi et al 1992; Lentz & Sadler 1991; Rogers & Conn 1990; Rogers & Kane 1986) and that continuous intravenous homocysteine infusion in primates results in patchy endothelial cell desquamation and focal proliferative intimal smooth muscle cell lesions *in vivo* (Harker et al 1976), which are similar in appearance to early atherosclerotic lesions in humans. Thus, homocysteine is thought to be an atherogenic agent.

CYTOKINES

Both interleukin-1 and tumour necrosis factor-α are potent modulators of endothelial cell functions relevant to haemostasis and thrombosis. In addition, interleukin-1 and tumour necrosis factor-α decrease the production of tissue-type plasminogen activator and increase type 1 plasminogen activator inhibitor, thereby suppressing net fibrinolytic activity (Bevilacqua et al 1986b; Emeis & Kooistra 1986; Nachman et al 1986; Schleef et al 1988), and induce the synthesis of platelet-activating factor (Bussolino et al 1988) and prostacyclin (Rossi et al 1985). These responses tend to tip the balance of the coagulant-anticoagulant molecules on the surface of the endothelium toward intravascular coagulation and thrombus formation. This leads to the hypothesis that anticoagulant mechanisms predominate on the surface of quiescent endothelium, whereas perturbed endothelium can promote clot formation (Stern et al 1985).

In our first study (Kobayashi et al 1990), we examined the effects of interleukin-1 and tumour necrosis factor-α on endothelial cell surface heparin-like compounds, which remain to be investigated among endothelial anticoagulant molecules. To achieve this goal, the effects of human recombinant cytokines on heparin-like molecules associated with the surface of porcine aortic endothelial cell cultures were examined.

Effect of cytokines on endothelial cell surface glycosaminoglycan biosynthesis

Incorporation of [^{35}S]-sulphate onto cultured porcine aortic endothelial cells was suppressed by human recombinant interleukin-1β (rIL-1β) or recombinant tumour necrosis factor-α (rTNF-α) in a dose- and time-dependent manner (Fig. 12.3). Maximal inhibition was achieved by incubation of cells with rIL-1β 100 ng/ml or rTNF-α 5 ng/ml for 12-24 h, resulting in an approximately 50% reduction in the synthesis of heparan sulphate on the cell surface. This inhibitory effect by cytokines occurred primarily in the synthesis of cell surface-associated sulphated glycosaminoglycans, approximately 80% of which consisted of heparan sulphate. The other cell surface sulphated glycosaminoglycans, i.e., chondroitin sulphates, were also affected to a similar extent to heparan sulphate. The reduction in incorporation of ^{35}S-radioactivity into

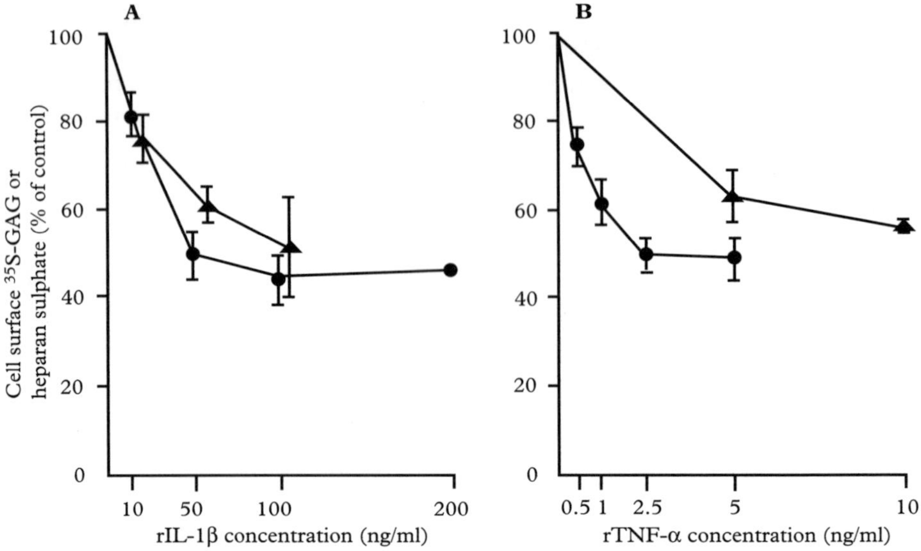

Fig. 12.3 Dose-dependent inhibition of endothelial cell surface glycosaminoglycan biosynthesis by cytokines. Endothelial cells were incubated with 50 mCi/ml of [^{35}S]-sulphate in the absence or presence of various concentration of recombinant interleukin-1β (rIL-1β) [**A**] or recombinant tumour necrosis factor-α (rTNF-α) [**B**] for 24 h. The radioactivity incorporated into total glycosaminoglycans (GAG, ●) or heparan sulphate (chondroitin ABC lyase-resistant materials, ▲) in cell surface fraction was expressed as percent of control. Data are given as means ± SEM of 3 separate experiments.

glycosaminoglycans appeared to result from reduced production rather than from increased degradation. Furthermore, the results obtained by isotopic incorporation methods agreed well with those shown by chemical techniques, such as affinity chromatography. These data make us confident that treatment of endothelial cells with cytokines resulted in a reduction of up to approximately 50% in the amount of cell surface-associated heparan sulphate, which serves as binding sites for antithrombin III, thereby inhibiting the interaction between the protease inhibitor (antithrombin III) and endothelial cells.

Characterization of heparan sulphate chains and proteoglycans derived from the cell surface revealed that either the size or net negative charge was not altered by cytokine treatment. Antithrombin III binding to endothelial cells treated with rIL-1β or rTNF-α seemed to be reduced somewhat less or more (to 60% or 40% of control) [Fig. 12.4], respectively, than the reduction in glycosaminoglycan production (to 50% of control) [Fig. 12.3]. In another series of parallel experiments on antithrombin III binding, however, glycosaminoglycan production in endothelial cells treated with rIL-1β was reduced to only 68 ± 5% (mean ± SEM), implying that the effects of rIL-1β (and possibly rTNF-α) were variable between cell cultures. The reduction in heparan sulphate production appeared to occur almost in parallel with the decrease in antithrombin III binding. This raises the possibility that cytokines affect the synthesis of both anticoagulant and nonanticoagulant heparan sulphate to a similar extent. The results of the fractionation of heparan sulphate by antithrombin affinity chromatography support this. Hence, the change in glycosaminoglycan metabolism of endothelial cells treated with cytokines is apparently quantitative rather than qualitative in nature.

Mechanism of inhibition of glycosaminoglycan production by cytokines

The mechanism by which cytokines inhibit glycosaminoglycan production is currently unknown. Nonspecific cytokine-induced suppression of

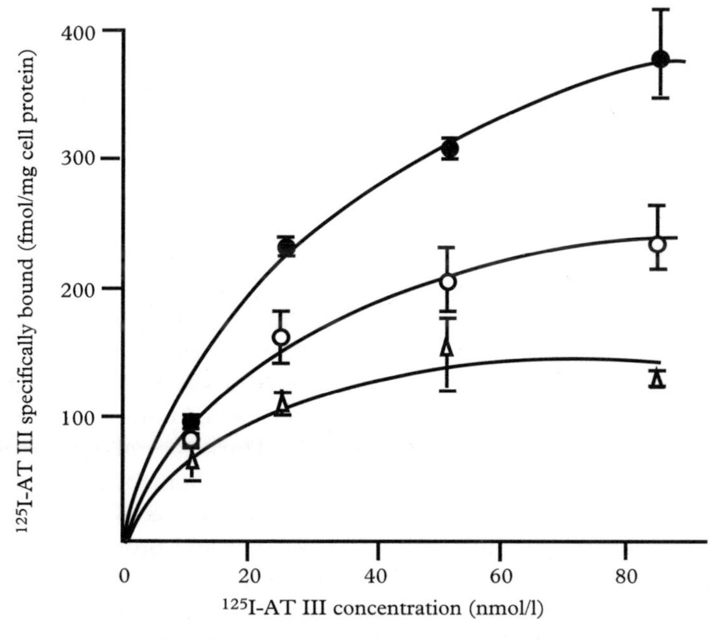

Fig. 12.4 Specific antithrombin III binding to control and cytokine-treated endothelial cells. Endothelial cells were incubated without (●) or with recombinant interleukin-1β (○) or recombinant tumour necrosis factor-α (△) for 48 hours. Increasing concentrations (10 to 85 nmol/l) of [^{125}I]-antithrombin III (AT III) were placed on the washed endothelial cell cultures in the presence or absence of a 100-fold excess of unlabelled AT III. Nonspecific binding is defined as the amount of [^{125}I]-AT III bound in the presence of an excess of unlabelled AT III, and accounted for less than 30% of total binding. Specific binding was obtained by subtracting nonspecific binding from total binding. Data are given as means ±SEM.

cellular metabolic activity is unlikely, as the number, protein content, and $[^3H]$-leucine incorporation rate of cells remained unchanged when the maximum reduction in glycosaminoglycan production occurred. Endothelial cell prostaglandins are not related to this cytokine effect, because the suppression of glycosaminoglycan synthesis by cytokines remained unchanged after the addition of indomethacin, an inhibitor of prostaglandin production. However, cytokines have been reported to inhibit glycosaminoglycan synthesis via an enhancement of prostaglandin production in certain cell types (Mitrovic et al 1981). Thus, when endothelial cells are exposed to cytokines, there may be a rapid and transient stimulation of procoagulant activity followed by a delayed and prolonged inhibition of anticoagulant mechanisms, including heparin-like activity. This indicates that various regulatory mechanisms in different phase of 'endothelial perturbation' may contribute to the shift of the haemostatic balance toward not only the generation but also to the maintenance of intravascular fibrin.

In conclusion, rIL-1β and rTNF-α reduced the synthesis of heparan sulphate on the endothelial cell surface, resulting in decreased antithrombin III binding and diminished heparin-like anticoagulant activity of endothelial cells. This mechanism is another cytokine-inducible endothelial effect on coagulation.

HOMOCYSTEINE

Homocysteinaemia caused by homozygous cystathionine β-synthase deficiency is associated with an increased incidence of vascular thrombosis and development of arteriosclerosis (Mudd et al 1985). Furthermore, elevated plasma homocysteine levels have been reported to be an independent risk factor for vascular disease (Clarke et al 1991; Malinow 1990; Stampfer et al 1992). The administration of homocysteine causes vascular injury and thrombosis in animals (Harker et al 1976). Recent studies using cell culture systems have shown that homocysteine enhances endothelial cell-associated factor V activity (Rogers & Kane 1986) and inhibits both thrombomodulin surface expression and protein C activation (Hayashi et al 1992; Lentz & Sadler 1991; Rogers & Conn 1990). Thus, endothelial cell coagulation properties were shown to be regulated by atherogenic stimuli. To our knowledge, however, no studies have yet reported the involvement of another important endothelial anticoagulant pathway, i.e. endothelial cell heparin-like glycosaminoglycan-antithrombin III anticoagulant mechanism, in this unique model of thrombosis and arteriosclerosis. Previous studies showed that homocysteine decreased cell surface thrombomodulin expression and protein C activation. These facts suggested that the perturbation of the vascular endothelial cell protein C mechanism by homocysteine may contribute to the thrombogenic tendency seen in patients with elevated blood levels of homocysteine.

In the following sections we describe some of the results of our recently published studies on homocysteine interaction with cultured endothelial cells (Nishinaga et al 1993).

Effects of homocysteine on antithrombin III binding to endothelial cell surface

Endothelial cells were grown in the absence or presence of various concentrations of homocysteine for 24 h. The binding of antithrombin III to the cell surface was assayed in parallel with the measurement of the incorporation of [^{35}S]-sulphate into heparan sulphate on the cell surface. Homocysteine-treated endothelial cells exhibited a large decrease in antithrombin III binding activity (Fig. 12.5). This did not result from either 'cellular injury' or nonspecific suppression of cellular metabolism caused by cytotoxic effects of homocysteine. In fact, unlike cytokines, which reduced antithrombin III binding primarily by inhibiting endothelial glycosaminoglycan metabolism rather nonspecifically, the overall biosynthesis of endothelial glycosaminoglycans, as judged by both [^{35}S]-sulphate incorporation into glycosaminoglycans and the proportion and the

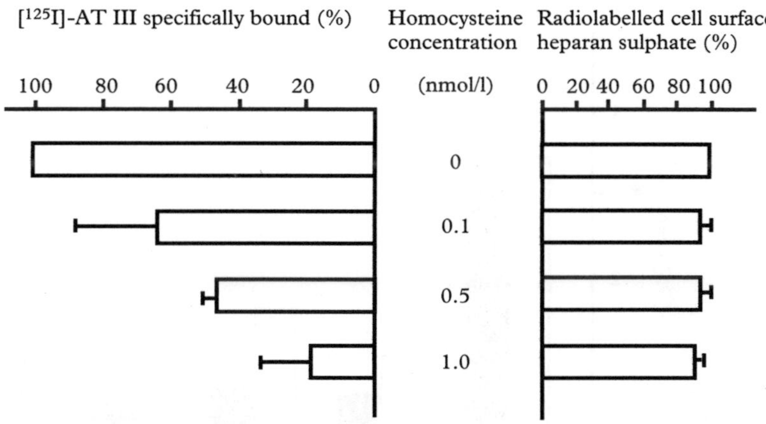

Fig. 12.5 Effects of increasing concentrations of homocysteine on [^{125}I]-antithrombin III (AT III) binding to endothelial cells and [^{35}S]-sulphate incorporation into cell surface heparan sulphate. Endothelial cell cultures, after treatment with various concentrations of homocysteine for 24 h, were incubated with 16 nmol/l of [^{125}I]-AT III. [^{125}I]-AT III specifically bound to the cell surface was determined as described in figure 12.4 and is shown on the left. In parallel with these experiments, endothelial cells under identical culture conditions were labelled with [^{35}S]-sulphate for 24 h, and the radioactivity incorporated into heparan sulphate (determined as chondroitin ABC lyase-resistant materials) in 'cell surface fractions' was determined as described in figure 12.4, and is shown on the right. Results are expressed as percent of those obtained in the absence of homocysteine. Data are given as means ± SEM.

net negative charge of heparan sulphate, remained almost intact (Fig. 12.5). In contrast, we found a substantial reduction in antithrombin III binding capacity of heparan sulphate isolated form homocysteine-treated endothelial cells using both affinity chromatography (Fig. 12.6) and dot-blot assay techniques (Fig. 12.7). It has been shown that only a small portion (a few percent) of endothelial cell surface-associated heparan sulphate possesses a specific oligosaccharide sequence with high affinity for antithrombin III and is almost exclusively involved in the binding of antithrombin III to the cells. This interaction between endothelial heparin-like compounds and the protease inhibitor is believed to contribute to the anticoagulant activity of endothelial cells. Thus, we demonstrated for the first time that homocysteine specifically inhibits the expression of endothelial anticoagulant heparin-like compounds, thereby perturbing an endothelial anticoagulant mechanism mediated by the interaction with antithrombin III.

Mechanisms of proteoglycan perturbation

The inhibition of antithrombin III binding to the cells requires free thiol groups. Hence, the mechanism by which homocysteine inhibits anticoagulant-active heparan sulphate appears to relate to the redox

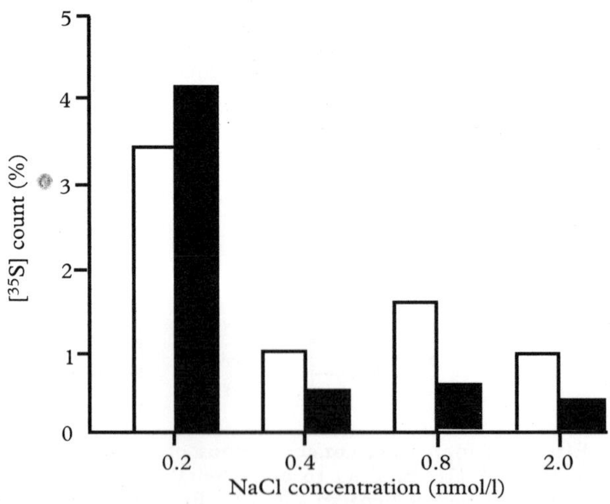

Fig. 12.6 Fractionation of ^{35}S-labelled cell surface heparan sulphate by antithrombin-affinity chromatography. ^{35}S-labelled cell surface heparan sulphate derived from control (□) and homocysteine-treated (■) cells were dissolved in Tris-HCl 0.01 mol/l (pH 7.4), applied to antithrombin-Affi-Gel and eluted stepwise by increasing the NaCl concentration (0.2, 0.4, 0.8 and 2.0 mol/l). Most of the radioactivity applied was unbound to the column. The fraction of NaCl 0.2 mol/l represents nonspecifically adsorbed radioactivity. The radioactivity in each fraction is expressed by percent of the total radioactivity applied to the column. Column recovery was >90%.

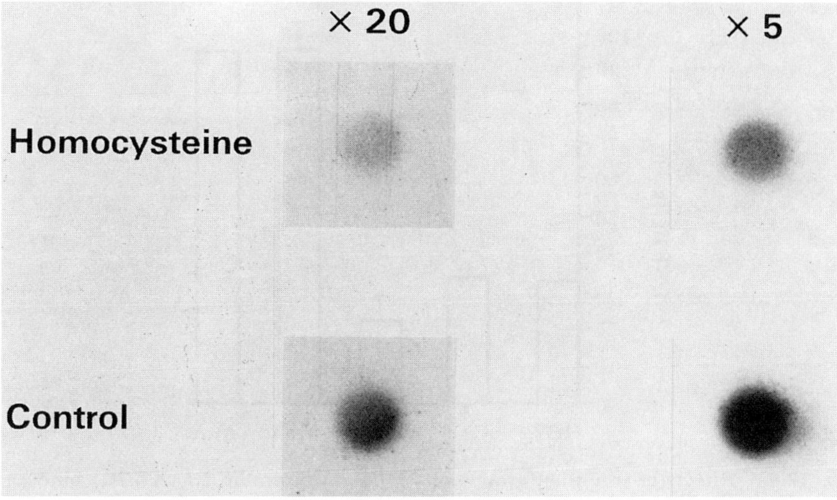

Fig. 12.7 Dot-blot autoradiography assay of [^{125}I]-antithrombin III (AT III) binding to cell surface from control and homocysteine-treated endothelial cells. Heparan sulphate from control and homocysteine-treated cells with equal amounts of ^{35}S-radioactivity was diluted 5 or 20 fold in phosphate-buffered saline and transferred onto the nitrocellulose membrane placed in a dot-blot apparatus. The blotted membrane was incubated with [^{125}I]-AT III and quantitated by autoradiography. No visible dots were detected in control membranes incubated without [^{125}I]-AT III.

potential of the sulphydryl-containing agent (Fig. 12.8). This sulphydryl effect may be caused by generation of hydrogen peroxide during thiol autooxidation, since incubation of catalase, but not superoxide dismutase, with homocysteine-treated endothelial cells prevented this response (Fig. 12.9).

In addition, the effect of homocysteine was enhanced in the presence of copper ions. This may be accounted for by copper-catalyzed hydrogen peroxide generation. These results are consistent with previous reports which showed that homocysteine and other sulphydryl agents could cause endothelial cell injury via hydrogen peroxide generation, as manifested by cell detachment or ^{51}Cr release (Dudman et al 1991; Saez et al 1982; Starkebaum & Harlan 1986; Wall et al 1980). It should be emphasized, however, that the inhibition of antithrombin III binding by homocysteine occurred without apparent 'cellular injury' and that this effect was evident only after at least 6 h of incubation in the present study, suggesting that hydrogen peroxide generation may have primarily affected the biosynthetic process of anticoagulant-active heparan sulphate in endothelial cells, but did not directly 'injure' those already present on the cell surface. On the other hand, it has been shown that homocysteine-induced suppression of protein C activation by endothelial cells is more rapid, i.e. >50% reduction within 0.5-3 h (Hayashi et al 1992; Rogers & Conn 1990) and that sulphydryl groups may (Lentz & Sadler 1991) or may not (Hayashi et al

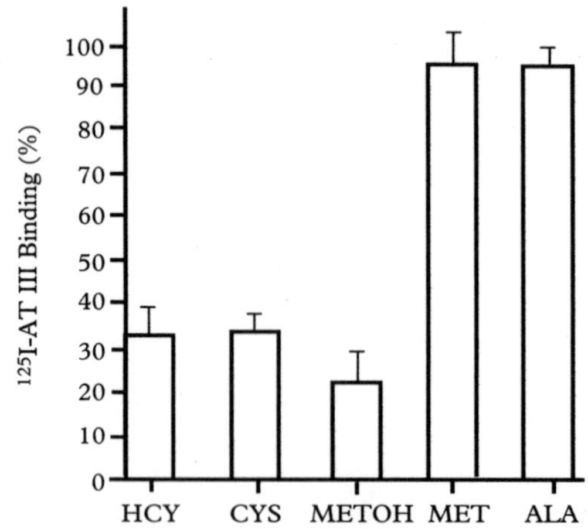

Fig. 12.8 Effects of free thiol groups on [^{125}I]-antithrombin III (AT III) binding to endothelial cells. Endothelial cell cultures after treatment with 1 mmol/l of sulphydryl agents, homocysteine (HCY), cysteine (CYS) and 2-mercaptoethanol (METOH), or nonsulphydryl agents, methionine (MET) and alanine (ALA) for 24 h were tested for [^{125}I]-AT III binding. Results are expressed as percent of the amount of AT III bound to control cells incubated without any agents. Data are given as means ± SEM.

1992; Rogers & Conn 1990) be required for this effect. The role of hydrogen peroxide was not evident in one of those studies (Rogers & Conn 1990). Instead, homocysteine may directly inhibit the thrombomodulin cofactor activity by reducing the disulphide-bound structures of the protein, with an increase in thrombomodulin mRNA and thrombomodulin protein synthesis as a compensatory mechanism (Hayashi et al 1992; Rogers & Conn 1990). Thus, homocysteine might inhibit two major anticoagulant pathways in endothelial cells by different mechanisms.

The inhibitory effect of homocysteine occurred at an 10-fold lower concentration of homocysteine in our study than that used in the previous experiments (0.1-1 *vs* 1-10 mmol/l, respectively) [Hayashi et al 1992; Rogers & Conn 1990]. Plasma concentrations of free homocysteine present in homocysteinuric patients are reported to be less than 1 mmol/l (Rogers & Kane 1986), while levels of homocysteine found in plasma of patients with premature vascular disease are considerably lower than those in homozygous homocysteinaemic patients, e.g. homocysteine 10-30 mmol/l (Clarke et al 1991; Malinow 1990; Stampfer et al 1992). Our data showing the inhibited expression of the antithrombin III-mediated anticoagulant system in endothelial cells by homocysteine concentrations as low as 0.1 mmol/l, or even at as low concentrations as 10 μmol/l in some conditions affecting redox potential such as the presence of copper ion, may be pathophysiologically relevant, at least in certain clinical situations. Furthermore, the inhibited expression of anticoagulant-active heparan sulphate may be a highly sensitive marker of 'endothelial cell perturbation' subsequent to alteration of the redox potential.

The mechanism of the synthesis and expression of anticoagulant heparan sulphate in endothelial cells is not well known. It requires: the production of a core protein; assembly of a linkage region of 4 monosaccharide units; generation of a precursor oligosaccharide chain; and subsequent polymer-modification reactions, including deacetylation of *N*-acetylglucosamine residues, *N*-sulphation of the resulting free amino groups, and conversion of D-glucuronic acid to L-iduronic acid units by epimerization at C-5, *O*-sulphation at C-2 of iduronic acid units and *O*-sulphation at C-6 of glucosamine units. The final step of this complex remodeling process is thought to be the glucosamine-3-*O*-sulphotransferase reaction, resulting in the generation of a region of a unique sequence of sulphated and nonsulphated uronic acid and glucosamine residues, which are required to complex with antithrombin III (de Agostini et al 1990a; Lindahl et al 1989). Homocysteine appears to perturb this biosynthetic pathway in a rather specific way and diminish cell-surface expression of anticoagulant-active heparan sulphate with high affinity for antithrombin III, without gross alternations of overall cellular glycosaminoglycan biosynthesis.

The mechanism by which cells treated with homocysteine are defective in the synthesis and/or subsequent expression on the cell surface of heparan

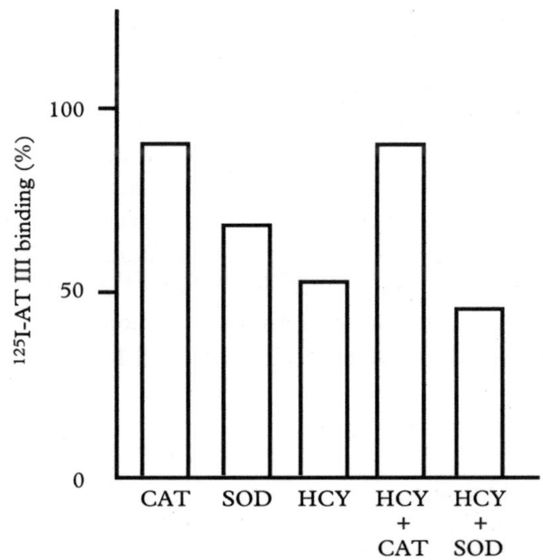

Fig. 12.9 Effects of catalase and superoxide dismutase on homocysteine-induced inhibition of [^{125}I]-antithrombin III (AT III) binding to endothelial cells. Endothelial cell cultures were incubated with homocysteine (HCY) in the presence or absence of catalase (CAT; 1000 U/ml) or superoxide dismutase (SOD; 200 U/ml) for 6 h, and tested for [^{125}I]-AT III binding. Results are expressed as mean percent of the amount of AT III bound to control cells incubated without any agents.

sulphate with the unique monosaccharide sequence required for the binding of antithrombin III remains to be determined. The synthesis of specific core proteins for anticoagulant-active heparan sulphate (Kojima et al 1992), if any, or the multimolecular arrays of biosynthetic enzymes that carry out post-translational modifications of the oligosaccharide chains within the Golgi complex might be perturbed by homocysteine. The latter concept is in accord with the recent study by Lentz and Sadler (1991) which showed that, in the presence of homocysteine, incorporation of [^{35}S]-sulphate into chondroitin sulphate glycosaminoglycan associated with thrombomodulin was decreased, suggesting that at least one of the direct or indirect target sites of homocysteine-induced perturbation could be a cytoplasmic process of proteins and/or proteoglycans within the Golgi complex.

Future investigation of the detailed molecular basis of the defective anticoagulant heparan sulphate expression in homocysteine-treated cells should help us to understand how cells synthesize and express different heparan sulphate proteoglycans with regions of defined monosaccharide sequence.

CONCLUSION

Anticoagulant-active heparan sulphate proteoglycans on the endothelial cell surface are decreased in response to atherothrombogenic stimuli such as cytokines and homocysteine. Cytokines appear to exert their effects through an overall inhibition of cellular glycosaminoglycan metabolism. Homocysteine, however, apparently perturbs this biosynthetic pathway in a more specific way, via the alteration of redox potential. Both result in the diminished endothelial cell-surface expression of heparin-like anticoagulant activity. It is not known whether endothelial cells in diabetes are also altered in this manner. There is, nevertheless, increasing evidence that the biosynthesis of heparan sulphate is indeed suppressed in diabetes. Further study should be directed toward this possible alteration of the expression of endothelial heparin-like compounds in diabetes, and its mechanism. This would help us to gain insight into another pathophysiological mechanism which may be involved in altered endothelial cell function during diabetes.

REFERENCES

Bevilacqua M P, Pober J S, Majeau G R 1986a Recombinant tumor necrosis factor induces procoagulant activity in cultured human vascular endothelium: characterization and comparison with the actions of interleukin 1. Proc Natl Acad Sci USA 83: 4533-4537

Bevilacqua M P, Schleef R R, Gimbrone M A et al 1986b Regulation of the fibrinolytic system of cultured human vascular endothelium by interleukin 1. J Clin Invest 78: 587-591

Boers G H J, Smals A G H, Trijbel F J H et al 1985 Heterozygosity for homocystiuria in premature peripheral and cerebral occlusive arterial disease. N Engl J Med 313: 709-715

Brattstrom L E, Hardebo J E, Hultberg B L 1984 Moderate homocysteinemia - A possible risk factor for arteriosclerotic cerebrovascular disease. Stroke 15: 1012-1016

Bussolino F, Camussi G, Baglioni C 1988 Synthesis and release of platelet-activating factor by human vascular endothelial cells treated with tumor necrosis factor or interleukin 1α. J Biol Chem 263: 11856-11861

Clarke R, Daly L, Robinson K et al 1991 Hyperhomocysteinemia: an independent risk factor for vascular disease. N Engl J Med 324: 1149-1155

Colucci M, Balconi G, Lorenzet R et al 1983 Cultured human endothelial cells generate tissue factor in response to endotoxin. J Clin Invest 71: 1893-1896

Damus P, Hicks M, Rosenberg R 1973 Anticoagulant action of heparin. Nature 246: 355

de Agostini A l, Lau H K, Leone C et al 1990a Cell mutants defective in synthesizing a heparan sulfate proteoglycan with regions of defined monosaccharide sequence. Proc Natl Acad Sci USA 87: 9784-9788

de Agostini A I, Watkins S C, Slayer H S et al 1990b Localization and anticoagulantly active heparan sulfate proteoglycans in vascular endothelium: antithrombin binding on cultured endothelial cells and perfused rat aorta. J Cell Biol 111: 1293-1304

Dudman N P B, Hicks C, Wang J et al 1991 Human arterial endothelial cell detachment *in vitro*: its promotion by homocysteine and cysteine. Atherosclerosis 91: 77-83

Emeis J J, Kooistra T 1986 Interleukin 1 and lipopolysaccharide induce an inhibitor of tissue-type plasminogen activator *in vivo* and in cultured endothelial cells. J Exp Med 163: 1260-1265

Esmon C T 1983 Protein C: biochemistry, physiology and clinical implications. Blood 62: 1155-1158

Esmon C T 1987 The regulation of natural anticoagulant pathways. Science 235: 1348-1352

Harker L A, Ross R, Slichter S J et al 1976 Homocysteine-induced arteriosclerosis. The role of endothelial cell injury and platelet response in its genesis. J Clin Invest 58: 731-741

Hayashi T, Honda G, Suzuki K 1992 An atherogenic stimulus homocysteine inhibits cofactor activity of thrombomodulin and enhances thrombomodulin expression in human umbilical vein endothelial cells. Blood 79: 2930-2936

Jackson R L, Busch S J, Cardin A D 1991 Glycosaminoglycans: molecular properties, protein interactions, and role in physiological processes. Physiol Rev 71: 481-539

Kobayashi M, Shimada K, Ozawa T 1990 Human recombinant interleukin-1β and tumor necrosis factor α-mediated suppression of heparin-like compounds on cultured porcine aortic endothelial cells. J Cell Physiol 144: 383-390

Kojima T, Leone C W, Marchildon G A et al 1992 Isolation and characterization of heparan sulfate proteoglycans produced by cloned rat microvascular endothelial cells. J Biol Chem 267: 4859-4869

Lentz S R, Sadler J E 1991 Inhibition of thrombomodulin surface expression and protein C activation by the thrombogenic agent homocysteine. J Clin Invest 88: 1906-1914

Lindahl U L F, Kusche M, Lindholt K et al 1989 Biosynthesis of heparin and heparan sulfate. Ann NY Acad Sci 556: 36-59

Loskutoff D J, Edgington T S 1977 Synthesis of a fibrinolytic activator and inhibitor. Proc Natl Acad Sci USA 74: 3903-3907

Malinow M R 1990 Hyperhomocyst(e)inemia. A common and easily reversible risk factor for occlusive atherosclerosis. Circulation 81: 2004-2006

Malinow M R, Kang S S, Taylor L M et al 1989 Prevalence of hyperhomocyst(e)inemia in patients with peripheral arterial occlusive disease. Circulation 79: 1180-1188

Mitrovic D, Lippiello L, Gruson F et al 1981 Effects of various prostanoids on the *in vitro* metabolism of bovine articular chondrocytes. Prostaglandins 22: 499-511

Moncada S, Vane J R 1979 The role of prostacyclin in vascular tissue. Fed Proc 38: 66-71

Moore K L, Esmon C T, Esmon N L 1989 Tumor necrosis factor leads to the internalization and degradation of thrombomodulin from the surface of bovine aortic endothelial cells in culture. Blood 73: 159-165

Mudd S H, Skovby F S, Levy K D et al 1985 The natural history of homocystinuria due to cystathionine β-synthase deficiency. Am J Hum Genet 37: 1-31

Nachman R L, Haijar K A, Silverstein R L et al 1986 Interleukin 1 induces endothelial cell synthesis of plasminogen activator inhibitor. J Exp Med 163: 1595-1604

Nawroth P P, Esmon C T, Stern D M 1986 Interleukin 1 induces endothelial cell procoagulant activity while suppressing cell-surface anticoagulant activity. Proc Natl Acad Sci USA 83: 3460-3464

Nawroth P P, Stern D M 1985 A pathway of coagulation on endothelial cells. J Cell Biochem 28: 253-264

Nawroth P P, Stern D M 1986 Modulation of endothelial cell hemostatic properties by tumor necrosis factor. J Exp Med 163: 740-745

Nishinaga M, Ozawa T, Shimada K 1993 Homocysteine, a thrombogenic agent, suppresses anticoagulant heparan sulfate expression in cultured porcine aortic endothelial cells. J Clin Invest 92: 1381-1386

Pejler G, Backstrom G, Lindahl U 1987 Structure and affinity for antithrombin of heparan sulfate chains derived from basement membrane proteoglycans. J Biol Chem 262: 5036-5043

Rogers G M, Shuman M A 1983 Prothrombin is activated on vascular endothelial cells by factor Xa and calcium. Proc Natl Acad Sci USA 80: 7001-7005

Rogers G M, Conn M T 1990 Homocysteine, an atherogenic stimulus, reduces protein C activation by arterial and venous endothelial cells. Blood 75: 895-901

Rogers G M, Kane W H 1986 Activation of endogenous factor V by a homocysteine-induced vascular endothelial cell activator. J Clin Invest 77: 1909-1916

Rosenberg R D, Rosenberg J S 1984 Natural anticoagulant mechanisms. J Clin Invest 74: 1-6

Rossi V, Breviario F, Ghezzi P et al 1985 Prostacyclin synthesis induced in vascular cells by interleukin-1. Science 229: 174-176

Saez G, Thornalley P J, Hill H A et al 1982 The production of free radicals during the autoxidation of cysteine and their effect on isolated rat hepatocytes. Biochem Biophys Acta 719: 24-31

Schleef R R, Bevilacqua M P, Sawdey M et al 1988 Cytokine activation of vascular endothelium. Effect on tissue-type plasminogen activator and type 1 plasminogen activator inhibitor. J Biol Chem 263: 5797-5803

Stampfer M J, Malinow M R, Willett W C et al 1992 A prospective study of plasma homocyst(e)ine and risk of myocardial infarction in US physicians. J Am Med Assoc 268: 877-881

Starkebaum G, Harlan J M 1986 Endothelial cell injury due to copper-catalyzed hydrogen peroxide generation from homocysteine. J Clin Invest 77: 1370-1376

Stern D, Nawroth P, Handley D et al 1985 An endothelial cell-dependent pathway of coagulation. Proc Natl Acad Sci USA 82: 2523-2527.

Wall R T, Harker L A 1980 The endothelium and thrombosis. Annu Rev Med 31: 361-371

Wall R T, Harlan J M, Harker L A et al 1980 Homocysteine-induced endothelial cell injury *in vitro*: a model for the study of vascular injury. Thromb Res 18: 113-121

Wight T N 1980 Vessel proteoglycan and thrombosis. Prog Hemost Thromb 5: 1-39

Wight T N 1989 Cell biology of arterial proteoglycans. Arteriosclerosis 9: 1-20.

13

Modulation of endothelial cell function by glycated proteins

H. Takeda, E. Yamaguchi, T. Nishikawa, M. Shichiri

INTRODUCTION

Glycation of cellular proteins induced by hyperglycaemia may play an important role in the development of diabetic macro- and microangiopathy. Glycated proteins are divided into two groups, early glycation products and advanced glycation end-products (AGEs). Early glycation products consist of Shiff base and Amadori products, which are closely related to products of oxidative protein modification because of their potency of autoxidation (Hunt et al 1990; Mullarkey et al 1990; Sakurai et al 1991). AGEs are obtained by advanced reaction of the Amadori products and are recognized by macrophages (Takata et al 1988). Both groups of glycated proteins may be closely related to the development of arteriosclerosis. It is well known that many kinds of Amadori products, e.g. haemoglobin A_{1c} and fructosamine, exist in diabetic patients and animals. Glycated low-density lipoproteins are also increased in diabetic subjects (Shinohara et al 1990). Using an enzyme-linked immunosorbent assay with specific anti-AGE antibody, several investigators have recently confirmed the existence of AGEs as well as early glycation products in various human and animal tissues, such as optic lens, red blood cells and renal cortex (Araki et al 1992; Makita et al 1992a, b; Mitsuhashi et al

Table 13.1 Effects of glycated lipoproteins on the arachidonic acid-induced synthesis of prostacyclin in cultured vascular endothelial cells. *Statistical significance:* *p <0.01 and **p <0.001 versus untreated controls, †p <0.01 versus nonglycated lipoprotein. (Reproduced with permission from Takeda et al 1992)

Addition	Mean (±SEM) 6-keto $PGF_{1\alpha}$ production (ng) per 10^6 cells (n = 8)
Untreated (control)	21.4 ± 1.8
LDL (0.2 mg/ml)	
nonglycated	12.6 ± 1.9*
glycated	8.8 ± 0.9**,†
HDL (0.2 mg/ml)	
nonglycated	13.6 ± 1.7*
glycated	10.9 ± 1.3**,†

1993; Nakayama et al 1993). Although these glycated proteins induce many reactions with various cells and substances, this review focus on the interaction between glycated proteins and vascular endothelial cells.

INTERACTION BETWEEN EARLY GLYCATION PRODUCTS AND ENDOTHELIAL CELLS

STIMULATION OF ENDOTHELIAL CELLS BY GLYCATED PROTEINS

There is little evidence that Amadori products directly affect the functions of endothelial cells. We therefore initially examined the effects of glycated low- or high-density lipoproteins (LDL or HDL) on arachidonic acid-induced prostacyclin synthesis in cultured endothelial cells following treatment for 5 min at 37°C (Table 13.1) [Takeda et al 1992]. The synthesis of 6-keto prostaglandin (PG) $F_{1\alpha}$ was similarly and significantly suppressed by glycated LDL and HDL compared with either the nonglycated native proteins or untreated control (buffer alone). The effects of the glycated lipoproteins on the spontaneous release of 6-keto $PGF_{1\alpha}$ and lactate dehydrogenase (LDH) from endothelial cells were then studied after incubation in Ham's F10 medium for 1-24 h at 37°C. The release of 6-keto $PGF_{1\alpha}$ was not significantly affected by these glycated lipoproteins.

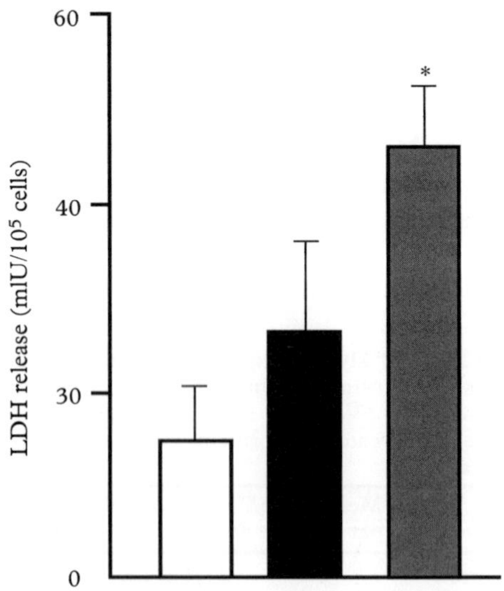

Fig. 13.1 Effects of glycated low-density lipoprotein (LDL) on the release of lactate dehydrogenase (LDH) from endothelial cells. Open column indicates the value obtained without LDL, hatched column that with native LDL and dotted column that with glycated LDL. Values are given as means ± SEM (n = 8). *Statistical significance:* *p <0.05 versus untreated control. (Reproduced with permission from Takeda et al 1992)

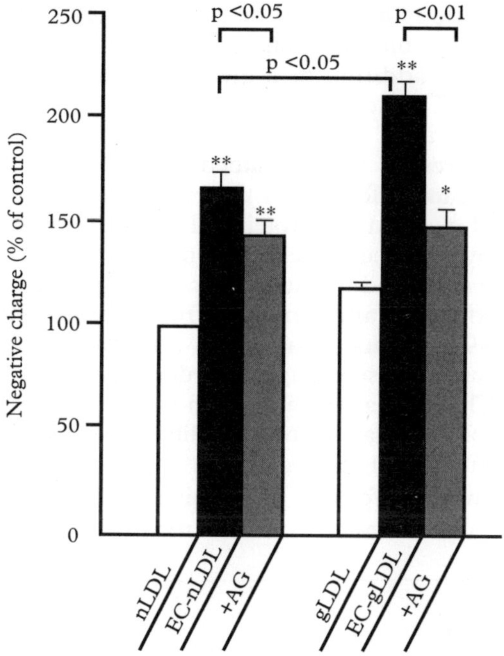

Fig. 13.2 Effect of aminoguanidine (AG) on the negative charge of endothelial cell-modified low-density lipoprotein (LDL). Values are given as means ± SEM (n = 6). *Abbreviations:* nLDL = native LDL; gLDL = glycated LDL; EC-nLDL = endothelial cell-modified nLDL; EC-gLDL = endothelial cell-modified gLDL. *Statistical significance:* *p <0.05, **p <0.01 versus nLDL control. (Reproduced with permission from Takeda et al 1993)

On the other hand, the release of LDH was increased gradually during incubation and was significantly increased by glycated LDL at 24 h compared with control (Fig. 13.1), but was unaffected by either native LDL or glycated HDL. These abnormalities were not observed when RPMI 1640 medium was used instead of Ham's F10 medium. In addition, there was no significant difference in thiobarbituric acid (TBA)-reacting substance content between the native LDL and glycated LDL in Ham's F10 medium. Similarly, there was no significant difference in the content of lipid hydroperoxides between the native LDL and glycated LDL in Ham's F10 medium. The content of lipid peroxides in LDLs in RPMI 1640 medium was also similar to that in Ham's F10 medium. Thus, glycated LDL, as well as oxidized LDL, may be cytotoxic for endothelial cells with respect to cellular LDH release (Kuzuya et al 1989, 1990).

OXIDATION OF GLYCATED LDL BY ENDOTHELIAL CELLS

Although oxidation of native LDL by endothelial cells under low Cu^{2+} ion concentration (Ham's F10 medium) is known to occur in some extent (EC-modified LDL), little is known in case of glycated LDL. We therefore examined the oxidative modification of glycated LDL by endothelial cells with and without the addition of a glycation inhibitor, aminoguanidine (Takeda et al 1993). The negative charge of glycated LDL was significantly increased by endothelial cell modification compared with EC-modified LDL (Fig. 13.2). Similar results were obtained for change in fluorescence, but there was no significant difference in the change in lipid peroxide contents between native and glycated lipoproteins. These data indicate that glycated LDL is oxidized by endothelial cells to a much greater extent than native LDL. This may be explained by the fact that early glycation products have a potency for autoxidation and generate free radicals (Hunt et al 1990; Mullarkey et al 1990; Sakurai et al 1991). As shown in figure 13.3, dose-dependent inhibition of these changes was demonstrated by the addition of aminoguanidine. This is in accordance with the data described by Picard et al (1992), who reported that aminoguanidine suppressed the oxidation of LDL induced by endothelial cells or low Cu^{2+} ion concentration.

Further studies were performed to examine the effects of these modified lipoproteins on cholesteryl ester accumulation in rat peritoneal

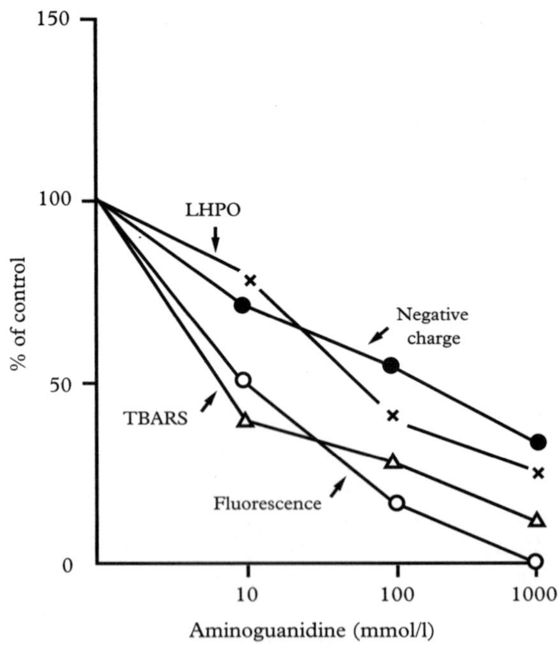

Fig. 13.3 Effect of aminoguanidine on oxidative modification of glycated low-density lipoprotein by vascular endothelial cells. Values are given as means of 3 duplicate determinations. *Abbreviations:* LHPO = lipid hydroperoxides; TBARS = thiobarbituric acid-reacting substances. (Reproduced with permission from Takeda et al 1993)

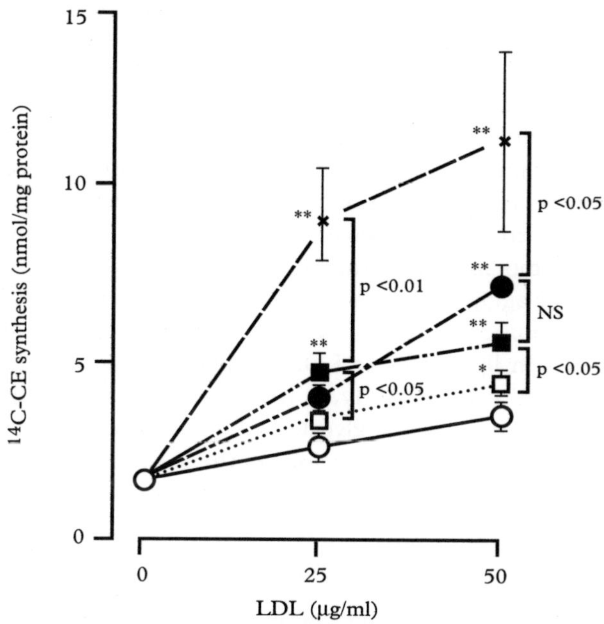

Fig. 13.4 Effects of modified low-density lipoproteins (LDL) on cholesteryl ester (CE) accumulation in rat peritoneal macrophages. Values are given as means ± SEM (n = 6). *Symbols:* ○ = native LDL; □ = glycated LDL; ● = endothelial cell-modified LDL; ■ = endothelial cell-modified glycated LDL; X = Cu^{2+}-oxidized LDL. *Statistical significance:* *p <0.05, **p <0.01 versus native LDL. (Reproduced with permission from Takeda et al 1993)

macrophages (Fig. 13.4) [Takeda et al 1993]. Cholesteryl ester synthesis was significantly stimulated by EC-modified glycated LDL compared with glycated LDL. These results suggested that glycated LDL may be more atherogenic than native LDL because of oxidative modification induced by endothelial cells, and that aminoguanidine may be able to inhibit such complicated LDL modifications.

INTERACTION BETWEEN AGES AND ENDOTHELIAL CELLS

EFFECTS OF AGES ON ENDOTHELIAL CELL FUNCTION

In contrast to the early glycation products, AGEs are known to induce variable endothelial cell responses. For example, it has been reported that AGEs induce increased endothelial cell permeability and modification of surface cell coagulation properties (Esposito et al 1989), transendothelial monocyte chemotaxis (Kirstein et al 1990), angiogenesis (Tezuka et al

1993), and defective vasodilation and antiproliferative effect of endothelium-dependent relaxing factor by quenching nitric oxide (Bucala et al 1991; Hogan et al 1992). In addition, Tilton et al (1993) have recently reported that aminoguanidine was able to prevent AGE formation and suppress nitric oxide synthetase activity, resulting in an improvement of the abnormal vascular permeability of early diabetic microangiopathy. Transendothelial monocyte chemotaxis might be induced when AGEs are recognized by scavenger receptors on the cell surface of monocyte/macrophages (Takata et al 1988). It has recently been shown that exogenous AGE administration in normal rats or rabbits induces complex vascular dysfunction resembling that seen in diabetes or aging (Vlassara et al 1992). Bucala et al (1993) proposed that AGE formation occurred not only at protein sites but also at membrane phospholipid sites in liposomes or LDL. Although their hypothesis remains to be confirmed by further study, it might suggest that endothelial cell functions are altered not only by glycated LDL (Amadori products) but also by AGE-LDL, or by AGE formation at the phospholipid sites on the endothelial cell membrane *per se*.

AGE RECEPTOR ON THE ENDOTHELIAL CELL SURFACE

It had been reported that AGEs are bound to endothelial cells (Bucala et al 1991) and macrophages (Takata et al 1988). However, it was not clarified until more recently whether or not specific receptors for AGEs exist. The question has been at least partially solved (Neeper et al 1992; Schmidt et al 1992). These studies described the isolation and characterization of two AGE binding proteins on the endothelial cell surface of bovine lung, receptor for AGE (RAGE) and lactoferrin-like polypeptide (LF-L). The RAGE is a 35-kDa polypeptide with a unique NH_2-terminal sequence, and may be closely associated with LF-L on the cell surface. Using an oligonucleotide probe based on the amino-terminal sequence of RAGE, an apparently full-length cDNA of 1.5 kb was isolated from a bovine lung cDNA library, which encoded a 394 amino acid mature protein. A partial clone encoding the human counterpart of RAGE, isolated from a human lung library, was found to be 90% homologous with the bovine molecule (Fig. 13.5). It has been further reported that human monocytes also have RAGE and LF-L, and that chemotaxis of human monocytes induced by soluble AGE-albumin was prevented in a dose-dependent manner by intact antibodies raised to these AGE-binding proteins (Schmidt et al 1993).

CONCLUSION

As mentioned above, glycated proteins may play an important role in the development of diabetic macro- and microangiopathy. However, several points still remain to be resolved in the AGE hypothesis. For example,

```
                 .          . +1        .          .          .
Bovine  MAAGAVVGAWMLVLSLGGTVTGDQNITARIGKPLVLNCKGAPKKPPQQLE    50
         |||..||||:||||| |.|.|.||||||||.||||.||||||||||.||
Human   GAAGTAVGAWVLVLSLWGAVVGAQNITARIGEPLVLKCKGAPKKPPQRLE    50

                 .          .          .          .          .
Bovine  WKLNTGRTEAWKVLSPQ.GDPWDSVARVLPNGSLLLPAVGIQDEGTFRCR    99
        |||||||||||||||||:||||||||||||||||:||||||||||.||||
Human   WKLNTGRTEAWKVLSPQGGGPWDSVARVLPNGSLFLPAVGIQDEGIFRCR   100

                 .          .          .          .          .
Bovine  ATSRSGKETKSNYRVRVYQIPGKPEIVDPASELMAGVPNKVGTCVSEGGY   149
        | .|.||||||||||||||||||||||||.|||| ||||||||||||||:|
Human   AMNRNGKETKSNYRVRVYQIPGKPEIVDSASELTAGVPNKVGTCVSEGSY   150

                 .          .          .          .          .
Bovine  PAGTLNWLLDGKTLIPDGKGVSVKEETKRHPKTGLFTLHSELMVTPARGG   199
        |||||.| ||||.|:|::||||||||:|:|||.||||||:||||||||||
Human   PAGTLSWHLDGKPLVPNEKGVSVKEQTRRHPETGLFTLQSELMVTPARGG   200

                 .          .          .          .          .
Bovine  ALHPTFSCSFTPGLPRRRALHTAPIQLRVWSEHRGGEGPNVDAVPLKEVQ   249
        . :|||||||.|||||:|||:||||| |||             ::|||.|||
Human   DPRPTFSCSFSPGLPRHRALRTAPIQPRVW...........EPVPLEEVQ   239

                 .          .          .          .          .
Bovine  LVVEPEGGAVAPGGTVTLTCEAPAQPPPQIHWIKDGRPLPLPPGPMLLLP   299
        ||||||||||||||||||||.||||.|||||:||| ||||||:|:|:||
Human   LVVEPEGGAVAPGGTVTLTCEVPAQPSPQIHWMKDGVPLPLPPSPVLILP   289

                 .          .          .          .          .
Bovine  EVGPEDQGTYSCVATHPSHGPQESRAVSVTIIETGEEGTTAGSVEGPGLE   349
        |:||:|||||||||||.|||||||||||:.|||.||||.||||||:|.||:
Human   EIGPQDQGTYSCVATHSSHGPQESRAVSISIIEPGEEGPTAGSVGGSGLG   339

                 .          .          .          .          .
Bovine  TLALTLGILGGLGTVALLIGVIVWHRRRQRKGQERKVPENQEEEEEERAE   399
        ||||.||||||||||.|||||||:|: ||||:|:|||.|||| ||||||||
Human   TLALALGILGGLGTAALLIGVILWQ.RRQRRGEERKAPENQ.EEEEERAE   387

                 .
Bovine  LNQPEEPEAAESSTGGP   416
        |||.|||||:|||||||
Human   LNQSEEPEAGESSTGGP   404
```

Fig. 13.5 Protein sequence alignment of bovine and human receptor for AGE (RAGE). Sequences were deduced from translation of the cDNAs, and alignments were made using the GAP program of the Genetics Computer Group. Vertical lines show sequence identity. Vertical rows of dots indicate threshold similarity. Gaps indicated by dots were introduced to produce optimal alignment. Underlining indicates conserved cysteines (bold underline), *N*-linked glycosylation sites (light underline), and transmembrane domain (dashed underline). (Reproduced with permission from Neeper et al 1992)

what is the chemical composition of AGE? Is it possible to use any chemical agent to inhibit the reaction of Amadori products sufficiently and safely for suppression of AGE formation? If these problems are solved, diabetic vascular complications may become preventable in the future.

REFERENCES

Araki N, Ueno N, Chakrabarti B et al 1992 Immunochemical evidence for the presence of advanced glycation end-products in human lens proteins and its positive correlation with aging. J Biol Chem 267: 10211-10214

Bucala R, Makita Z, Koschinsky T et al 1993 Lipid advanced glycosylation: pathway for lipid oxidation *in vivo*. Proc Natl Acad Sci USA 90: 6434-6438

Bucala R, Tracey K J, Cerami A 1991 Advanced glycosylation products quench nitric oxide and mediate defective endothelium-dependent vasodilation in experimental diabetes. J Clin Invest 87: 432-438

Esposito C, Gerlach H, Brett J et al 1989 Endothelial receptor-mediated binding of glucose-modified albumin is associated with increased monolayer permeability and modulation of cell surface coagulant properties. J Exp Med 170: 1387-1407

Hogan M, Cerami A, Bucala R 1992 Advanced glycosylation end-products block the antiproliferative effect of nitric oxide: role in the vascular and renal complications of diabetes mellitus. J Clin Invest 90: 1110-1115

Hunt J V, Smith C C T, Wolff S P 1990 Autoxidative glycosylation and possible involvement of peroxides and free radicals in LDL modification by glucose. Diabetes 39: 1420-1424

Kirstein M, Brett J, Radoff S et al 1990 Advanced protein glycosylation induces transendothelial human monocyte chemotaxis and secretion of platelet-derived growth factor: role in vascular disease of diabetes and aging. Proc Natl Acad Sci USA 87: 9010-9014

Kuzuya M, Naito M, Funaki C et al 1989 Protective role of intracellular glutathione against oxidized low density lipoprotein in cultured endothelial cells. Biochem Biophys Res Commun 163: 1466-1472

Kuzuya M, Naito M, Yamada K et al 1990 Involvement of intracellular iron in the toxicity of oxidized low density lipoprotein to cultured endothelial cells. Biochem Int 22: 567-573

Makita Z, Vlassara H, Cerami A et al 1992a Immunochemical detection of advanced glycosylation end products *in vivo*. J Biol Chem 267: 5133-5138

Makita Z, Vlassara H, Rayfield E et al 1992b Hemoglobin-AGE: a circulating marker of advanced glycosylation. Science 58: 651-653

Mitsuhashi T, Nakayama H, Itoh T et al 1993 Immunochemical detection of advanced glycation end-products in renal cortex from STZ-induced diabetic rat. Diabetes 42: 826-832

Mullarkey C J, Edelstein D, Brownlee M 1990 Free radical generation by early glycation products: a mechanism for accelerated atherogenesis in diabetes. Biochem Biophys Res Commun 173: 932-939

Nakayama H, Mitsuhashi T, Kuwajima S et al 1993 Immunochemical detection of advanced glycation end-products in lens crystallins from streptozotocin-induced diabetic rat. Diabetes 42: 345-350

Neeper M, Schmidt A M, Brett J et al 1992 Cloning and expression of a cell surface receptor for advanced glycosylation end-products of proteins. J Biol Chem 267: 14998-5004

Picard S, Parthasarathy S, Fruebis J et al 1992 Aminoguanidine inhibits oxidative modification of low density lipoprotein protein and the subsequent increase in uptake by macrophage scavenger receptors. Proc Natl Acad Sci USA 89: 6876-6880

Sakurai T, Kimura S, Nakano M et al 1991 Oxidative modification of glycated low density lipoprotein in the presence of iron. Biochem Biophys Res Commun 177: 433-439

Schmidt A M, Vianna M, Gerlach M et al 1992 Isolation and characterization of two binding proteins for advanced glycosylation end-products from bovine lung which are present on the endothelial cell surface. J Biol Chem 267: 14987-14997

Schmidt A M, Yan S D, Brett J et al 1993 Regulation of human mononuclear phagocyte migration by cell surface-binding proteins for advanced glycation end-products. J Clin Invest 92: 2155-2168

Shinohara M, Takeda H, Kishikawa H et al 1990 Glycation of serum high- and low-density lipoproteins in diabetic subjects. Journal of the Japanese Diabetes Society 33: 799-803

Takata K, Horiuchi S, Araki N et al 1988 Endocytic uptake of nonenzymatically glycosylated proteins is mediated by a scavenger receptor for aldehyde-modified proteins. J Biol Chem 263: 14819-14825

Takeda H, Yamaguchi E, Kobori S et al 1993 Investigation on the acceleration of atherogenesis by glycated lipoproteins and its prevention: effect of aminoguanidine on the oxidative modification of glycated low-density lipoproteins induced by vascular endothelial cells. Journal of the Japanese Atherosclerosis Society 21: 361-365

Takeda H, Yano T, Kishikawa H et al 1992 Abnormalities in platelets and vascular endothelial cells induced by glycated lipoproteins. Intern Med 31: 746-751

Tezuka M, Koyama N, Morisaki N et al 1993 Angiogenic effects of advanced glycation end-products of the Maillard reaction on cultured human umbilical cord vein endothelial cells. Biochem Biophys Res Commun 193: 674-680

Tilton R G, Chang K, Hasan K S et al 1993 Prevention of diabetic vascular dysfunction by guanidines: inhibition of nitric oxide synthetase versus advanced glycation end-product formation. Diabetes 42: 221-232

Vlassara H, Fuh H, Makita Z et al 1992 Exogenous advanced glycosylation end-products induce complex vascular dysfunction in normal animals: a model for diabetic and aging complications. Proc Natl Acad Sci USA 89: 12043-12047

SECTION 5

Accelerated Permeability and Angiogenesis

14

Abnormal endothelial cell permeability in diabetes

O. Tokunaga, J. L. Fan, T. Yamada

INTRODUCTION

This article is aimed at looking at the general changes in endothelial cells which occur over the life span of an individual, not specifically in patients with diabetes mellitus. Vascular endothelial cells have long been thought to be polygonal and to comprise a homogeneous population forming an 'en face' pavement arrangement. Although giant endothelial cells were found in Hautchen preparations in the 1940s and 1950s, this topic has not been reviewed until recently. Multinucleated variant endothelial cells have been demonstrated to emerge in accordance with atherosclerotic severity and ageing in the human aorta. These findings prompted us to investigate the functional alterations of these cells during the course of their life span. We describe the capability of prostacyclin (PGI_2) and endothelin-1 (ET-1) synthesis by human endothelial cells deriving from infancy to elderly subjects using a biosynthetic assay and immunohistology. In additon, the general concept of increased permeability by endothelial injury in diabetes mellitus, which causes retinopathy and nephropathy, is reviewed. A 3-demensional *in vitro* model system for vascular system is proposed for future investigation.

MULTINUCLEATED VARIANT ENDOTHELIAL CELLS

PRESENCE OF VARIANT ENDOTHELIAL CELLS IN PRIMARY CULTURE FROM HUMAN AORTA

We have cultured endothelial cells from human aortae and inferior venae cavae of autopsied subjects ranging in age from infancy to 85 years (Tokunaga et al 1989). The cultured endothelial cells could be classified into 2 types: the typical small type and the larger type. The typical endothelial cells were small, round to polygonal and arranged uniformly. Their diameter ranged from 50-70 μm (Fig. 14.1). On the other hand, endothelial cells of the second type were more varied in size and shape. They were larger than the typical cells, ranging from 100-200 μm in diameter and had more than 2 nuclei. Giant endothelial cells >250 μm in diameter were intermingled among the typical endothelial cells in primary cultures, even from adolescent aortae, and were usually multinucleated,

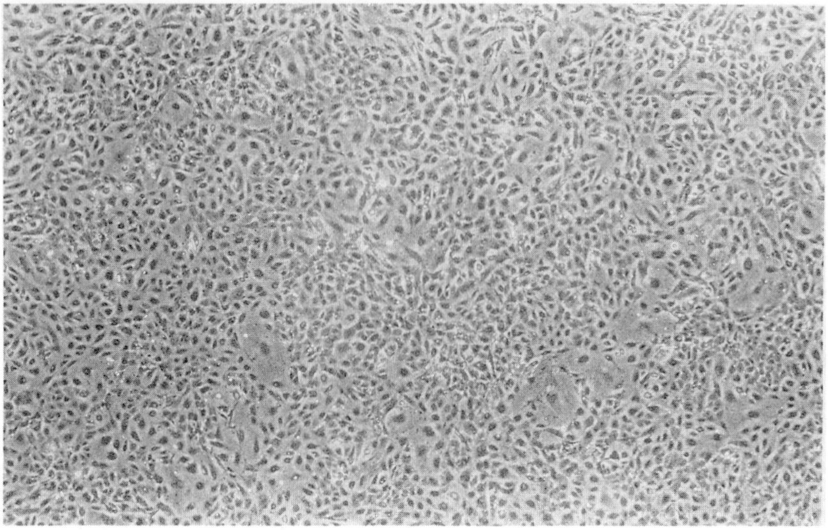

Fig. 14.1 Mixture of typical endothelial cells and variant endothelial cells in primary culture.

occasionally with ≥10 nuclei. Multinucleated cells containing more than 3 nuclei, which contained von Willebrand factor (vWF), were designated as 'variant endothelium'. Various other groups have successfully cultured endothelial cells from human arteries but they did not find any morphologically unusual cells (Fryer et al 1966; Glassberg et al 1982; Hoshi & McKeehan 1986). The presence of multinucleated giant cells in cultured endothelial cells from human aorta was first but only briefly reported by Repin et al (1984), and then by Antonov et al (1986).

VARIANT CELLS ARE ENDOTHELIAL CELLS AND HAVE NO MITOTIC ACTIVITY

Multinucleated variant cells were positive for vWF by immunofluorescence (Fig. 14.2) or immunoenzymatic methods, and contained Weibel-Palade bodies in the cytoplasm when observed by transmission electron microscopy. Both of these are specific markers for endothelial cells. [^{3}H]-Thymidine autoradiography revealed uptake by the nuclei of mononuclear endothelial cells, but not by the multinuclei of variant cells. This ruled out the possibility of intracytoplasmic nuclear multiplication without cell division.

IN VIVO PRESENCE OF VARIANT ENDOTHELIAL CELLS IN HUMAN AORTA

Endothelial cells of aortae from infants and children were small, round and regular in size when observed by scanning electron microscopy (Fig. 14.3).

In young adults in their twenties, large endothelial cells were occasionally seen. In adults, colonies of giant endothelial cells were scattered throughout the aorta (Fig. 14.3). The giant endothelial cells were extremely large, occasionally 10 times as large as the surrounding typical small ones. Advanced atherosclerotic lesions, such as fibrous plaques and calcified lesions, were almost invariably covered by large and giant endothelial cells. The *in vivo* presence of multinuclei in variant endothelial cells was also confirmed by transmission electron microscopy.

MULTINUCLEATED VARIANT ENDOTHELIAL CELLS ARE WELL CORRELATED WITH ATHEROSCLEROSIS AND LESS WITH AGEING

The ratio of variant endothelial cell to total endothelial cell numbers was analyzed in relation to atherosclerotic index (Gore & Tajada 1957) and age. Atherosclerotic index ranged from 0.01 in a 14-year-old boy to 21.17 in an 81-year-old man. The variant endothelial cell ratio from primary culture was significantly correlated with the severity of atherosclerosis (Fig. 14.4). However, the relationship between variant endothelial cell ratio and ageing was not as significant as that to atherosclerotic index.

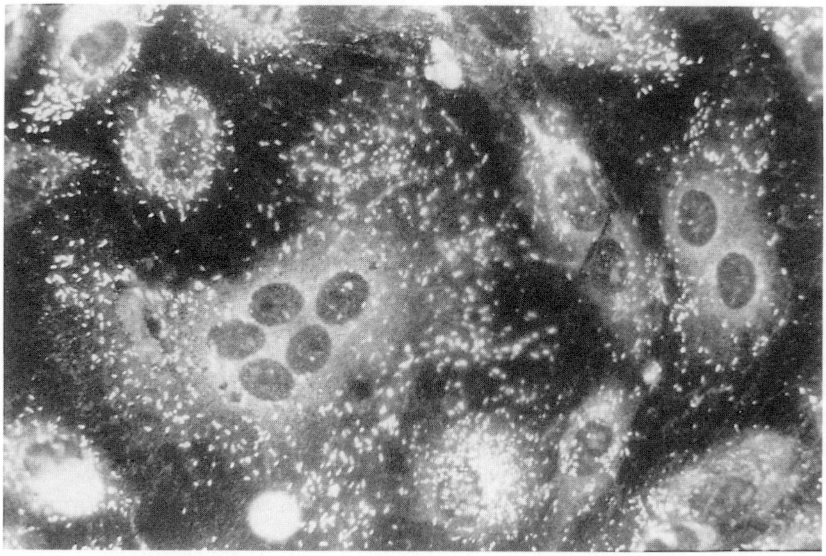

Fig. 14.2 Endothelial cells in primary culture from the aorta of diabetic patient, which are positive for von Willebrand factor (vWF). Multinucleated giant endothelial cells with 5 nuclei are positive for vWF as well as the surrounding typical endothelial cells.

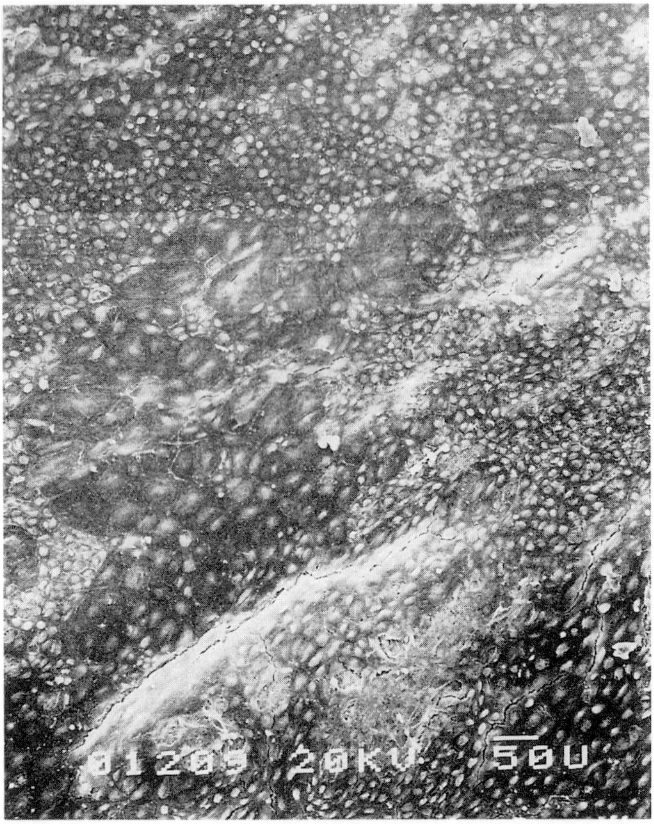

Fig. 14.3 Colony of giant endothelial cells are seen in the centre lying on the intima-thickened aorta from a 69-year-old male, which are surrounded by the small typical endothelial cells.

MORPHOGENESIS AND THE ROLE OF VARIANT ENDOTHELIAL CELLS

The *in vivo* presence of colonies made up of giant cells gave rise to questions regarding their mechanism of formation. As intracytoplasmic nuclear multiplication without cell division could be ruled out, an adhesive mechanism seemed more probable, which might possibly be caused by injury to the cell membrane. Numerous factors are known to cause endothelial injury, such as mechanical, chemical, toxic, viral or immunological agents, extracellular matrices and more recently cytokines (Jorgensen et al 1986). Since enlarged cells with or without multinuclei are often formed *in vitro* as they cease growing, senescence seemed to contribute to the formation of variant endothelial cells to some extent. However, the exact morphogenic process and the role of variant endothelial cells in various vascular diseases remain unclear.

INCREASED PERMEABILITY CAUSED BY ENDOTHELIAL INJURY

Most investigations of endothelial permeability have studied capillary and venular endothelium obtained from tissue affected by diabetic retinopathy and nephropathy, while studies of large artery endothelium are less frequent.

PERMEABILITY IN LARGE ARTERIES

Schwartz and colleagues (1978) have carried out studies of transendothelial passage using Evans' Blue dye. When the dye was injected intravenously, a characteristic and consistent pattern of uptake was obtained. They showed that the areas of increased permeability might represent areas of spontaneous haemodynamic injury (Caplan et al 1974). In some instances, dead or severely injured cells were partially or completely lifted into the lumen and occasional microthrombi were also noted. In silver nitrate-stained Häutchen preparations of endothelium, the injured or dead cells show intense silver staining and such cells were found much more often in blue areas than those in nonstained areas (Gerrity et al 1977).

It has been reported that oxygen radicals are synthesized in endothelial cells, and these cells are extremely sensitive to the cytotoxic effect of active oxygen radicals. In order to protect endothelial cells from injury, oxygen radicals are scavenged by the endothelial cells themselves. The glutathione redox cycle, one of the scavenger mechanisms for oxygen radicals, is

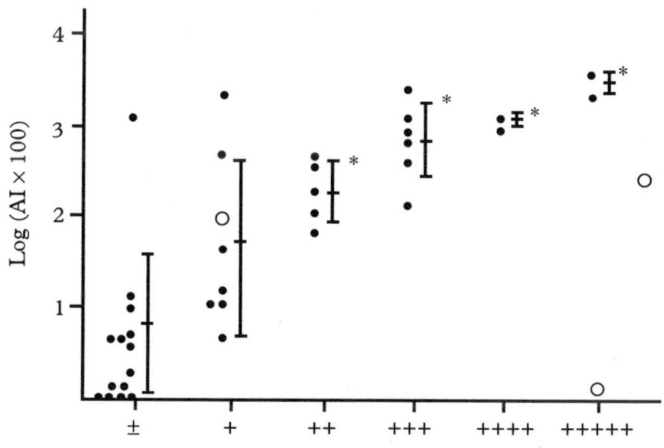

Fig. 14.4 Scattergram of atherogenic index (AI) and the degree of variant endothelial cells. Lines show means ± SD. The number of concomitant variant endothelial cells is graded as follows: ± = 0-5; + = 5-10; ++ = 10-15; +++ = 15-30; and ++++ = >30. Cases marked by open circle indicate a specific form of arteritis, polyarteritis nodosum. *Statistical significance:* *p <0.01 versus ± grade.

impaired in high glucose conditions. This may therefore be associated with a potentiation of oxygen radical-induced endothelial cell injury in diabetics (Kashiwagi et al 1993).

PERMEABILITY IN CAPILLARIES

Diabetic retinopathy

Retinopathy is the most common form of the vascular damage in diabetic patients and the pathophysiological defect in diabetic retinopathy appears to lie at the level of the retinal capillaries. Two general categories of retinopathy exist: nonproliferative retinopathy and proliferative retinopathy. Nonproliferative retinopathy can include venous abnormalities, microaneurysms, and retinal haemorrhage, oedema and exudates. This may progress to proliferative retinopathy, characterized by neovascularization, glial proliferation and vitreo-retinal traction (Olesky 1992). Probably, the earliest retinal change is increased capillary permeability. This abnormality can be readily reversed by effective glycaemic control, but the relationship of this form of capillary permeability to retinopathy is unknown. Oedema of the retina is caused by abnormal capillary permeability and ischaemia.

Retinal studies in streptozotocin-induced diabetic rats have revealed that endothelial cell tight junction permeability to lanthanum and luminal surface area were normal. However, several alterations in the diabetic retinal microvessels were observed: abnormal membrane turnover, an alteration in endothelial cell luminal membrane composition, a change in pericyte-endothelial cell interaction and alteration in extracellular matrix turnover (Caldwell & Slapnick 1992). A glucose-intolerant genetically obese (fa/fa) rat may be a suitable model for studying the pathophysiology of ocular complications. In this rat, retinal microangiopathy is observed, which is characterized by an increase in focal thickenings and in nodules of the basement membrane, an increase in pinocytic activity indicative of changes in vascular permeability, and an increase in the number of intercellular endothelial junctions (Dosso et al 1990).

The primary pathogenic events underlying the changes of nonproliferative retinopathy in human diabetics are unclear, but loss of supporting capillary pericytes, endothelial proliferation and hyperviscosity with red cell aggregation, together or alone, have all been proposed.

Diabetic nephropathy

Kidney disease is common, and renal failure is one of the major causes of death in diabetes. The dominant form of diabetic nephropathy is microvascular disease, affecting the renal glomerulus (Olesky 1992). A number of distinct morphologic and functional abnormalities characterize diabetic glomerulopathy, one of which is the hyalinosis lesion synonymous to exudative lesion or fibrin cap (Barrie et al 1952; Hall 1952). The initial change characteristic of this lesion is the accumulation of hyaline eosinophilic homogeneous material between endothelial cells and the glomerular basement membrane of the capillary loops (Olson 1992). This lesion is not specific for diabetic nephropathy, although it is seen in approximately 60% of diabetic kidneys (Bloodworth 1978). The pathogenesis of the lesion is not well understood, although its early development has been associated with endothelial injury and possible haemodynamic alterations. Its prevalence in diabetic kidneys increases with the severity of the nephropathy and correlates with the degree of arteriosclerosis, and it has been suggested that it is associated with ischaemia (Bloodworth 1978; Nakamoto et al 1980).

ABNORMAL FUNCTION OF HUMAN ENDOTHELIAL CELLS

Among the many functions of human vascular endothelium which can be altered, in this section we will specifically discuss the qualitative and quantitative changes in PGI_2 and endothelin synthesis in relation to atherosclerosis and ageing. Endothelial cells were cultured from human aortas obtained from infants through to elderly subjects as previously mentioned (Tokunaga et al 1989).

PROSTACYCLIN STAINING ON TISSUE SECTIONS BY THE ABC METHOD

Blood vessels are a major source of the antithrombotic agent, prostacyclin (Moncada et al 1976). This major prostaglandin (PG) product of arachidonic acid metabolism in the vascular wall is synthesized primarily by the endothelium. Recent advances in immunohistochemical techniques have made it possible to determine the location and degree of PGI_2 synthesis using the ABC method (Harold et al 1988). Generally, endothelial cells from young subjects were intensely positive for PGI_2. Endothelial cells from the aorta of a 24-year-old male subject revealed less immunoreactivity than those from younger subjects. Endothelial cells from subjects over 30 years of age revealed weak staining, except for a 73-year-old female showing moderate staining intensity. Some of the smooth muscle cells in the diffusely thickened intima or in atherosclerotic lesions were also faintly positive for PGI_2, but no medial smooth muscle cells were positive in any of the subjects.

DIFFERENCE IN PROSTACYCLIN SYNTHESIS BETWEEN YOUNG, MIDDLE-AGED AND ELDERLY SUBJECTS

Fifteen subjects were selected for examination of PGI_2 synthesis in relation to age. They were divided into 3 groups each spanning 3 decades and were designated as young, middle-aged and elderly groups, respectively. The stable end-metabolite of prostacyclin, 6-keto-$PGF_{1\alpha}$, released into the supernatant of the cultured cells was measured with a radioimmunoassay kit. Although PGI_2 synthesis markedly decreased with cell passage, the relative synthetic rate between donor ages was maintained during the course of passages. Analysis was carried out at the 5th to the 7th passage. The young group synthesized the greatest amount of PGI_2, the middle-aged group less, and the elderly group least (Fig. 14.5). The difference was statistically significant between the young and the other 2 groups, but did not attain significance between middle-aged and elderly groups (Tokunaga et al 1991).

Recent studies have demonstrated that atherosclerotic vascular tissue and serum from elderly people generate less PGI_2 (Sinzinger et al 1979, Umeda et al 1989). An age-related decline in PGI_2 synthesis was clearly demonstrated by our biosynthetic and immunohistological analyses (Tokunaga et al 1991), and reduced PGI_2 production by the vascular wall can therefore be proposed as one possible pathogenic mechanism of atherosclerosis. The immunohistological method clearly demonstrated that not only endothelial cells but also intimal smooth muscle cells, to a lesser degree, were immunoreactive to PGI_2. This immunohistological

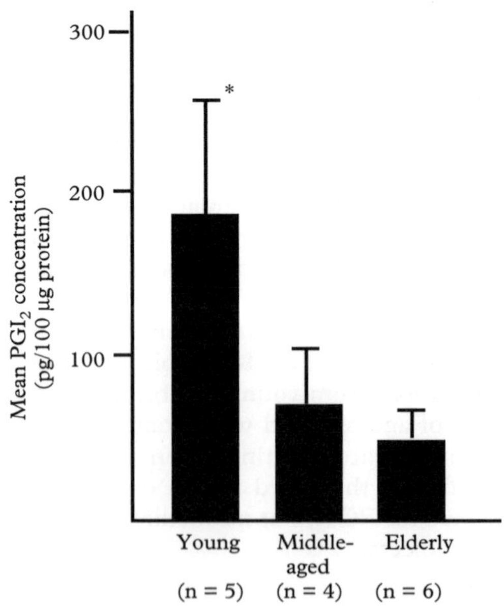

Fig. 14.5 Prostacyclin (PGI_2) synthesis by aortic endothelial cells from young, middle-aged and elderly subjects. Aortic endothelial cells from the young group released the largest amount of PGI_2. Endothelial cells from the middle-aged group released less PGI_2 followed by the elderly group which released the least amount of PGI_2. *Statistical significance:* *$p < 0.01$ for young versus middle-aged or elderly groups.

demonstration supports previous reports that vascular smooth muscle cells synthesized PGI_2, though the quantity was not as large as that synthesized by endothelial cells. Combined PGI_2 immunostaining analysis on the aortic tissue sections with PGI_2 bioassay by the cultured aortic endothelial cells revealed a higher productivity of young endothelial cells and the age-related decline in PGI_2 productivity. It is thus concluded that a decreased capability of PGI_2 synthesis with age could play an important role in the development and advancement of thrombosis and atherosclerosis.

ENDOTHELIN IMMUNOSTAINING OF AORTA

ET, a 21-amino acid peptide purified from the supernatant of endothelial cell culture, is a novel and potent vasoconstrictor (Yanagisawa et al 1988). Genomic DNA analysis of ET has revealed that there is an ET gene family comprising 3 types (Hartter & Woloszczuk 1989; Ishida et al 1989). ET-1 exists in many organs, e.g. lung, kidney and brain, and has various biological functions including vasoconstriction (Itoh et al 1988; Koseki et al 1989). The functions of ET-2 and ET-3, except for vasoconstriction, have not been fully elucidated.

Human aorta was obtained at autopsy (<2-h postmortem) from subjects ranging in age from an aborted foetus to elderly. Specimens were fixed in either conventional 10% formalin or 3% paraformaldehyde. After deparaffinization, 4-μm thick sections were subjected to an immunohistochemical examination for ET-1. Aortic endothelial cells of the fetus were ovoid in shape and not immunoreactive to anti-ET-1 antibody. Medial smooth muscle cells from the fetus were negative. However, endothelial cells in the vasa vasorum were positive with anti-ET-1. The aortic endothelial cells and smooth muscle cells from adolescent subjects were positive for ET-1 (Fig. 14.6). The immunoreactivity of ET-1 did not decrease with ageing, and was as intense as that of a 20-year-old subject even in the most elderly subject. The intensity of immunoreactive ET-1 was always much greater in the endothelial cells than that in the smooth muscle cells (Tokunaga et al 1992).

Hybridization signals by ^{35}S-labelled antisense probe RNA were most intense on the endothelial cells from the elderly subject. Foetal aortic endothelial cells revealed the least signal, indicating a developing but still immature gene translation system. Interestingly, milder but positive signals were noted in most of the intimal and medial smooth muscle cells and appeared distinct when less stringent hybridization conditions were employed.

ET-1 BIOSYNTHESIS ASSAY BY ENDOTHELIAL AND SMOOTH MUSCLE CELLS

Human aortic endothelial cells were cultured by a method which has been previously described (Tokunaga et al 1989). ET-1 released into the

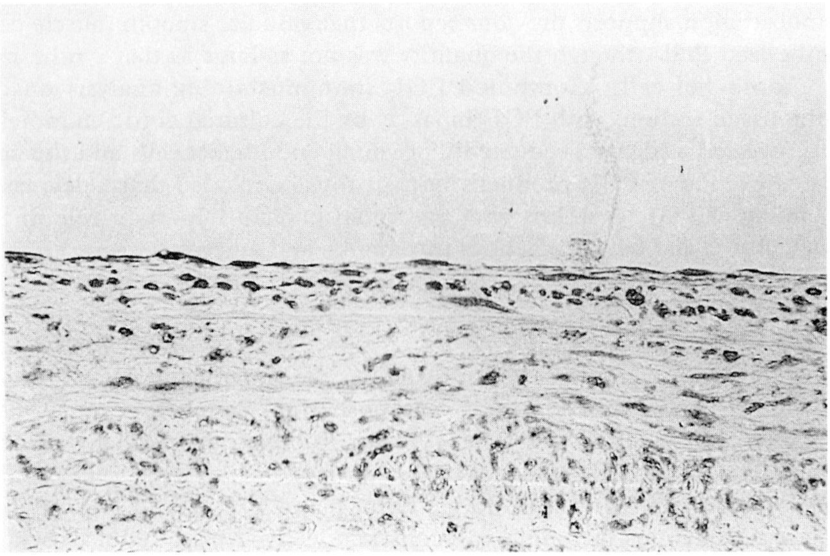

Fig. 14.6 Endothelin-1 immunostaining of aortic cells from a 14-year-old male. Intense immunostaining was noted in the endothelial cell layer and lesser immunoreaction occurred in intimal or medial smooth muscle cells.

supernatant of the cultured endothelial cells was measured by radioimmunoassay. ET-1 synthesis was invariably low in subjects under the age of 50 years. ET-1 synthesis by the older group over 50 years of age was significantly ($p < 0.05$) higher than that of the younger group (Fig. 14.7). Smooth muscle cells appeared to synthesize ET-1, but their synthetic rate was much less than that of endothelial cells. The immunostaining intensity of endothelial cells on aortic tissue sections from elderly subjects was equal to that from the younger subjects. This is a sharp contrast to PGI_2 synthesis in that the aortic endothelial cells of the young group synthesized the largest amount of prostacyclin *in vitro* and were most intensely immunostained, with a progressive decrease in the older groups.

CULTURE MODEL SYSTEM SIMULATING VASCULAR WALL

Most vascular research using cell culture has been performed in a conventional 2-dimensional culture system in dishes. Recently, a number of studies have been performed in an attempt to elucidate endothelial cell behaviour using a 3-dimensional culture system. Foltz et al (1982) and Furie et al (1984) improved an amnion model system, originally designed by Russo et al (1981), and developed an *in vitro* vessel model that consisted of amnion connective tissue lined by cultured endothelial cells instead of amnion epithelium. Migliorisi et al (1987) and Yamada et al (1992) used the same model system and showed leucocytic interaction across the endothelium. However, this model is actually a 2-dimensional model system.

A practical 3-dimensional model system was developed using collagen gel matrix (Yang et al 1980). Smooth muscle cells, which are first grown and pelleted by centrifugation, are gently mixed with and embedded in acidic type I collagen solution. The mixture of cells and collagen gel is seeded on a nitrocellulose filter dish which is specifically designed for cell culture, and the dish is placed in a larger plastic dish, in which culture medium is poured. The medium gradually diffuses into the acidic collagen solution and turns its pH neutral, which allows the collagen solution to solidify. The solidified collagen gels, in which smooth muscle cells are embedded, are ready for endothelial culture. The endothelial cells are seeded on the solidified collagen gels (Fig. 14.8). If leucocytes are placed in the upper chamber, interaction between leucocytes and endothelial cells, leucocytes and smooth muscle cells, and even endothelial cells and smooth muscle cells can be sequentially observed (Fig. 14.9). This model can also be used for transport studies of various molecular sizes.

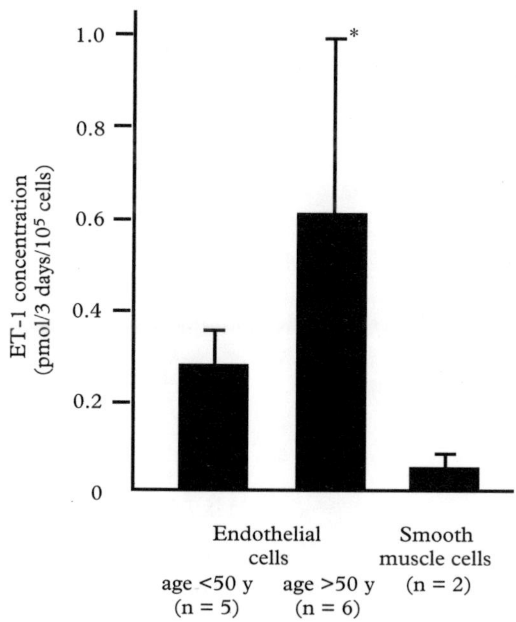

Fig. 14.7 Endothelin-1 (ET-1) biosynthesis (mean ± SD) by cultured human aortic endothelial cells obtained from subjects of different ages. ET-1 synthesis was invariably low in the subjects under the age of 50 years, but was significantly increased (* $p < 0.05$) in those over the age of 50 years. Smooth muscle cells produced minimal ET-1. Values are given as means ± SD.

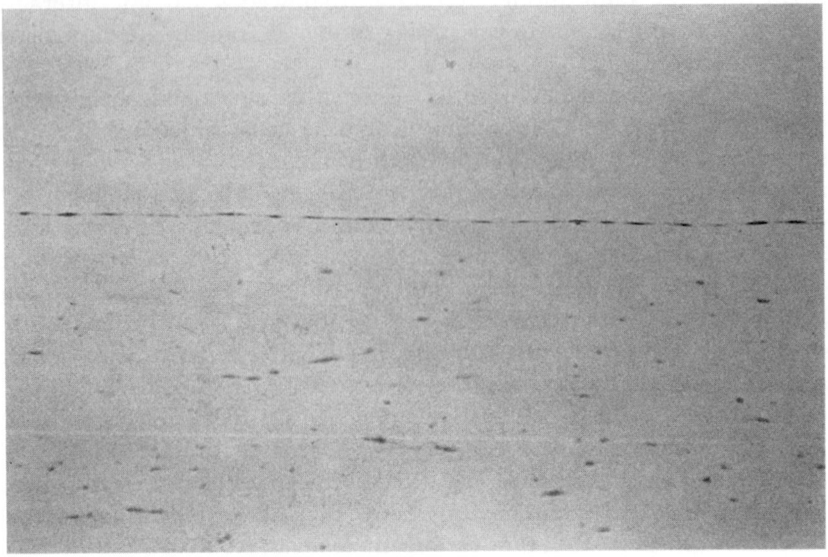

Fig. 14.8 Three-dimensional culture model system. The endothelial cells are cultured on a collagen gel matrix in which smooth muscle cells are preliminarily grown.

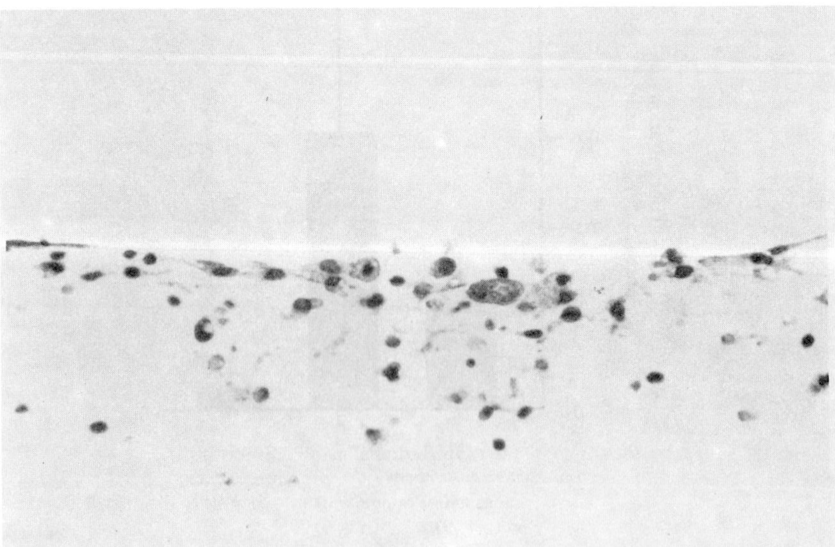

Fig. 14.9 Interaction of endothelial cells in a 3-dimensional culture model system with leucocytes being poured in the upper chamber. The leucocytes disrupt the endothelial cell layer and migrate underneath.

CONCLUSION

Human endothelial cells were analyzed using a cell culture technique and electronmicroscopy. The presence of multinucleated endothelial cells, called variant endothelial cells, were found *in vitro* and *in vivo*. Variant endothelial cells are thought to be formed by adhesion of activated or injured cells. Endothelial functions generally decline with age, as seen with the reduction in PGI_2 synthesis. However, ET-1 synthesis in endothelial cells goes contrary to this decline: it is invariably low in subjects under 50 years of age but is significantly higher in those aged over 50 years.

In diabetes, blood vessels are systematically affected, and retinal, renal and cerebral microangiopathies play an especially important role in the prognosis of the disease. The latter two microangiopathies are often fatal. For future detailed studies of the vascular changes in various conditions including diabetes, an *in vitro* 3-dimensional culture system is proposed.

REFERENCES

Antonov M A, Nikolaeva M A, Klueva T S et al 1986 Primary culture of endothelial cells from atherosclerotic human aorta. Part 1. Identification, morphological and ultrastructural characteristics of two endothelial cell subpopulations. Atherosclerosis 59: 1-19

Barrie H J, Askanazy C L, Smith G W 1952 More glomerular changes in diabetics. Can Med Assoc J 66: 428-435

Bloodworth J M B 1978 A re-evaluation of diabetic glomerulosclerosis 50 years after the discovery of insulin. Hum Pathol 9: 439-453

Caldwell R B, Slapnick S M 1992 Freeze-fracture and lanthanum studies of the retinal microvasculature in diabetic rats. Invest Ophthalmol Vis Sci 33: 1610-1619

Caplan B A, Gerrity R G, Schwartz C J 1974 Endothelial cell morphology in focal areas *in vitro* Evans blue uptake in the young pig aorta. I. Quantitative light microscopic findings. Exp Mol Pathol 21: 102-117

Dosso A, Rungger B E, Rohner J F et al 1990 Ocular complications in the old and glucose-intolerant genetically obese (fa/fa) rat. Diabetologia. 33:137-144

Foltz C M, Russo R G, Siegel G P et al 1982 Interactions of tumor cells with whole basement membrane in the presence or absence of endothelium. Prog Clin Biol Res 89: 353-371

Fryer D G, Birnbaum G, Luttrell C N 1966 Human endothelium in cell culture. J Atheroscler Res 6: 151-163

Furie M B, Cramer E B, Naprstek B L et al 1984 Cultured endothelial cell monolayers that restrict the transendothelial passage of macromolecules and electrical current. J Cell Biol 98: 1033-1041

Gerrity R G, Richardson M, Somer J B et al 1977 Endothelial morphology in areas of *in vivo* Evans blue uptake in the aorta of young pigs. II. Ultrastructure of the intima in areas of differing permeability to proteins. Am J Pathol 89: 313-334

Glassberg M K, Bern M M, Coughlin C C et al 1982 Cultured endothelial cells derived from the human iliac arteries. In Vitro 18: 859-866

Gore I, Tajada C 1957 The quantitative appraisal of atherosclerosis. Am J Pathol 33: 875-882

Hall G M F 1952 The significance of atheroma of the renal arteries in Kimmerlstiel-Wilson's syndrome. J Pathol Bacteriol 64: 103-120

Harold J G, Siegel R J, Fitzgerald G A et al 1988 Differential prostacyclin production by human umbilical vasculature. Arch Pathol Lab Med 112: 43-46

Hartter E, Woloszczuk W 1989 Radioimmunoassay of endothelin-1. Lancet 1: 909

Hoshi H, McKeehan W L 1986 Isolation, growth requirements, cloning, prostacyclin production and life-span of human adult endothelial cells in low serum culture medium. In Vitro 22: 51-56

Ishida N, Tsujioka K, Tomoi M et al 1989 Differential activities of two distinct endothelin family peptide on ileum and coronary artery. FEBS Lett 247: 337-340

Itoh Y, Yanagisawa M, Ohkubo S et al 1988 Cloning and sequence analysis of cDNA encoding the precursor of a human endothelium-derived vasoconstrictor peptide, endothelin: identity of human and porcine endothelin. FEBS Lett 231: 440-444

Jorgensen A G T, Larsen R L, Kinlough-Rathbone B G et al 1986 Injury to cultured endothelial cells by thrombin-stimulated platelets. Lab Invest 54: 408-415

Kashiwagi A, Hidaka H, Shigeta Y 1993 Abnormal radical scavenger function and cell injury in endothelial cell cultured in high glucose media. Journal of the Japanese Atherosclerosis Society 21: 373-377

Koseki C, Imai M, Hirata M et al 1989 Autoradiographic distribution in rat tissues of binding sites for endothelin: a neuropeptide. Am J Physiol 256: R858-866

Migliorisi G, Folkes E, Pawlowski N et al 1987 *In vitro* studies of human monocyte migration across endothelium in response to leukotriene B4 and f-Met-Leu-Phe. Am J Pathol 127: 157-167

Moncada S, Gryglewski R J, Bunting S et al 1976 An enzyme isolated from arteries transforms prostaglandin endoperoxides to an unstable substance that inhibits platelet aggregation. Nature 263: 663-665

Nakamoto Y, Takazaki E, Hayakawa H et al 1980 Intrarenal microaneurysms in diabetic nephropathy. Lab Invest 42: 433-439

Olesky J 1992 Diabetes mellitus. In: Wyngaarden J B et al (eds) Cecil Textbook of Medicine. Saunders, Philadelphia, pp 1307-1308

Olson J L 1992 Diabetes mellitus. In: Heptinstall R H (ed.) Pathology of the Kidney, Vol. III. Little Brown, Boston, pp 1722-1724

Repin V S, Dolgov O E, Zaikina I D et al 1984 Heterogeneity of endothelium in human aorta. A quantitative analysis by scanning electron microscopy. Atherosclerosis 50: 35-52

Russo R G, Liotta L A, Thorgeirsson U et al 1981 Polymorphonuclear leukocyte migration through human amnion membrane. J Cell Biol 91: 459-467

Schwartz C J, Gerrioty R G, Lewis L J 1978 Arterial endothelial structure and function with particular reference to permeability. Paoletti R & Gotto Jr A M (eds) Atherosclerosis Review, 3rd ed. Raven Press, New York, pp 109-124

Sinzinger H, Feigel W, Silberbauer K 1979 Prostacyclin generation in atherosclerotic arteries. Lancet 2: 469

Tokunaga O, Fan J, Watanabe T 1989 Atherosclerosis- and age-related multinucleated variant endothelial cells in primary culture from human aorta. Am J Pathol 135: 967-976

Tokunaga O, Yamada T, Fan J et al 1991 Age-related decline in prostacyclin synthesis by human aortic endothelial cells. Am J Pathol 138: 941-949

Tokunaga O, Fan J, Watanabe T et al 1992 Endothelin. Immunohistologic localization in aorta and biosynthesis by cultured human aortic endothelial cells. Lab Invest 67: 210-217

Umeda F, Inoguchi T, Nawata H 1989 Reduced stimulatory activity on prostacylin production by cultured endothelial cells in serum from aged and diabetic patients. Atherosclerosis 75: 61-66

Yamada T, Fan J, Shimokama T et al 1992 Induction of fatty streak-like lesions *in vitro* using a culture model system simulating arterial intima. Am J Pathol 141: 1435-1444

Yanagisawa M, Kurihara K, Tomobe Y et al 1988 Endothelin: a novel potent vasoconstrictor peptide produced by vascular endothelial cells. Nature 332: 411-415

Yang J, Guizman R, Richards J et al 1980 Primary culture of mouse mammary tumor epithelial cells embedded in collagen gels. In Vitro 16: 502-506

15

Angiogenesis in diabetes

H. Ito

INTRODUCTION

Angiogenesis, the growth of vessels and their components (e.g. endothelial cells, pericytes, extracellular matrix) has been gaining increasing attention from a number of different points of views, because of the fundamental role of this process in reproduction, embryonic development, wound healing, and pathological conditions such as tumour growth, tumour metastasis formation, diabetic retinopathy, rheumatoid arthritis and atherosclerosis (Folkman & Shing 1992).

Angiogenesis can be beneficial in the formation of collateral circulation under conditions of limited blood supply, ischaemia, induced by stenosis or occlusion of vessels in various organs or tissues. Cardiac performance might be improved by capillary growth in the hypertension-induced hypertrophic heart. On the other hand, prevention of capillary growth might enable regulation of irregular capillary growth in conditions such as proliferative retinopathy, rheumatoid arthritis or growth of tumours.

Recent progress in angiogenesis research is briefly reviewed in this article, especially in relation to diabetes mellitus. Possible new therapeutic modalities are discussed from the viewpoint of angiogenesis regulation.

REGULATION OF ANGIOGENESIS

Angiogenesis is a complex process, involving five major steps (Fig. 15.1): 1) proteolysis of the basement membrane by proteases secreted by endothelial cells, which alters cell adhesiveness to the basement membrane and adjacent cells; 2) proliferation of endothelial cells; 3) migration of endothelial cells; 4) tube formation; and 5) fusion of the tube at its leading edge to form a loop. Further sprouting of cells then develops from the distal portion of the loop to form secondary loops and a new capillary network (Forrester 1987). The various steps in this process of angiogenesis is highly regulated.

Recent advances in research have revealed specific molecules which either stimulate or inhibit angiogenesis. However, details of the interactions of these molecules with opposing functions have not well elucidated. Table 15.1 summarizes the properties of representative angiogenic polypeptides. Basic fibroblast growth factor (bFGF), acidic FGF (aFGF), epidermal growth factor (EGF), vascular endothelial cell growth factor (VEGF), platelet-derived growth factor (PDGF), transforming growth factor-α (TGF-α) and insulin-like growth factor I (IGF-I) are mitogenic for endothelial cells. IGF-I is mitogenic specifically for microvessel endothelial cells and not for macrovessel endothelial cells (Bar et al 1988; King et al 1985). All these molecules (except VEGF, whose effect remains to be determined) also stimulate endothelial cell migration. Tumour necrosis factor-α (TNF-α) and transforming growth factor-β (TGF-β) inhibit endothelial cell proliferation. Angiogenin, TGF-β and TNF-α have no effect on endothelial cell migration, but the latter two molecules stimulate migration of monocytes, including macrophages.

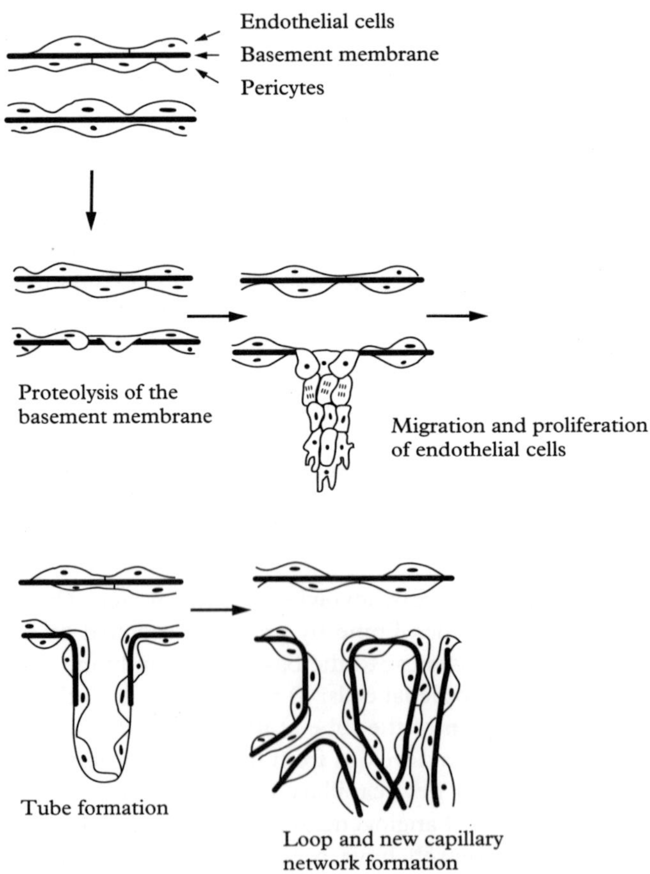

Fig. 15.1 Sequential steps in the formation of a new capillary (angiogenesis).

Table 15.1 Angiogenic polypeptides.

Angiogenic factor	Molecular weight	Stimulatory effect on endothelial cells	
		proliferation	migration
Acidic fibroblast frowth factor (aFGF)	18,000	+	+
Basic fibroblast growth factor (bFGF)	16,400	+	+
Epidermal growth factor (EGF)		+	+
Vascular endothelial cell growth factor (VEGF)	45,000	+	?
Platelet-derived growth factor (PDGF)	45,000	+	+
Transforming growth factor-α (TGF-α)	5,500	+	+
Insulin-like growth factor I (IGF-I)	7,600	+	+
Angiogenin	14,100	0	0
Transforming growth factor-β (TGF-β)	25,000	–	0 (+ for monocytes)
Tumour necrosis factor-α (TNF-α)	55,000	–	0 (+ for monocytes)

+ = stimulates; – = inhibits; 0 = no effect; ? = not determined.

Activated macrophages have known to secrete several angiogenic factors, and the angiogenic action of these two factors can therefore be explained by their stimulatory activities for monocyte migration. Although the precise mechanisms of how angiogenin stimulates angiogenesis is unknown, it has a unique ribonucleolytic activity (Shapiro et al 1986) essential for angiogenesis. It also stimulates prostacyclin secretion (Bicknell & Vallee 1989) and phospholipase C activity (Bicknell & Vallee 1988) in endothelial cells. These activities of angiogenin might correlate with its potency for neovascularisation.

In addition to the above-mentioned polypeptides, there are nonpeptide molecules which have also been demonstrated to stimulate angiogenesis. These include: prostacyclin (Ohtsu et al 1988), prostaglandin E_1 (Ziche et al 1982), prostaglandin E_2 (Form & Auerbach 1983), leukotriene C_4 (Kanayasu et al 1989), nicotinamide (Kull et al 1987), adenosine (Dusseau et al 1986), high glucose concentrations (Hayashi et al 1991) and advanced glycation end-products (Tezuka et al 1993).

ANGIOGENESIS AND DISEASES

Folkman and Klagsbrun (1987) proposed a new entity for certain morbid states, which they termed ‘angiogenic disease’. Some of these morbid states were previously thought to be unrelated, but persistent angiogenesis appears to be the dominant pathology. These conditions include: solid neoplastic tumours; chronic rheumatoid arthritis; haemangioma and angiofibroma; psoriasis; capillary proliferation within atherosclerosis; and various ophthalmological diseases, including proliferative diabetic retinopathy, retrolental fibroplasia, rubeosis iridis, retinitis proliferans due to sickle cell disease, obstruction of the central retinal artery or vein, senile disciform macular degeneration and various other ischaemic diseases.

The process of angiogenesis is analogous in these morbid states, although it is not clear whether the same angiogenic factors have a role in the pathological growth of capillary blood vessels for each morbid state. Since understanding of the mechanisms involved in angiogenesis has progressed rapidly, it may be possible to develop new therapeutic modalities for these diseases in which capillary growth is insufficient, including delayed wound healing, chronic skin ulceration, insufficient development of collaterals in ischaemic heart disease and ischaemic peripheral vascular disease, and nonhealing fractures. At present, there are no effective therapeutic agents for these morbid states. Further progress in understanding the mechanisms of angiogenesis should provide new ideas for the treatment of these pathological conditions.

MECHANISMS OF NEW VESSEL FORMATION IN DIABETIC PATIENTS

Neovascularization of the retina is the major risk factor for severe visual loss in diabetic retinopathy, and decreases quality of life in diabetics patients profoundly. The growth of new capillary vessels in the retina involves alterations in the behaviour of retinal capillary endothelial cells. Systemic metabolic and haemodynamic abnormalities in diabetes (hyperglycaemia, hypercoagulability, dyslipidaemia, disturbance of microcirculation, hypertension, etc.) induce endothelial cell abnormalities in the retina.

The capillaries of the retina contain two types of cells: endothelial cells and intramural pericytes. Endothelial cells line the capillary lumen and form a permeability (blood-retinal) barrier. They produce and are surrounded by a basement membrane. Pericytes are selectively lost early in the course of diabetic retinopathy. The ratio of endothelial cells to

Table 15.2 Effect of high glucose levels on endothelial cell proliferation as a function of foetal bovine serum (FBS) concentration. Endothelial cells dissociated from bovine carotid artery were cultured in medium supplemented with various FBS concentrations and low or high glucose concentration for 6 days. The number of cells on the day following inoculation was $2.335 \pm 0.147 \times 10^4$ cells/well. Values are given as means ± SEM. Statistical significance: *$p < 0.05$, **$p < 0.01$ versus control. (Adapted from and reproduced with permission from Hayashi et al 1991)

FBS concentration (%)	No. of cells ($\times 10^4$/well) glucose 5.6 mmol/l	glucose 16.7 mmol/l	% of control
0.05	4.49 ± 0.35	7.79 ± 0.57**	173.3
0.10	7.50 ± 0.51	10.20 ± 1.16	136.6
0.25	13.52 ± 0.89	17.79 ± 0.70**	131.6
0.50	22.21 ± 2.11	26.65 ± 1.15*	120.0
1.00	34.77 ± 1.72	31.68 ± 0.71	91.1
10.00	56.33 ± 0.85	50.31 ± 1.99*	89.3

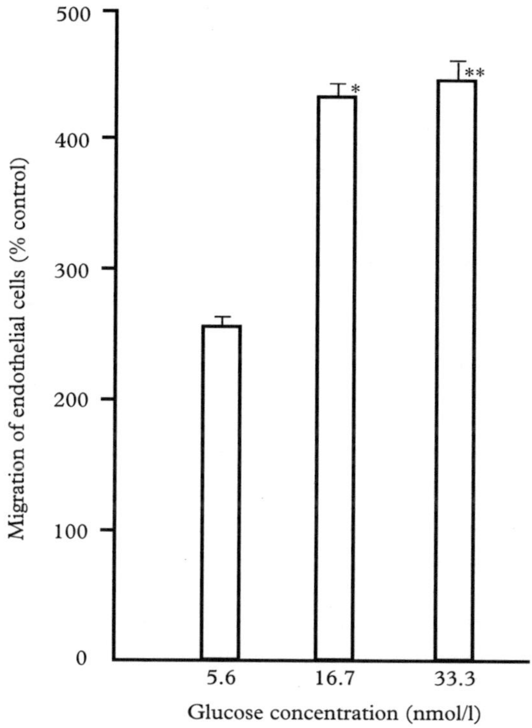

Fig. 15.2 Effects of glucose treatment on migration of endothelial cells. Endothelial cells derived from bovine carotid artery were pretreated with various concentrations of glucose for 6 days and endothelial cell migration was assayed by Boyden chamber method using 10% foetal bovine serum as a stimulator. Each value represents the mean ± SEM of 6 replicate wells. Treatment with high glucose significantly stimulated migration of endothelial cells (F ratio = 4.640, $p < 0.05$ by ANOVA; and *$p < 0.05$, **$p < 0.01$ versus glucose 5.6 mmol/l by Student's t-test). (Reproduced with permission from Hayashi et al 1991)

pericytes in normal retinal capillaries is 1:1. However, the ratio is increased to 1:4 after several years of diabetes and reaches 1:10 with an even longer duration of diabetes (Kuwabara & Cogan 1963). This specific loss of pericytes is one of the primary events contributing to the retinopathic process.

Breakdown of the blood-retinal barrier is another early feature of diabetic retinopathy. Dilatation and proliferation of endothelial cells occur in the capillaries where there is a loss of pericytes. Adjacent capillaries develop diminished perfusion and eventually become acellular tubes consisting solely of basement membrane (Wise et al 1971). Dilated capillaries develop microaneurysmal outpouchings (which are clusters of endothelial cells lacking pericytes), leak intravascular fluid and may eventually give rise to the growth of new capillaries (neovascularization-angiogenesis).

The precise mechanism of pericyte loss is still unclear. The specific localization of aldose reductase in pericytes (Akagi et al 1983; Gabbay 1972) suggests an important role for the polyol pathway, at least partly, in pericyte loss in diabetes. In fact, pericytes maintained in culture with medium containing a high glucose concentration have been demonstrated to undergo degenerative changes (Buzney et al 1977). However, further experimental and clinical studies will be necessary to confirm the relationship between pericyte loss and activation of the polyol pathway.

In vitro experiments by various authors (Orlidge & D'Amore 1987; Sato & Rifkind 1989) have shown that physical contact of endothelial cells and pericytes is necessary for pericytes to exhibit an inhibitory effect on endothelial cells proliferation. Furthermore, only when these cells are in contact do endothelial cells release the active form of TGF-β, which has been shown to inhibit endothelial cell proliferation (Antonelli-Orlidge et al 1989; Sato & Rifkind 1989). These results suggest that the loss of pericytes as a result of hyperglycaemia prevents the expression of active TGF-β by endothelial cells, which are then prone to proliferate and form microaneurysms and new vessels.

We have recently demonstrated that high glucose levels can also stimulate endothelial proliferation when cells are cultured in medium containing foetal bovine serum at concentrations of less than 0.5% (Table 15.2) [Hayashi et al

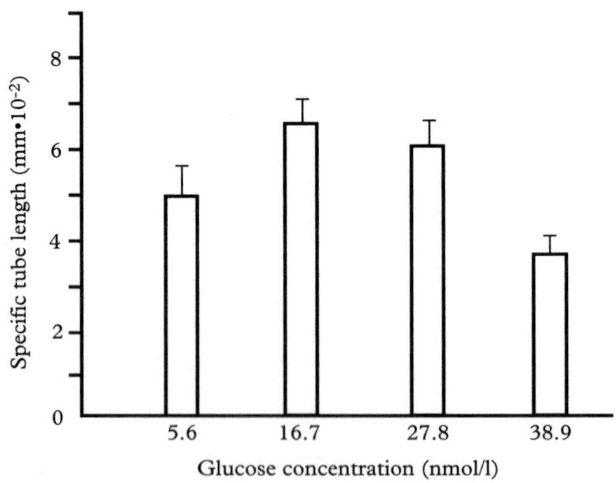

Fig. 15.3 Effect of various concentrations of glucose on tube formation of endothelial cells. Endothelial cells derived from bovine carotid artery were incubated within collagen gels with 2% foetal bovine serum containing various concentrations of glucose for 4 days and tube length per unit area (specific tube length) was measured using an image analyzer. Each value represents the mean ± SEM of 6 replicate wells. A significant difference was observed by ANOVA (F ratio = 3.803, $p < 0.05$), and the specific tube lengths in cultures containing glucose 16.7 and 27.8 mmol/l were significantly longer than that in culture containing glucose 5.6 mmol/l ($p < 0.05$ by Student's t test). (Reproduced with permission from Hayashi et al 1991)

Table 15.3 Endothelial cell growth modulators identified in the retina and concentration changes in the eyes of diabetic animals. (Reproduced with permission from King et al 1993)

Endothelial cell growth modulaor identified in the retina	Concentration changes in the eyes of diabetic animals
Fibroblast growth factor (aFGF + bFGF)	↑ →
Epidermal growth factor (EGF)	→
Transforming growth factor-β (TGF-β)	↑
Platelet-derived growth factor (PDGF)	?
Insulin	→
Insulin-like growth factor I (IGF-I)	↑ →
Insulin-like growth factor II (IGF-II)	↑
Growth hormone (GH)	↑
Endothelial cell-stimulating angiogenesis factor (ECAF)	?
Tumour necrosis factor-α (TNF-α)	→
Vascular endothelial cell growth factor (VEGF)	?

↑ = increased; → = not changed; ? = unknown.

1991]. Elevated levels of glucose also stimulate both endothelial cell migration and tube formation (Figs 15.2 and 15.3) [Hayashi et al 1991]. In addition, high glucose levels and experimental diabetes increase membranous protein kinase C (PKC) activity, which represents the active pool of PKC, in retinal capillary endothelial cells (Lee et al 1989a) and in the retina (Lee et al 1989b). Since PKC activation has been considered as taking part in the effector mechanisms of various growth factors (e.g. FGF, PDGF, EGF and IGF-I) enhanced PKC activity might have a important role in endothelial cell proliferation and neovascularization in the diabetic retina.

The exact angiogenic factor, or factors, which is, or are, responsible for the development of neovascularization and fibrosis in the diabetic retina has, or have, not been identified. However, various types of growth factors have been identified in the retina and their concentrations measured in the diabetic eye (Table 15.3) [King et al 1993]. FGF polypeptides are considered to be some of most potent angiogenic factors. Two types of FGF, aFGF and bFGF, have been found in the retina. Both molecules have no signal sequence and are therefore considered to be released during cell destruction, e.g. following ischaemia. Their role in proliferative diabetic retinopathy is still unclear. However, several reports have demonstrated elevated bFGF levels in ocular fluid (Baird et al 1985) and vitreous (Sivalingam et al 1990) of diabetic patients with proliferative retinopathy. It is well known that ischaemia precedes the development of proliferative retinopathy and that neovascularization occurs at the border of the avascular area. As previously described, ischaemia can induce FGF release. Therefore, it is reasonable to postulate that FGF has some important role in the development of proliferative diabetic retinopathy. With respect to the cellular sources of FGF in the retina, capillary endothelial cells have been shown to produce bFGF (Schweigerer et al 1987b) and retinal pigment epithelial cells have been shown to produce

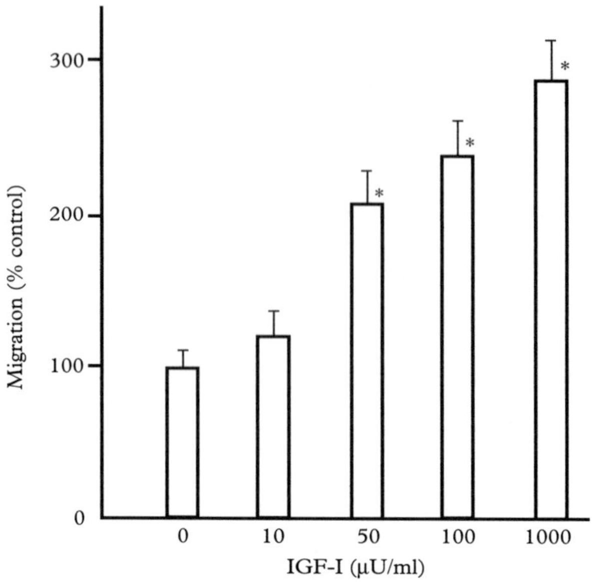

Fig. 15.4 Effects of various concentrations of insulin-like growth factor I (IGF-I) on endothelial migration. Migration of endothelial cells derived from bovine carotid artery was assayed by Boyden chamber method. Each value represents the mean ± SEM. A significant dose-dependent stimulation on cellular migration was found by ANOVA (F ratio = 18.84, $p < 0.01$) and by Student's t-test (*$p < 0.01$ versus control). (Reproduced with permission from Nakao-Hayashi et al 1992)

both aFGF and bFGF (Schweigerer et al 1987a). Furthermore, intravitreal injection of bFGF and the placement of chambers which release bFGF slowly have been demonstrated to cause retinal fibrovascular proliferation (Grant et al 1993). These results suggest that FGF might have an important role in the pathogenesis of proliferative diabetic retinopathy.

Growth hormone (GH) has been postulated as playing an important role in the development of proliferative diabetic retinopathy, since pituitary ablation can effectively treat proliferative retinopathy (Kohner et al 1972; Poulsen 1953). Most of the mitogenic actions of GH are mediated by IGF-I (Underwood & Van Wyke 1992). Although a majority of diabetic patients have normal serum IGF-I levels, elevated levels can be seen in diabetics with rapid accelerating proliferative retinopathy (Merimee et al 1983). A large population-based study has demonstrated that higher serum levels of IGF-I correlated with a higher frequency of proliferative diabetic retinopathy (Dills et al 1991). It has also been noted that in patients with preproliferative retinopathy who subsequently developed neovascularization serum IGF-I levels at the time of the first appearance of neovascularization were higher than those measured at 3 months before the development of neovascularization (Hyer et al 1989). Furthermore, intravitreal concentrations of IGF-I were higher in diabetics with proliferative retinopathy than in nondiabetic patients (Grant et al 1986). *In vitro* studies have demonstrated that IGF-I stimulates endothelial cell proliferation (King et al 1985), migration (Fig. 15.4) [Nakao-Hayashi et al 1992], tube formation (Fig. 15.5) [Nakao-Hayashi et al 1992] and production of proteases associated with basement membrane degradation (Grant & Guay 1991). Intravitreal injection of IGF-I and the placement of chambers from which IGF-I released slowly caused retinal fibrovascular proliferation in a similar manner to that previously noted with bFGF (Grant et al 1993). Taken together, these results also suggest that IGF-I might have some crucial role in the development of proliferative diabetic retinopathy.

TGF-β has been also postulated to have important role in the development of proliferative diabetic retinopathy. TGF-β has been found in the retina and is produced by retinal pigment epithelial cells (Glaser 1988). It has been recently reported that total TGF-β levels measured using a radioreceptor assay in vitreous were 3-times higher in patients with proliferative vitreoretinopathy than in patients without (Connor et al

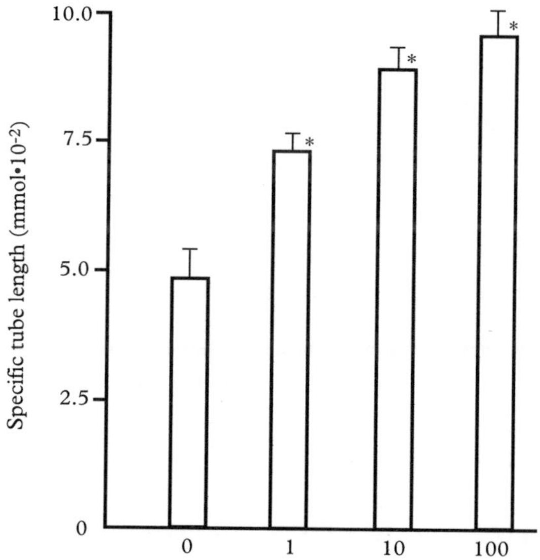

Fig. 15.5 Effects of various concentration of IGF-I on tube formation of endothelial cells. Endothelial cells derived from bovine carotid artery were cultured within collagen gels in culture medium containing 2% foetal bovine serum and various concentrations of IGF-I. The specific length, length of tubular structure per unit area, was determined on day 4 of culture using an image analyzer. Each value represents the mean ± SEM. A significant dose-response relationship was found by ANOVA (F ratio = 20.07, $p < 0.05$) and by Student's t-test (*$p < 0.001$ versus control). (Reproduced with permission from Nakao-Hayashi et al 1992)

1989). Since proliferative vitreoretinopathy frequently occur in advanced proliferative diabetic retinopathy, TGF-β may play a role in the development of proliferative diabetic retinopathy.

Endothelial cell-stimulating angiogenesis factor (ESAF) is a nonprotein angiogenic factor with a low molecular weight (approximately 400 daltons), which has been isolated from both retina and vitreous fluid (Taylor et al 1989). ESAF levels have been demonstrated to be higher in the anoxic retina than in the normal retina (Taylor et al 1986). ESAF activates prometalloproteinases and dissociates collagenase from its complex with tissue inhibitor of metalloproteinases (Weiss et al 1987). ESAF activity in vitreous aspirates of patients with extraretinal neovascularization appeared to be higher than those in vitreous humor taken from autopsied normal eyes (Taylor et al 1989). These findings suggest possible importance of ESAF in the development of proliferative diabetic retinopathy.

As described earlier, the disruption of the balance between factors stimulating and inhibiting angiogenesis plays a crucial role in the development of neovascularization. However, there are few reports available on angiogenic inhibitors in the ocular tissues. It has been reported that vitreous from normal eyes inhibited angiogenesis (Raymond & Jacobson 1982). Several molecules which inhibit endothelial cell proliferation have been partially purified from vitreous (Jacobson et al 1985; Raymond & Jacobson 1982). Recently, Taylor and Weiss (1985) also partially purified an inhibitor of angiogenesis from vitreous, which proved to be a 5,700-dalton glycoprotein and an inhibitor of collagenase activity. The nature of this inhibitor is interesting, because at least one of the angiogenic inhibitors derived from cartilage, which also inhibits angiogenesis in vitreous, has been identified as molecule with high homology to tissue inhibitor of metalloprteinases (Moses et al 1990). An angiogenic inhibitor with molecular weight of less than 100,000 daltons has also been partially purified from the ocular lens (Williams et al 1984). However, no inhibitor has been completely purified and chemically identified. Thus, the role of angiogenic inhibitor(s) in the development of proliferative diabetic retinopathy has not been clearly established.

THERAPEUTIC APPLICATION OF FGF FOR ISCHAEMIC DISEASES

Diabetes mellitus is one of major risk factors for cardiovascular disease, which is a major cause of morbidity in patients with diabetes mellitus. Despite recent advances in invasive therapeutic modalities for atherosclerotic cardiovascular diseases, these techniques are often not able to be applied to diabetics because of the intensive and diffuse development of atherosclerosis. One of the potential therapeutic approaches is to

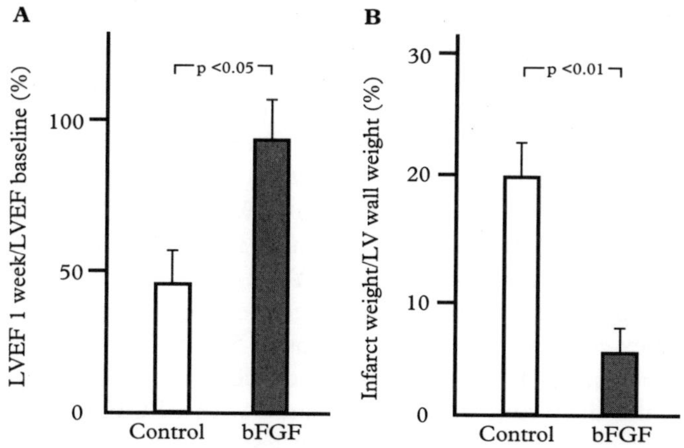

Fig. 15.6 Effects of intracoronary bFGF treatment on left ventricular ejection fraction (LVEF) [**A**] and infarct weight (**B**) 1 week after occlusion of the left anterior descending coronary artery in dogs. Values represent means ± SEM. (Reproduced with permission from Yanagisawa-Miwa et al 1992)

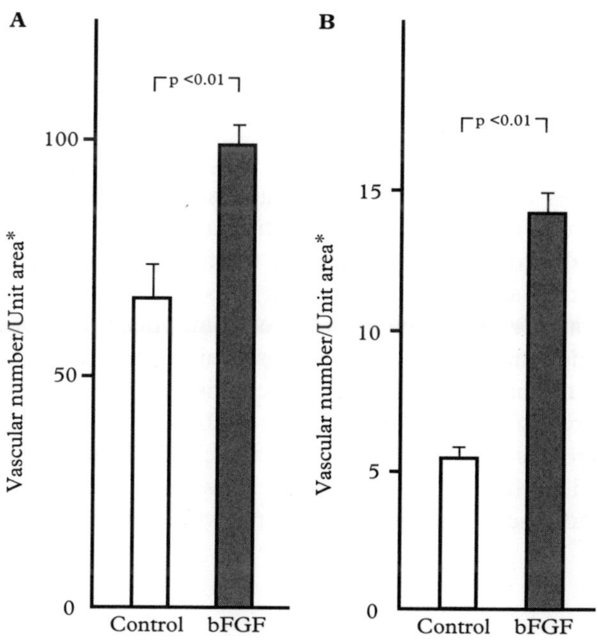

Fig. 15.7 Effects of intracoronary bFGF treatment on the number of capillaries (**A**) and arterioles (**B**) in infarcted area bordering a noninfarct area 1 week after occlusion of the left anterior descending coronary artery in dogs. Values represent means ± SEM. (Reproduced with permission from Yanagisawa-Miwa et al 1992)

stimulate the formation of collateral vessels, but the precise mechanisms of collateral vessel formation are still not clearly established. However, it has been shown that endothelial cell growth-stimulating factor(s) play an important role in the development of coronary collateral vessel formation (Schaper et al 1988). In addition, high concentrations of FGF are present in myocardial tissue (Casscells et al 1990; Kardami & Frandich 1989; Quinkler et al 1989; Sasaki et al 1989; Weiner & Swain 1989). We therefore studied the effects of intracoronary injection of bFGF in a canine experimental myocardial infarct model (Yanagisawa-Miwa et al 1992).

bFGF (10 μg) in 10 ml of saline or vehicle alone were injected into the left circumflex coronary artery in 2 groups of 5 dogs 30 min after and again 6 h after occlusion of the left anterior descending coronary artery. One week after the occlusion the group treated with bFGF showed a greater recovery of cardiac systolic function and lesser infarct size (Fig. 15.6), as well as an higher number of arterioles and capillaries in the infarct that was bordered by a noninfarct area (Fig. 15.7). The development of collateral capillaries has been also demonstrated *in vivo* following bFGF administration in rabbit (Baffour et al 1992) and rat (Chelboun et al 1992) models of acute lower limb ischaemia.

These results suggest that angiogenic factors also have an important role in the development of collateral circulation. The use of angiogenic factors might therefore bring about a new therapeutic modality for atherosclerotic ischaemic diseases.

CONCLUSION

Recent advances in research into angiogenesis are reviewed, especially in relation to the pathogenesis of proliferative diabetic retinopathy. Furthermore, the role of angiogenesis in the formation of collateral vessels, which have a crucial role for the salvage of ischaemic tissue, are discussed briefly in this article. Although a variety of compounds have been identified as potent angiogenic factors and also as inhibitors of angiogenesis, their precise role in the pathogenesis of neovascularisation for different angiogenic diseases is currently unclear. However, research in the field of angiogenesis is now rapidly progressing. In the future we can expect fruitful results from this research field which will bring about new therapeutic modalities for retinopathy and macroangiopathy in patients with diabetes mellitus.

REFERENCES

Akagi Y, Kador P F, Kuwabara T et al 1983 Aldose reductase localization in human retinal mural cells. Invest Ophthalmol Vis Sci 24: 1516-1519

Antonelli-Orlidge A, Saunders K B, Smith S R et al 1989 An activated form of transforming growth factor β is produced by cocultures of endothelial cells and pericytes. Proc Natl Acad Sci USA 86: 4544-4548

Baffour R, Berman J, Garb J L et al 1992 Enhanced angiogenesis and growth of collaterals by *in vivo* administration of recombinant basic fibroblast growth factor in a rabbit model of acute lower limb ischemia: dose-response effect of basic fibroblast growth factor. J Vasc Surg 16: 181-191

Baird A, Culler F, Jones K L et al 1985 Angiogenic factor in human ocular fluid. Lancet 2: 563

Bar R S, Siddle K, Dolash S et al 1988 Actions of insulin and insulin-like growth factors I and II cultured microvessel endothelial cells from bovine adipose tissue. Metabolism 37: 714-720

Bicknell R, Vallee B L 1988 Angiogenin activates endothelial cell phospholipase C. Proc Natl Acad Sci USA 85: 5961-5965

Bicknell R, Vallee B L 1989 Angiogenin stimulates endothelial cell prostacyclin secretion by activation of phospholipase A2. Proc Natl Acad Sci USA 86: 1573-1577

Buzney S M, Frank R N, Varma S D et al 1977 Aldose reductase in retinal mural cells. Invest Ophthalmol Vis Sci 16: 392-396

Casscells W, Speir E, Sasse J et al 1990 Isolation, characterization, and localization of heparin-binding growth factors in the heart. J Clin Invest 85: 433-441

Chelboun J O, Martins R N, Mitchell C A et al 1992 bFGF enhances the development of the collateral circulation after acute arterial occlusion. Biochem Biophys Res Commun 185: 510-516

Connor Jr T B, Roberts A B, Sporn M B et al 1989 Correlation of fibrosis and transforming growth factor-beta type 2 levels in the eye. J Clin Invest 83: 1661-1666

Dills D G, Moss S E, Klein R et al 1991 Association of elevated IGF-I levels with increased retinopathy in late-onset diabetes. Diabetes 40: 1725-1730

Dusseau J W, Hutchins P M Malbasa D S 1986 Stimulation of angiogenesis by adenosine on the chick choriallantoic membrane. Circ Res 59: 163-170

Folkman J Shing Y 1992 Angiogenesis. J Biol Chem 267: 10931-10934

Folkman J, Klagsbrun M 1987 Angiogenic factors. Science 235: 442-447

Form D M, Auerbach R 1983 PGF_2 and angiogenesis. Proc Exp Biol Med 172: 214-218

Forrester J V 1987 Mechanisms of new vessel formation in the retina. Diabet Med 4: 423-430

Gabbay K H 1972 Purification and immunological identification of bovine retinal aldose reductase. Isr J Med Sci 8: 162-1628

Glaser B M 1988 Extracellular modulating factors and control of intraocular neovascularization: an overview. Arch Ophthalmol 106: 603-607

Grant M B, Mames R N, Fitzgerald C et al 1993 Insulin-like growth factor I acts as an angiogenic agent in rabbit cornea and retina: comparative studies with basic fibroblast growth factor. Diabetologia 36: 282-291

Grant M B, Guay C 1991 Plasminogen activator production by human retinal endothelial cells of non-diabetic and diabetic origin. Invest Ophthalmol Vis Sci 32: 53-64

Grant M B, Russel B, Fitzgerald C et al 1986 Insulin-like growth factors in vitreous: studies in controls and diabetics with neovascularization. Diabetes 35: 416-420

Hayashi J N, Ito H, Kanayasu T et al 1991 Effects of glucose on migration, proliferation and tube formation by vascular endothelial cells. Virchows Arch B Cell Pathol 60: 245-252

Hyer S L, Sharp P S, Brooks R A et al 1989 A two-year follow-up study of serum insulin-like growth factor-I in diabetics with retinopathy. Metabolism 38: 586-589

Jacobson B, Dorfman T, Basu P K et al 1985 Inhibition of vascular endothelial cell growth and trypsin activity by vitreous. Exp Eye Res 41: 581-595

Kanayasu T, Nakao-Hayashi J, Asuwa N et al 1989 Leukotriene C_4 stimulate angiogenesis in bovine carotid artery endothelial cells *in vitro*. Biochem Biophys Res Commun 159: 572-578

Kardami E, Frandrich R R 1989 Basic fibroblast growth factor in atria and ventricles of the vertebrate heart. J Cell Biol 109: 1865-1875

King G L, Banskota N K, Shiba T et al 1993 Endothelial cell abnormalities in diabetes. In: Draznin B, Eckel R H (eds) Diabetes and Atherosclerosis: Molecular Basis and Clinical Aspects. Elsevier, New York, pp 191-211

King G L, Goodman A D, Buzney S et al 1985 Receptors and growth-promoting effects of insulin and insulin-like growth factors on cells from bovine retinal capillaries and aorta. J Clin Invest 75: 1028-1036

Kohner E M, Joplin G F, Cheng H et al 1972 Pituitary ablation in the treatment of diabetic retinopathy. Trans Ophthalmol Soc UK 92: 79-90

Kull Jr F C, Brent D A, Parikh I et al 1987 Chemical identification of tumor-derived angiogenic factor. Science 236: 843-845

Kuwabara T, Cogan D G 1963 Retinal vascular patterns IV. Mural cells at the retinal capillaries. Arch Ophthalmol 69: 492-502

Lee T S, MacGregor L C, Fluharty S J et al 1989a Differential regulation of protein kinase C and (Na,K)-adenosine triphosphate activities by elevated glucose levels in retinal capillary endothelial cells. J Clin Invest 83: 90-94

Lee T S, Saltsman K A, Ohashi H et al 1989b Activation of protein kinase C by elevation of glucose concentration: proposal for a mechanism in the development of diabetic vascular complications. Proc Natl Acad Sci USA 86: 5141-5145

Merimee T J, Zapf J Froesch E R 1983 Insulin-like growth factors: studies in diabetics with and without retinopathy. N Engl J Med 309: 527-530

Moses M A, Sudhalter J, Langer R 1990 Identification of an inhibitor of neovascularization from cartilage. Science 248: 1408-1410

Nakao-Hayashi J, Ito H, Kanayasu T, et al 1992 Stimulatory effects of insulin and insulin-like growth factor I on migration and tube formation by vascular endothelial cells. Atherosclerosis 92:141-149

Ohtsu A, Fujii K, Kurozumi S 1988 Induction of angiogenic response by chemically stable prostacyclin analogs. Prostaglandins Leukot Essent Fatty Acid 33: 35-39

Orlidge A, D'Amore P A 1987 Inhibition of capillary endothelial cell growth by pericytes and smooth muscle cells. J Cell Biol 105: 1455-1462

Poulsen J E 1953 The Houssay phenomenon in man: recovery from retinopathy in a case of diabetics with Simmons disease. Diabetes 2: 7-12

Quinkler W, Maasberg M, Bernotat-Danielowski S et al 1989 Isolation of heparin-binding growth factors from bovine, porcine and canine hearts. Eur J Biochem 181: 67-73

Raymond L, Jacobson B 1982 Isolation and identification of stimulatory and inhibitory cell growth factor in bovine vitreous. Exp Eye Res 34: 267-286

Sasaki H, Hoshi H, Hong Y-M et al 1989 Purification of acidic fibroblast growth factor from bovine heart and its localization in the cardiac myocytes. J Biol Chem 264: 17606-17612

Sato Y, Rifkind D B 1989 Inhibition of endothelial cell movement by pericytes and smooth muscle cells: activation of a latent transforming growth factor-β_1-like molecule by plasmin during co-culture. J Cell Biol 109: 309-315

Schaper W, Gorge G, Winkler B et al 1988 The collateral circulation of the heart. Prog Cardiovasc Dis 31: 57-77

Shapiro R, Riordan J F, Vallee B L 1986 Characteristic ribonucleolytic activity of human angiogenin. Biochemistry 25: 3527-3532

Schweigerer L, Malerstein B, Neufeld G et al 1987a Basic fibroblast growth factor is synthesized in cultured retinal pigment epithelial cells. Biochem Biophys Res Commun 143: 934-940

Schweigerer L, Neufeld G, Friedman J et al 1987b Capillary endothelial cells express basic fibroblast growth factor, a mitogen promotes their own growth. Nature 325: 257-259

Sivalingam A, Kenney J, Brown G C et al 1990 Basic fibroblast growth factor levels in the vitreous of patients with proliferative diabetic retinopathy. Arch Ophthalmol 108: 869-872

Taylor C M, Kissun R D, Schor A M et al 1989 Endothelial cell-stimulating angiogenesis factor in vitreous from extraretinal neovascularization. Invest Ophthalmol Vis Sci 30: 2174-2178

Taylor C M, Weiss J B, Kissun R D et al 1986 Effects of oxygen tension on the quantities of procollagenase activating angiogenic factor present in the developing kitten retina. Br J Ophthalmol 70: 162-165

Taylor C M, Weiss J B 1985 Partial Purification of a 5.7 kd glycoprotein from bovine vitreous. Biochem Biophys Res Commun 133: 911-926

Tezuka M, Koyama N, Morisaki N et al 1993 Angiogenic effects of advanced glycation end products of the Maillard reaction on cultured human umbilical cord vein endothelial cells. Biochem Biophys Res Commun 193: 674-680

Underwood L E, Van Wyke J J 1992 Normal and aberrant growth. In: Wilson J D, Foster D W (eds) Williams Textbook of Endocrinology, 8th edition. W B Saunders, Philadelphia, pp 1079-1138

Weiner H L, Swain J L 1989 Acidic fibroblast growth factor mRNA is expressed by cardiac myocytes in culture and the protein is located to the extracellular matrix. Proc Natl Acad Sci USA 86: 2683-2687

Weiss J B, Odedra R, McLaughlin B 1987 Low molecular mass angiogenesis factor: their role in angiogenesis. In: Tsuchiya M et al (eds) Microcirculation - An Update, vol. 2. Elsevier, Amsterdam, pp 777-780

Williams G A, Eisenstein R, Schumacher B et al 1984 Inhibitor of vascular endothelial cell growth in the lens. Am J Ophthalmol 97: 366-371

Wise G N, Dollerly G T, Henkind P 1971 The retinal circulation. Harper & Row, New York, pp 290-420

Yanagisawa-Miwa A, Uchida Y, Nakamura F et al 1992 Salvage of infarcted myocardium by angiogenic action of basic fibroblast growth factor. Science 257: 1401-1403

Ziche M, Jones J, Gullino P M 1982 Role of prostaglandin in E_1 and copper in angiogenesis. J Nat Canc Inst 69: 475-482

16

Transforming growth factor-β: interaction of endothelial cells and pericytes/smooth muscle cells

Y. Sato

INTRODUCTION

It is recognized that cytokines and growth factors play important roles in the physiology and pathophysiology of the vascular system. Vascular wall is primarily composed of endothelial cells and mural pericytes or smooth muscle cells. Pericytes are cells that surround endothelial cells in capillary vessels or post-capillary venules, while smooth muscle cells are present in large vessels. Endothelial cells and mural pericytes/smooth muscle cells are able to produce certain cytokines or growth factors, and these factors may affect the functions of vascular cells in autocrine and/or paracrine manners. Transforming growth factor-β (TGF-β) is one of the cytokines which is secreted from both endothelial cells and pericytes/smooth muscle cells, and it has potent effects on vascular cell motility, growth and differentiation.

Diabetic retinopathy is a common vascular complication of diabetes and is the major cause of blindness in adulthood. It is known that the disappearance of pericytes from retinal capillaries precedes proliferative exacerbation (angiogenesis), and that haemorrhage from fragile neovessels leads to blindness. It is therefore speculated that pericytes have some protective function against the proliferative change of diabetic retinopathy. In this article, a possible role of pericytes modulating the progress of angiogenesis via the effect of TGF-β will be described.

ANGIOGENESIS AND PROTEINASE ACTIVITY

Angiogenesis is a process by which a new vascular network is formed from pre-existing vessels. Angiogenesis is a complex phenomenon which includes at least four distinct properties of endothelial cells (Folkman 1986): degradation of vascular basement membrane and interstitial matrices; migration; proliferation; and tube formation (differentiation). The initial event in angiogenesis is the degradation of extracellular matrices by proteinases. Proteinases, which are involved in the degradation of extracellular matrices, are plasminogen activator-plasmin and matrix metalloproteinases, such as collagenase and stromelysin (for review see Moscatelli & Rifkin 1988). Endothelial cells synthesize two types of plasminogen activator, urokinase-type (uPA) and tissue-type (tPA) plasminogen activator, as well as their specific inhibitor, plasminogen activator inhibitor 1 (PAI-1). Moreover, endothelial cells synthesize latent matrix metalloproteinases and their specific inhibitor, tissue inhibitor of metalloproteinase 1 (TIMP-1). Plasminogen activators convert plasminogen to plasmin, and plasmin converts latent matrix metalloproteinases to their active form. This proteinase cascade is therefore required for the expression of their activity. Furthermore, proteinase activity is determined by the balance between proteinases and their specific inhibitors (Fig. 16.1).

However, it is not simply a matter of amounts of proteinases and their inhibitors. There are cell-surface receptors for uPA and tPA, and cell-surface binding sites for plasminogen and plasmin (Fig. 16.2). The uPA receptor is a glycosyl-phosphatidylinositol-anchored membrane protein (Roldan et al 1990), and uPA binds to the receptor with its N-terminal noncatalytic domain (Appella et al 1987). Although the presence of a tPA receptor was once controversial, an endothelial cell membrane protein (molecular weight ~40,000) has now been purified as a tPA receptor protein, which also binds plasminogen (Hajjar 1991). PAI-1 promptly binds plasminogen activators, quenching their activity in the fluid phase. However, once bound to their receptors, plasminogen activators become relatively resistant to inhibition by PAI-1 and express their proteinase activity at the pericellular milieu, converting cell-surface-bound plasminogen to plasmin. Cell-surface-bound plasmin degrades laminin, fibronectin, and proteoglycan: components of extracellular matrices. Plasmin also activates latent matrix metalloproteinases, and activated

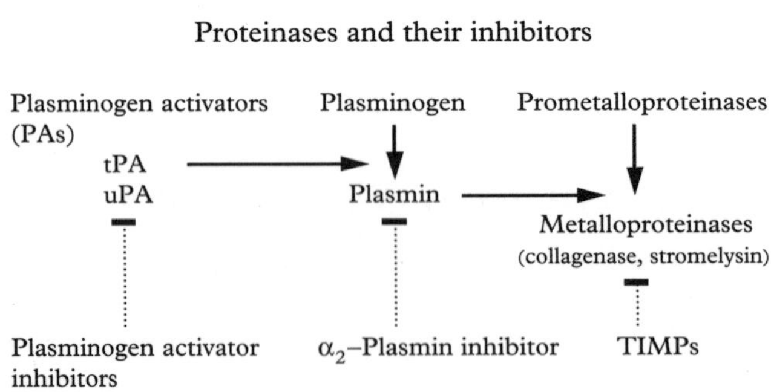

Fig. 16.1 Proteinases for matrix degradation and their specific inhibitors. Endothelial cells produce 2 types of plasminogen activator, tPA and uPA, and their specific inhibitor PAI-1. Endothelial cells also a produce latent form of matrix metalloproteinases and their specific inhibitor TIMP-1. Plasminogen activators convert plasminogen to plasmin. Plasmin activates latent metalloproteinases. *Abbreviations:* PAI-1 = plasminogen activator inhibitor 1; TIMP-1 = tissue inhibitor of metalloproteinase 1; tPA = tissue-type plasminogen activator; uPA = urokinase-type plasminogen activator.

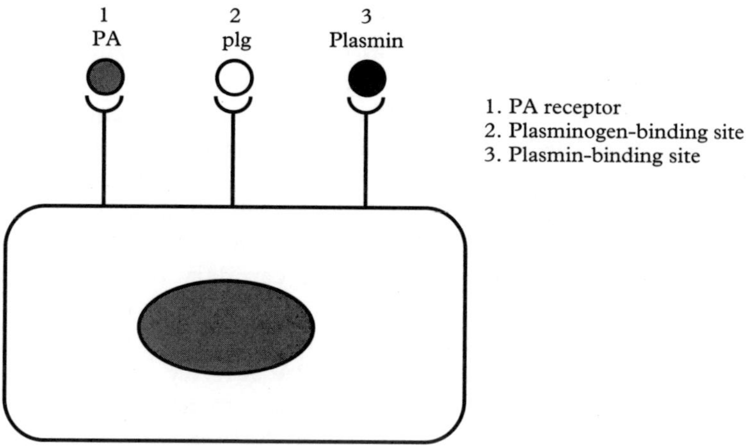

Fig. 16.2 Cell-associated plasminogen activator (PA), plasminogen (plg) and plasmin. Endothelial cells express receptors for plasminogen activators, and binding sites for both plasminogen and plasmin. This cell-associated plasminogen activator-plasmin system is involved in pericellular proteolysis.

matrix metalloproteinases degrade collagen, a major component of extracellular matrices. In this way, cell-surface plasminogen activator-plasmin plays a fundamental role in the degradation of vascular basement membrane and interstitial matrices.

Polypeptide growth factors are the most important inducers of angiogenesis, and fibroblast growth factors (FGFs), epidermal growth factor/ transforming growth factor-α (EGF/,TGF-α) and vascular endothelial growth factor (VEGF) are characterized as angiogenic growth factors. The FGF family contains 9 growth factors or proto-oncogene products with high affinities for heparin, and acidic FGF (aFGF) and basic FGF (bFGF), two prototypes of the family, are well known angiogenic factors. The concentration of bFGF in vitreous fluid is elevated in patients with diabetic proliferative retinopathy (Sivalingam et al 1990). However, bFGF lacks a signal sequence for secretion. The mode of release of bFGF from a cell is therefore currently obscure. EGF and TGF-α display a 38 % homology with conservation of all 6 cysteine residues. They share the same cell-surface receptor, and their biological effects are similar. VEGF is a homodimeric polypeptide and 4 different sizes of peptide molecules originate from a single VEGF gene by alternative splicing. Although FGFs and EGF/TGF-α act on not only endothelial cells but also other cell types, VEGF is known to act specifically on endothelial cells. Recently, PlGF (placenta growth factor), isolated from a human placenta cDNA library, has been shown to have 53% homology with VEGF (Maglione et al 1991). These growth factors stimulate proteinase synthesis, migration, and proliferation of endothelial cells, and induce angiogenesis (Grotendorst et al 1989; Leung et al 1989; Mawatari et al 1989; Montesano et al 1986; Pepper et al 1991; Presta et al 1986; Schreiber et al 1986).

bFGF is produced by a variety of cell types including endothelial cells (Schweigerer et al 1987). bFGF produced by endothelial cells stimulates plasminogen activator synthesis, endothelial cell migration and DNA synthesis, and tube formation by endothelial cells in an autocrine manner (Odekon et al 1992; Sato & Rifkin 1988; Sato et al 1991). When a confluent monolayer of bovine aortic or capillary endothelial cells is wounded by mechanical damage, endothelial cells at the wound edge express uPA activity and migrate into the denuded area. Anti-bFGF antibody blocked the expression of uPA activity and migration of endothelial cells, indicating that these phenomena are dependent on endogenous bFGF (Odekon et al 1992; Sato & Rifkin 1988). The induction of uPA activity in migrating endothelial cells is derived from increased expression of both uPA and uPA receptors, and this expression is dependent on endogenous bFGF (Odekon et al 1992; Pepper et al 1993). Bovine capillary endothelial cells spontaneously form tube-like structures in type I collagen gel, and antibody to bFGF blocks this tube-like formation (Sato et al 1991).

IGF-I (insulin-like growth factor I), another growth factor, has been implicated in the development of diabetic proliferative retinopathy (Grant et al 1986; Merimee et al 1983). However, the effect of IGF-I on angiogenesis has not been fully characterized. We therefore compared the effect of IGF-I on cultured human microvascular endothelial cells with that of EGF/TGF-α, one of the known angiogenic growth factors (Sato et al 1993). Both EGF/TGF-α and IGF-I stimulated migration and proliferation of endothelial cells, phenomena required for angiogenesis. EGF/TGF-α induced tPA mRNA expression in endothelial cells, while IGF-I did not. We predominantly detected tPA mRNA in our human endothelial cell system. We did detect a small amount of uPA mRNA, but there was no increase in response to EGF/TGF-α treatment. The effects of EGF/TGF-α and IGF-I on tube formation by endothelial cells were further compared. When endothelial cells on type 1 collagen gel were treated with EGF/TGF-α, endothelial cells invaded the gel and formed numerous tube-like structures in the gel. The effect of EGF/TGF-α on tube formation was markedly inhibited by the simultaneous addition of anti-tPA antibody or aprotinin, a serine protease inhibitor. On the other hand, IGF-I had no such inducible effect on tube formation by endothelial cells. However, when tPA was added simultaneously with IGF-I, there was a significant induction of tube formation in the gel, and the combined effect of tPA and IGF-I was comparable to that of EGF/TGF-α. These observations clearly demonstrate that the induction of PA in endothelial cells in response to growth factors is required for the initiation of angiogenesis.

TGF-β AND ANGIOGENESIS

TGF-β composes a family of 25-kDa homodimeric polypeptides. Five isoforms (TGF-β1-5) have been identified, and three of them (TGF-β1, 2, and 3) are present in mammals. TGF-β is considered as a multifunctional cytokine influencing cell motility, growth, differentiation, proteinase activity and extracellular matrix production (for reviews see Lyons & Moses 1990; Massegue 1990; Sporn & Robert 1992). TGF-β is produced by almost all cell types, and receptors for TGF-β have a ubiquitous distribution. Therefore, this cytokine is capable of affecting the physiology and/or pathophysiology of many cell types and many organs.

Endothelial cells respond to TGF-β1 very well, while they fail to respond to TGF-β2 (Qian et al 1992). TGF-β1 decreases plasminogen activator activity of endothelial cells by inducing PAI-1 (Saksela et al 1987), inhibits the migration and proliferation of endothelial cells (Heimark et al 1986; Sato & Rifkin 1988), and inhibits the angiogenic effect of bFGF *in vitro* (Pepper et al 1990). Thus, TGF-β1 was at first proposed as an inhibitor of angiogenesis. On the other hand, TGF-β1 was found to induce fibrosis and angiogenesis *in vivo* (Roberts et al 1986). This angiogenic effect of TGF-β1 *in vivo* is considered to be indirect and mediated by factors released from fibroblasts or macrophages, because TGF-β1 is a potent chemoattractant for these cells (Yang & Moses 1990). However, a recent observation suggests that TGF-β1 may act on endothelial cells and support the progress of angiogenesis under certain conditions. High concentrations (5 ng/ml) of TGF-β1 inhibited the *in vitro* angiogenic effect of bFGF, and this effect was mediated by the inhibition of plasminogen activator activity of endothelial cells via the induction of PAI-1 (Pepper et al 1990). In contrast, low concentrations (200-500 pg/ml) of TGF-β1 potentiated the *in vitro* angiogenic effect of bFGF or VEGF (Pepper et al 1993). It is thus suggested that TGF-β may have bidirectional effects on angiogenesis, whose effect is dependent on the concentration of TGF-β or the level of PA activity of endothelial cells.

ACTIVATION OF LATENT TGF-β BY ENDOTHELIAL CELLS AND PERICYTES/SMOOTH MUSCLE CELLS INTERACTION

ROLE OF ENDOTHELIAL CELLS

Almost all cell types including endothelial cells and pericytes/smooth muscle cells produce and secrete TGF-β, and most cells have receptors for TGF-β. As TGF-β expresses profound effects on most cells even at a very low concentrations, the expression of its effects must be tightly regulated. The characteristic feature of TGF-β is that it is always secreted as a biologically inactive latent form (Pircher et al 1984; Wakefield et al 1987). Thus, the activation of latent TGF (LTGF-β) is a limiting step for

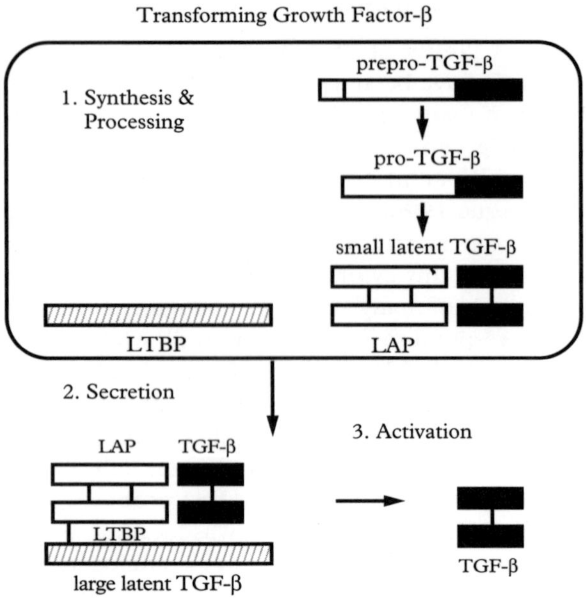

Fig. 16.3 Synthesis, secretion and activation of transforming growth factor-β (TGF-β). TGF-β is synthesized and secreted in a latent form. Therefore, post-secretion activation is required for the expression of its activity. *Abbreviations:* LAP = latency-associated peptides; LTBP = latent TGF-β binding protein.

expression of its activity (Fig. 16.3). There are three components of the LTGF-β complex: mature TGF-β, TGF-β latency-associated peptides (LAP), and the latent TGF-β binding protein (LTBP) (Miyazono et al 1988; Wakefield et al 1988). Mature TGF-β is a 25-kDa homodimeric polypeptide. LAP is a 75-kDa homodimer representing the NH_2-terminal remnant of pro-TGF-β. LAP determines the latency of the complex by binding to the mature TGF-β through noncovalent interactions. LTBP, a 125-160-kDa protein derived from a distinct gene, is attached to LAP by a disulphide bond, and is required for the assembly and secretion of LTGF-β from cells (Miyazono et al 1991). LTGF-β composed of mature TGF-β, LAP and LTBP is denoted as the large LTGF-β complex, whereas the complex composed of the mature TGF-β and LAP is denoted as the small LTGF-β complex. Both endothelial cells and pericytes/smooth muscle cells have been shown to secrete large LTGF-β (Flaumenhaft et al 1993).

Although the mechanism for activation of LTGF-β *in vivo* is poorly understood, we found that LTGF-β is activated quite efficiently by the interaction of endothelial cells and pericytes/smooth muscle cells in tissue culture conditions (Sato & Rifkin 1989). When a confluent monolayer of bovine aortic or capillary endothelial cells was wounded, and bovine retinal pericytes or bovine aortic smooth muscle cells were co-cultured immediately after the wounding, pericytes or smooth muscle cells inhibited endothelial cell migration (Fig. 16.4). This inhibition was abrogated by anti-TGF-β antibody. While endothelial cells and pericytes/smooth muscle cells secreted LTGF-β in homotypic culture conditions, it was found that active TGF-β was generated during co-culture of endothelial cells and pericytes/smooth muscle cells with contact between the two cell types. Antonelli-Orlidge et al (1989) independently reported that the inhibition of endothelial cell proliferation by co-culture with pericytes/smooth muscle cells was mediated by activated TGF-β. While LTGF-β can be activated by transient acidic or basic conditions, heat or chaotrophic agents like urea *in vitro*, these conditions are not the likely mechanisms for LTGF-β activation during co-culture. It is reported that LTGF-β is activated by proteolysis of the latent complex with plasmin and cathepsin D (Lyons et al 1988), or by alteration of carbohydrate structures within LAP (Miyazono & Heldin 1989). Plasmin cleaves LAP and releases mature TGF-β from the LTGF-β complex (Lyons et al 1990). Since migrating endothelial cells express plasminogen activator activity, it is possible that the activation of LTGF-β during co-culture is dependent on the plasminogen activator-plasmin activity of endothelial cells. This idea was proved by the following observations. Simultaneous addition of serine

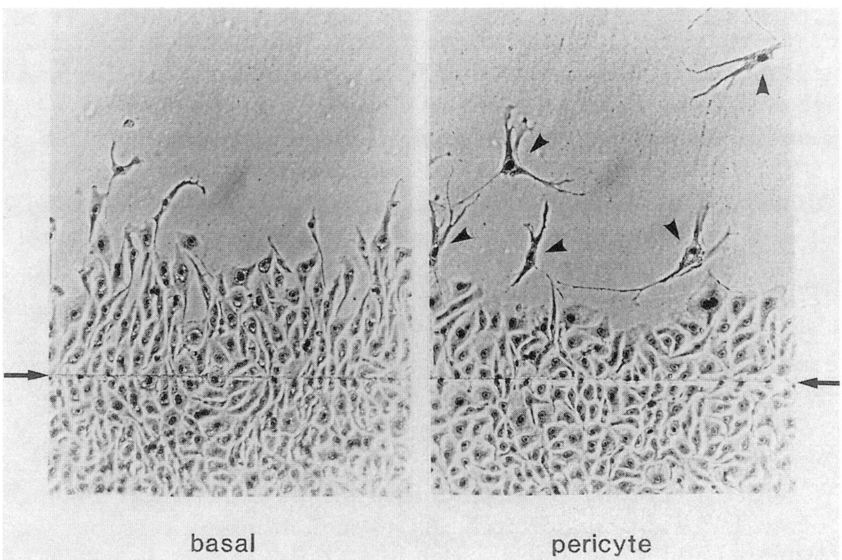

Fig. 16.4 Inhibition of endothelial cell migration by pericytes. Confluent monolayers of bovine endothelial cells were wounded with a razor blade, and further incubated in the serum-free medium for overnight. Retinal pericytes were plated immediately after the wounding. Pericytes (arrows) inhibited the migration of endothelial cells.

protease inhibitors (aprotinin; ε-aminocaproic acid; or a rather specific inhibitor for plasmin, α_2-plasmin inhibitor) almost completely neutralized the inhibitory effect of pericytes/smooth muscle cells on endothelial cell migration (Sato & Rifkin 1989). Moreover, removal of plasminogen from the tissue culture conditions or the addition of lipoprotein(a), which competes with plasminogen, blocked the activation of LTGF-β during co-culture (Kojima et al 1991). Therefore, the activation of LTGF-β by the interaction of endothelial cells and pericytes/smooth muscle cells appears to be mediated by plasminogen activator-plasmin activity expressed on the surface of endothelial cells.

ROLE OF PERICYTES/SMOOTH MUSCLE CELLS

Since LTGF-β is activated by plasmin during co-culture of endothelial cells and pericytes/smooth muscle cells and plasminogen activator-plasmin is localized on the cell surface, it is reasonable to assume that the targeting of LTGF-β to the cell surface is required for its activation. LAP contains two potential cellular binding domains: mannose-6-phosphate and an Arg-Gly-Asp sequence (Derynck et al 1985; Kovacina et al 1989). It has been shown that LTGF-β is able to bind to the cell surface via cation-independent mannose-6-phosphate/insulin-like growth factor II (IGF-II) receptor (Kovacina et al 1989). Dennis and Rifkin (1991) reported that excess amounts of mannose-6-phosphate or antibody to IGF-II receptor prevented the activation of LTGF-β during co-culture of endothelial cells and smooth muscle cells. Therefore, they speculated that the LTGF-β complex binds to the cell surface via IGF-II receptor, and that this binding is required for its activation during co-culture.

Another factor that may be involved in the targeting of LTGF-β is LTBP. LTBP contains 16 EGF-like common repeats and 3 copies of a motif with 8 cysteine residues (Kanzaki et al 1990; Tsuji et al 1990). The EGF-like domain repeats are proposed to be involved in protein-protein interaction. Flaumenhaft et al (1993) showed that antibody to LTBP or an excess amount of free LTBP inhibited the activation of LTGF-β during co-culture of endothelial cells and smooth muscle cells. Thus, they speculated that LTBP directs LTGF-β to the activation site on the surface with these EGF-like domain repeats. However, these two observations did not directly show the cellular targeting of LTGF-β.

We examined the targeting of LTGF-β by the binding of ^{125}I-large LTGF-β1 to endothelial cells or smooth muscle cells. It was found that ^{125}I-large LTGF-β1 bound specifically to smooth muscle cells, but not to endothelial cells. Thus, the targeting of LTGF-β appears to be cell-type specific to mural smooth muscle cells. Schatchard analysis revealed that there were high-affinity and low-affinity binding sites on smooth muscle cells: a high-affinity site with a dissociation constant of about 140 pmol/l

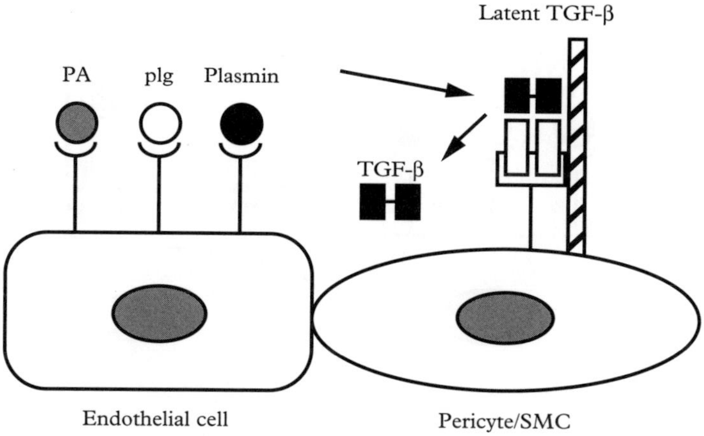

Fig. 16.5 Activation of latent transforming growth factor-β (TGF-β) during co-culture of endothelial cells and pericytes/smooth muscle cells. Endothelial cells express plasminogen activator-plasmin on their cell surface. Latent TGF-β is specifically targeted to pericytes/smooth muscle cells. During co-culture of endothelial cells and pericytes/smooth muscle cells, plasmin localized on the surface of endothelial cells activates latent TGF-β targeted on pericytes/smooth muscle cells. *Abbreviations:* PA = plasminogen activator; plg = plasminogen; SMC = smooth muscle cell.

and 1264 sites per cell and a low-affinity site with a dissociation constant of about 5.1 nmol/l and 13,850 sites per cell.

In order to understand the precise roles of LAP and/or LTBP on the targeting and activation of LTGF-β during co-culture of endothelial cells and pericytes/smooth muscle cells, we developed 10 monoclonal antibodies (mAbs) that recognized either LAP or LTBP (Sato et al 1993). Each mAb was added to the co-culture wound migration assay, and we found that one of the mAbs against LAP (KM704) neutralized the inhibitory effect of smooth muscle cells on the migration of endothelial cells. We did not observe any mAbs against LTBP capable of blocking the activation of LTGF-β during co-culture. Furthermore, we found that KM704, which prevented the activation of LTGF- during co-culture, blocked the binding of ^{125}I-large LTGF-β1 to smooth muscle cells. Our demonstration is the first to show that LTGF-β is selectively targeted to smooth muscle cells but not to endothelial cells, and that elimination of targeting of LTGF-β to smooth muscle cells appears to block the activation of LTGF-β during co-culture of endothelial cells and smooth muscle cells. This implies a unique mechanism for the activation of LTGF-β during co-culture (Fig. 16.5).

Endothelial cells express plasminogen activator-plasmin activity on their cellular surface. However, as LTGF-β is not targeted to endothelial cells, the activation of LTGF-β is not efficient in homotypic culture conditions. In contrast, LTGF-β is targeted to pericytes/smooth muscle cells, but pericytes/smooth muscle cells do not express enough plasminogen activator

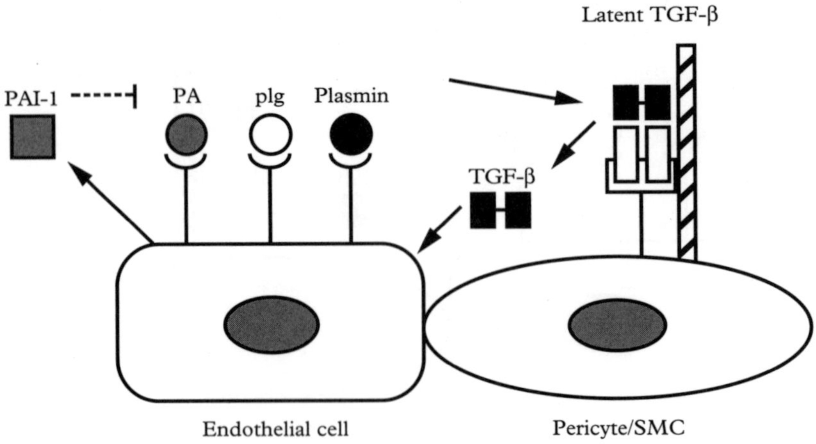

Fig. 16.6 Regulation of the activation of latent transforming growth factor-β (TGF-β). Once latent TGF-β is activated, TGF-β induces PAI-1. PAI-1 inhibits PA activity of endothelial cells, and prevents the further activation of latent TGF-β. Thus, the activation of latent TGF-β is regulated by the balance between PA and PAI-1. *Abbreviations:* PA = plasminogen activator; PAI = plasminogen activator inhibitor; plg = plasminogen; SMC = smooth muscle cells.

activity to activate LTGF-β in homotypic culture conditions. During co-culture of endothelial cells and pericytes/smooth muscle cells with cell contact, plasminogen activator-plasmin localized on the surface of endothelial cells efficiently activates LTGF-β targeted to pericytes/smooth muscle cells. It is possible that a cell which possesses both plasminogen activator activity and the binding sites for LTGF-β could activate LTGF-β in homotypic culture conditions.

As described previously, LAP contains two potential cellular binding domains: mannose-6-phosphate and an Arg-Gly-Asp sequence. Therefore, we examined whether mannose-6-phosphate or an Arg-Gly-Asp sequence in LAP might be responsible for the targeting of LTGF-β to smooth muscle cells (Sato et al 1993). The binding of ^{125}I-large LTGF-β to smooth muscle cells showed no competitive inhibition by either mannose-6-phosphate or the synthetic peptide Arg-Gly-Asp-Ser. These results suggest that neither the mannose-6-phosphate nor an Arg-Gly-Asp sequence in LAP is involved in the targeting of LTGF-β to smooth muscle cells, and that KM704 might recognize an entirely different domain of LAP responsible for the targeting of LTGF-β to smooth muscle cells.

REGULATION OF THE ACTIVATION OF LATENT TGF-β BY THE INDUCTION OF PAI-1

Once active TGF-β is generated during co-culture of endothelial cells and pericytes/smooth muscle cells, active TGF-β inhibits the migration and proliferation of endothelial cells (Antonelli-Orlidge et al 1989; Sato & Rifkin 1989). Moreover, there is a more than 20-fold increase in the level of PAI-1 protein, and the plasminogen activity of endothelial cells is inhibited during co-culture (Sato et al 1990). Therefore, the generation of active TGF-β by the interaction of endothelial cells and pericytes/smooth muscle cells may protect against the initiation of angiogenesis.

It was found that less than 10% of LTGF-β was activated during co-culture of endothelial cells and pericytes/smooth muscle cells (Sato et al 1990). Since plasminogen activator-plasmin is responsible for the activation of LTGF-β and TGF-β induces PAI-1 during co-culture of endothelial cells and pericytes/smooth muscle cells, it is possible that TGF-β may regulate its own generation by interfering with plasminogen activator-plasmin activity via the induction of PAI-1. Conditioned Medium (CM) was collected every 12 hours and the TGF-β activities in CM were determined. Active TGF-β was found only in the first 12 h of co-culture CM, and no active TGF-β was found during subsequent 12 to 36 h. However, when CM was collected in the presence of antibody to PAI-1, the generation of active TGF-β during co-culture proceeded at a constant rate for at least 36 h. When antibody to PAI-1 was removed at the 24-h point, the generation of active TGF-β was lost during 24 to 36 h. Therefore, the activation of LTGF-β by the interaction of endothelial cells and pericytes/smooth muscle cells appears to be self-regulated and determined by the levels of plasminogen activator and PAI-1 (Fig. 16.6).

CONCLUSION

LTGF-β can be efficiently activated at the cell surface where plasminogen activator-plasmin and LTGF-β are targeted, and the activation is self regulated via the induction of PAI-1 by activated TGF-β. Furthermore, activated TGF-β is easily captured and inactivated by ubiquitous α_2-macroglobulin (O'Connor-McCourt & Wakefield 1987). Therefore, expression of the effect of TGF-β is limited spaciotemporally in the immediate vicinity where it is generated. LTGF-β is specifically targeted to mural pericytes/smooth muscle cells and is efficiently activated by plasminogen activator-plasmin on the surface of endothelial cells, which are stimulated by angiogenic growth factors. Hence, the disappearance of pericytes from retinal capillaries in diabetic retinopathy may be caused the deficiency of active TGF-β generation.

ACKNOWLEDGMENT

A part of the studies presented here was supported by Grant-in-Aid 03268108 from the Japanese Ministry of Education, Science and Culture.

REFERENCES

Antonelli-Orlidge A A, Saunders K B, Smith S R et al 1989 An activated form of transforming growth factor beta is produced by co-culture of endothelial cells and pericytes. Proc Natl Acad Sci USA 86: 4544-4548

Appella E E A, Robinson S J, Ullrich M P et al 1987 The receptor-binding sequence of urokinase. A biological function for the growth factor module of proteases. J Biol Chem 262: 4437-4440

Dennis P, Rifkin D B 1991 Cellular activation of latent transforming growth factor-β requires binding to the cation-independent mannose-6-phosphate/insulin-like growth factor type II receptor. Proc Natl Acad Sci USA 88: 580-584

Derynck R, Jarrett J A, Chen E Y et al 1985 Human transforming growth factor-β complementary DNA sequence and expression in normal and transformed cells. Nature 316: 701 -705

Flaumenhaft R, Abe M, Sato Y et al 1993 Role of the latent TGF-β binding protein in the activation of latent TGF-β by the co-culture of endothelial cells and smooth muscle cells. J Cell Biol 120: 995-1002

Folkman J 1986 How is blood vessel growth regulated in normal and neoplastic tissue? - G H A Clowes memorial award lecture. Cancer Res 46: 467-473

Grant M, Russell B, Fitzgerald C et al 1986. Insulin-like growth factors in vitreous. Studies in control and diabetic subjects with neovascularization. Diabetes 35: 416-420

Grotendorst G R, Soma Y, Takehara K et al 1989 EGF and TGF-alpha are potent chemoattractants for endothelial cells and EGF-like peptides are present at sites of tissue regeneration. J Cell Physiol 139: 617-623.

Hajjar K A 1991 The endothelial cell tissue plasminogen activator receptor. Specific interaction with plasminogen. J Biol Chem 266: 21962-21970

Heimark R L, Twardzik D R, Schwartz S M 1986 Inhibition of endothelial regeneration by type-beta transforming growth factor from platelets. Science 233: 1078-1080

Kanzaki T, Olofsson A, Moren A et al 1990 TGF-β1 binding protein: a component of the large latent complex of TGF-β1 with multiple repeat sequences. Cell 61: 1051-1061

Kojima S, Harpel P C, Rifkin D B 1991 Lipoprotein(a) inhibits the generation of transforming growth factor: an endogenous inhibitor of smooth muscle cell migration. J Cell Biol 113: 1439-1445

Kovacina K S, Steele-Perkins G, Purchio A F et al 1989 Interactions of recombinant and platelet transforming growth factor-β1 precursor with the insulin-like growth factor II/mannose-6-phosphate receptor. Biochem Biophys Res Commun 160: 393-403

Leung D W, Cachianes G, Kuang W-J et al 1989 Vascular endothelial growth factor is a secreted angiogenic mitogen. Science 246: 1306-1309

Lyons R M, Keski-Oja J, Moses H L 1988 Proteolytic activation of latent transforming growth factor-β from fibroblast conditioned medium. J Cell Biol 106: 1659-1665

Lyons R M, Gentry L E, Purchio A F et al. 1990 Mechanism of activation of latent recombinant transforming growth factor-l by plasmin. J Cell Biol 110: 1361-1367

Lyons R M, Moses H L 1990 Transforming growth factor-β and the regulation of cell proliferation. Eur J Biochem 187: 467-473

Maglione D, Guerriero V, Viglietto G et al 1991 Isolation of a human placenta cDNA coding for a protein related to the vascular permeability factor. Proc Natl Acad Sci USA 88: 9267-9271

Massague J 1990 The transforming growth factor-beta family. Ann Rev Cell Biol 6: 597-641

Mawatari M, Kohno K, Mizoguchi H et al 1989 Effects of tumor necrosis factor and epidermal growth factor on cell morphology, cell surface receptors, and the production of tissue inhibitor of metalloproteinases and IL-6 in human microvascular endothelial cells. J Immunol 143: 1619-1627

Merimee T J, Zapf J, Froesch E R 1983 Insulin-like growth factors. Studies in diabetics with and without retinopathy. N Engl J Med 309: 527-530

Miyazono K, Hellman U, Wernstedt C et al 1988 Latent high molecular complex of transforming growth factor 1. J Biol Chem 263: 6407-6415

Miyazono K, Heldin C-H 1989 Role for carbohydrate structure in TGF-β1 latency. Nature 338: 158-160

Miyazono K, Olofsson A, Colosetti P et al 1991 A role of the latent TGF-β1 in the assembly and secretion of TGF-β1. EMBO J 10: 1091-1101

Montesano R, Vassali J-D, Baird A et al 1986 Basic fibroblast factor induces angiogenesis *in vitro*. Proc Natl Acad Sci USA 83: 7297-7301

Moscatelli D, Rifkin D B 1988 Membrane and matrix localization of proteinases: a common theme in tumor cell invasion and angiogenesis. Biochem Biophys Acta 948: 67-85

O'Connor-McCourt M D, Wakefield L M 1987 Latent transforming growth factor-beta in serum. A specific complex with $alpha_2$-macroglobulin. J Biol Chem 262: 14090-14099

Odekon L E, Sato Y, Rifkin D B 1992 Urokinase-type plasminogen activator mediates basic fibroblast growth factor-induced bovine endothelial cell migration independent of its proteolytic activity. J Cell Physiol 150: 258-263

Pepper M S, Belin D, Montesano R et al 1990 Transforming growth factor-beta1 modulates basic fibroblast growth factor induced proteolytic and angiogenic properties of endothelial cells *in vitro*. J Cell Biol 111: 743-755

Pepper M S, Ferrara N, Orci L et al 1991. Vascular endothelial growth factor (VEGF) induces plasminogen activators and plasminogen activator inhibitor-1 in microvascular endothelial cells. Biochem Biophys Res Commun 181: 902-906

Pepper M S, Vassalli J-D, Orci L et al 1993 Biphasic effect of transforming growth factor-1β on *in vitro* angiogenesis. Exp Cell Res 204: 356-363

Pircher R, Lawrence D A, Jullien P 1984 Latent β-transforming growth factor in nontransformed and Kirsten sarcoma virus-transformed normal kidney cells, clone 49F. Cancer Res 44: 5538-5543

Presta M, Moscatelli D, Joseph-Silverstein J et al 1986 Purification from a human hepatoma cell line of a basic fibroblast growth factor-like molecule that stimulates capillary endothelial cell plasminogen activator production, DNA synthesis, and migration. Mol Cell Biol 6: 4060-4066

Qian S W, Burmester J K, Merwin J R et al 1992 Identification of a structural domain that distinguishes the action of the type 1 and type 2 isoforms of transforming growth factor beta on endothelial cells. Proc Natl Acad Sci USA 89: 6290-6294

Roldan A L, Cubellis M V, Masucci M T et al 1990 Cloning and expression of the receptor for human urokinase plasminogen activator, a central molecule in cell surface, plasmin-dependent proteolysis. EMBO J 9: 467-474

Roberts A B, Sporn M B, Assoian R K et al 1986 Transforming growth factor type β: rapid induction of fibrosis and angiogenesis *in vivo* and stimulation of collagen formation *in vitro*. Proc Natl Acad Sci USA 83: 4167-4171

Saksela O, Moscatelli D, Rifkin D B 1987 The opposing effects of basic fibroblast growth factor and transforming growth factor beta on the regulation of plasminogen activator activity in capillary endothelial cells. J Cell Biol 105: 957-963

Sato Y, Rifkin D B 1988 Autocrine activities of basic fibroblast growth factor: regulation of endothelial cell movement, plasminogen activator synthesis, and DNA synthesis. J Cell Biol 107: 1199-1205

Sato Y, Rifkin D B 1989 Inhibition of endothelial cell movement by pericytes and smooth muscle cells: activation of a latent transforming growth factor-β1-like molecule by plasmin during co-culture. J Cell Biol 109: 309-315

Sato Y, Tsuboi R, Lyons R et al 1990 Characterization of the activation of latent TGF-β by co-culture of endothelial cells and pericytes or smooth muscle cells: a self-regulating system. J Cell Biol 111: 757-763

Sato Y, Shimada T, Takaki R 1991 Autocrinological role of basic fibroblast growth factor on tube formation of vascular endothelial cells *in vitro*. Biochem Biophys Res Commun 180: 1098-1102

Sato Y, Okamura K, Morimoto A et al 1993 Indispensable role of tissue-type plasminogen activator in growth factor-dependent tube formation of human microvacular endothelial cells *in vitro*. Exp Cell Res 204: 223-229

Sato Y, Okada F, Abe M, et al 1993 The mechanism for the activation of latent TGF-β during co-culture of endothelial cells and smooth muscle cells: cell-type specific targeting of latent TGF-β to smooth muscle cells. J Cell Biol 123: 1249-1254

Schreiber A B, Winkler M E, Derynck R 1986 Transforming growth factor-alpha: a more potent angiogenic mediator than epidermal growth factor. Science 233: 1250-1253

Schweigerer L, Neufeld G, Friedman J et al 1987 Capillary endothelial cells express basic fibroblast growth factor, a mitogen that promotes their own growth. Science 325: 257-259

Sivalingam A, Kennedy J, Brown G C et al 1990 Basic fibroblast growth factor levels in the vitreous of patients with proliferative diabetic retinopathy. Arch Ophthalmol 108: 869-872

Sporn M B, Robert A B 1992 Transforming growth factor-β: recent progress and new challenges. J Cell Biol 119: 1017-1021
Tsuji T, Okada F, Yamaguchi K et al 1990 Molecular cloning of the large subunit of transforming growth factor type b masking protein and expression of the mRNA in various tissues. Proc Natl Acad Sci USA 267: 19482-19488
Wakefield L M, Smith D M, Masui T et al 1987 Distribution and modulation of the cellular receptor for transforming growth factor-beta. J Cell Biol 105: 965-975
Wakefield L M, Smith D M, Flanders K C et al 1988 Latent transforming growth factor-β from human platelets. J Biol Chem 263: 7646-7654
Yang E Y, Moses H L 1990 Transforming growth factor-β1 induced changes in cell migration, proliferation, and angiogenesis in the chicken chorioallantoic membrane. J Cell Biol 111: 731-741

17

Inhibition of vascular endothelial cell proliferation by the protein kinase C pathway: a possible mechanism underlying the pathogenesis of diabetic vascular complications

T. Sasaguri, C. Kosaka

INTRODUCTION

Diabetes mellitus accelerates the formation of atherosclerotic lesions, and vascular complications are the prominent clinical manifestations of this disease. The reason for this cannot be explained solely by the fact that diabetes is frequently accompanied by hypertension and hyperlipidaemia, which are well established atherogenic factors. Other mechanisms associated with the diabetic state certainly contribute to the process of atherogenesis.

According to the response-to-injury hypothesis (Ross 1993), atherogenesis is initiated by 'injury' of vascular endothelial cells, which play an important role as a dynamic interface between circulating blood and the vascular wall. The earliest manifestations of injured endothelial cells are alterations in one or more of their physiological properties. In diabetes, hyperglycaemia or some other metabolic abnormalities may alter endothelial cell function. For example, prostacyclin production has been reported to be impaired in diabetic patients (Johnson et al 1979), diabetic rats (Harrison et al 1978) and in endothelial cells exposed to high concentrations of glucose (Ono et al 1988), the alteration of which would stimulate platelet aggregation. Endothelium-dependent aortic relaxation was lower in diabetic than in normal rats (Meraji et al 1987), and, moreover, high concentrations of glucose stimulated endothelial cells to produce endothelin, a potent vasoconstrictor (Yamauchi et al 1990).

The initial injurious events in atherogenesis do not necessarily lead to endothelial cell death. Fatty streaks, the early lesions of atherosclerosis, can develop at sites covered with morphologically intact endothelium. Nevertheless, cellular desquamation may happen more frequently in injured than in normal endothelium. In fact, endothelial denudation has been observed even during the early phases of atherogenesis in humans (Davies et al 1988), hypercholesterolaemic nonhuman primates (Masuda & Ross 1990) and diabetic rabbits (Dolgov et al 1982). When endothelial cells are wounded and contact with neighbouring cells is disrupted, the surrounding cells migrate into the wounded area to re-establish cell-to-cell connections (Reidy 1985). However, if the wound is too large to be covered by these cells, cells surrounding the denuded area may begin to proliferate to repair the intima. If recovery from the wound is delayed for any reason, the loss of the endothelial barrier may allow plasma components to infiltrate the intima, and platelets may adhere to the exposed subendothelial tissue and release active substances, such as platelet-derived growth factor and thromboxane A_2, which may stimulate smooth muscle cell migration and proliferation. Therefore, rapid endothelial regeneration after wound formation should prevent the progression of atherosclerotic lesions. It is therefore important to study the way in which endothelial cell growth is regulated under both physiological and pathological (including diabetic) conditions.

Proliferation of cultured endothelial cells is inhibited in the presence of high concentrations of glucose (Lorenzi et al 1985; Stout 1982). Retinal vascular endothelium of hyperglycaemic mice manifests a delay in replication (Naeser 1986). Therefore, hyperglycaemia may interrupt endothelial cell turnover, resulting in an exacerbation of vascular lesions. However, the underlying mechanism by which excess glucose inhibits endothelial cell growth remains unknown. In some cultured cells, such as bovine retinal capillary endothelial cells (Lee et al 1989) and rat renal mesangial cells (Ayo et al 1991), protein kinase C (PKC) has been reported to be activated in the presence of high concentrations of glucose, and, in parallel, the level of 1,2-diacylglycerol (DAG), a PKC activator, to be elevated. PKC activation and DAG elevation have also been shown *in vivo* in glomeruli (Craven & DeRubertis 1989), aorta and heart (Inoguchi et al 1992) of streptozotocin-induced diabetic rats. Endothelial cells can take in glucose independently of insulin (Corkey et al 1981; King et al 1983), although insulin-dependent glucose uptake has also been shown in some endothelial cells (Abe et al 1990; King et al 1983). Therefore, the intracellular glucose concentration can be elevated in proportion to excess extracellular glucose. An excess of intracellular glucose may lead to activation of the polyol pathway to generate fructose via sorbitol, elevating the $NADH/NAD^+$ ratio, which may result in an increase in *de novo* synthesis of DAG, via glycerol-3-phosphate formation (Lee et al 1989). An elevation of sorbitol content has been demonstrated in diabetic rat endothelium (Brolin & Naeser 1988).

We therefore wondered whether activation of the PKC pathway is involved in excess glucose-induced impairment of endothelial cell growth, since PKC has been shown to inhibit proliferation of a variety of cells, including vascular smooth muscle cells (Huang & Ives 1987; Sasaguri et al 1993). However, the effects of PKC on endothelial cell proliferation have not been investigated sufficiently.

Progression of the eukaryotic cell cycle is controlled by several cyclins and cyclin-dependent kinases (Hunter & Pines 1991; Norbury & Nurse 1992; Sherr 1993). Cyclin A is expressed from the late G_1 to S phase and has been suggested to play role in G_1/S progression, activating Cdk2 (a cyclin-dependent kinase), which might subsequently phosphorylate a putative substrate that initiates DNA synthesis (Elledge et al 1992; Girard et al 1991; Pagano et al 1992, 1993; Rosenblatt et al 1992; Tsai et al 1991). The retinoblastoma gene product (pRB) might also be involved in G_1/S regulation (Levine 1993). pRB activity is controlled by phosphorylation; the underphosphorylated (active) form is able to suppress G_1/S transition and the hyperphosphorylated (inactive) form loses this ability, allowing cells to enter the S phase. However, G_2/M transition is controlled by B-type cyclins forming a complex with Cdc2 (Cdk1), which phosphorylates several proteins including nuclear lamins, vimentin, caldesmon, and histone H1, both *in vitro* and *in vivo* (Norbury & Nurse 1992).

Against this background, we attempted to determine the role of the PKC pathway in the regulation of endothelial cell proliferation with regard to factors controlling the cell cycle, such as cyclins, cyclin-dependent kinases and pRB (Kosaka et al 1993a, b).

MATERIALS AND METHODS

CELL CULTURE AND CELL CYCLE SYNCHRONIZATION

Endothelial cells, obtained from human umbilical vein by collagenase digestion, were cultured in Dulbecco's modified Eagle's medium containing 20% (v/v) foetal bovine serum (FBS) and 10 ng/ml human recombinant basic fibroblast growth factor (bFGF) [Amersham], and used within 7 passages. G_0 synchronization was achieved by serum starvation for 48 h; G_1/S synchronization was achieved by treatment of cells released from G_0 with 1 μg/ml aphidicolin for 20 h; and M-phase arrest was achieved by treatment of cells released from G_1/S arrest with 0.5 μg/ml nocodazole or 0.5μg/ml colcemide for 48 h. The number of cells was determined with a Coulter counter.

FLOW CYTOMETRY

Cells fixed with 70% (v/v) ethanol were stained with propidium iodide (0.005%, w/v) following treatment with RNase (2 mg/ml), or with acridine orange (6 μg per 1 ml of 0.1 mol/l sodium citrate/Na_2HPO4 [pH 2.6]) following treatments with RNase and 0.1 mol/l KCl/HCl (pH 1.4). Fluorescence was analyzed with a flow cytometer (Cyto ACE-150, Japan Spectroscopic Co.).

DNA SYNTHESIS ASSAY

Growing cells were trypsinized and seeded in 24-multiwell plates at a density of 1 x 10^4 cells/well. After G_0 or G_1/S synchronization, cells were labelled with 37 kBq/ml [6-^{3}H]-thymidine (Amersham). At indicated times, the medium was removed and cells were washed with Dulbecco's phosphate-buffered saline (PBS) supplemented with Ca^{2+} and Mg^{2+}. Cells were treated with 5% (w/v) trichloroacetic acid for 10 min followed by removal of the acid with ethanol:diethyl ether (3:1, v/v). The precipitates were then lysed with 0.3 mol/l NaOH. After neutralization with HCl, the lysates were counted for radioactivity in a liquid scintillation counter.

PHORBOL ESTER BINDING ASSAY

Cells were incubated in the presence of various concentrations of phorbol 12-myristate, 13-acetate (PMA) labelled with tritium (New England Nuclear) at 37°C for 15 min. Incubation was terminated by rapid washes with ice-cold PBS, followed by lysis with 0.1 mol/l NaOH and 0.1% (w/v) sodium dodecylsulphate (SDS). Radioactivity in the lysates was determined by liquid scintillation counting. Nonspecific binding was determined by incubating cells in the presence of a 1,000-fold higher concentration of unlabelled PMA.

PKC ENZYME ASSAY

Cells scraped from dishes were sonicated in the buffer containing 50 mmol/l Tris/HCl (pH 7.4), 5 mmol/l EDTA, 10 mmol/l EGTA, 0.3% (w/v) 2-mercaptoethanol, 20 μg/ml leupeptin, 50 μg/ml phenylmethylsulphonyl fluoride (PMSF), and 10 mmol/l benzamidine hydrochloride (lysis buffer). The suspension was centrifuged at 100,000 ×g for 1 h and the resultant supernatant was used as the soluble fraction. After removal of contaminating soluble proteins by re-centrifugation, the pellet was sonicated in lysis buffer containing 1% (v/v) Triton X-100 and centrifuged again. The supernatant was used as the particulate fraction. PKC activity in these fractions was measured using the 'Protein Kinase C Assay System' (Amersham).

CYCLIN-DEPENDENT KINASE ASSAY

Cells were lysed in 10 mmol/l Tris/HCl (pH 7.4), 1 mmol/l EDTA, 1 mmol/l EGTA, 100 mmol/l NaF, 200 μmol/l Na_3VO_4, 20 μg/ml leupeptin, 20 μg/ml PMSF and 0.1% (v/v) Nonidet P-40 (buffer A), and centrifuged at 16,000 ×g to remove insoluble pellets. After the addition of 120 mmol/l NaCl, the lysate (1 ml) was incubated with 50 μl of 50% (v/v) protein A Sepharose (Pharmacia) for 30 min at 4°C followed by centrifugation. The supernatant was incubated with a polyclonal antibody to the carboxyl terminal sequence of Cdc2 kinase (Oncogene Science) for 1 h at 4°C. Then, 30 μl of 50% protein A Sepharose was added and incubation was continued for 1 h at 4°C. The precipitates were washed 5 times with buffer

A, after which it was suspended in 20 mmol/l Tris/HCl (pH 7.4) and 10 mmol/l $MgCl_2$. The reaction mixture (75 μl), containing 25 μl of the suspension, 20 mmol/l Tris/HCl (pH 7.4), 10 mmol/l $MgCl_2$, 1 mmol/l dithiothreitol, 100 μg/ml histone H1 (Boehringer) and 50 μmol/l [γ-^{32}P]-ATP (Amersham) was incubated for 30 min at 30°C. The reaction was stopped with 30 μl of 300 mmol/l H_3PO_4, and the mixture was then absorbed to Whatman p81 binding paper (9 cm^2). After 4 washes with 200 ml of 75 mmol/l H_3PO_4, radioactivity was determined by liquid scintillation counting. Cdc2-specific activity was calculated by subtracting control values, obtained by reactions in the absence of histone H1 from the activity obtained as outlined above.

WESTERN BLOTTING

Cells were sonicated in the buffer containing 50 mmol/l Tris/HCl (pH 7.4), 120 mmol/l NaCl, 5 mmol/l EDTA, 5 mmol/l EGTA, 100 mmol/l NaF, 200 μmol/l Na_3VO_4, 10 μg/ml aprotinin, 20 μg/ml PMSF, 1 mmol/l dithiothreitol and 0.5% (v/v) Nonidet P-40 followed by centrifugation at 16,000 ×g. The supernatant (60 μg) was applied to SDS polyacrylamide gel electrophoresis. Proteins were transferred to a vinylidene fluoride membrane and probed with antibodies to human cyclin-dependent kinases or pRB followed by detection using the 'ECL Western blotting detection system' (Amersham). When immunoprecipitates were examined, they were prepared as described above. When PKC isoforms were examined, subcellular fractions were prepared as described above .

NORTHERN BLOTTING

Total cellular RNA was isolated by the method described previously by Chomczynski and Sacchi (1987) with some modifications. Equal amounts of RNA quantified by spectrophotometry were size-fractionated by electrophoresis on 1% (w/v) agarose gel containing 20 mmol/l 3-(*N*-morpholino)propanesulphonic acid buffer (pH 7.0), 5 mmol/l sodium acetate, 0.5 mmol/l EDTA and 6% (v/v) formaldehyde. RNA was then transferred to a nylon membrane filter with a solution containing 3 mol/l NaCl and 0.3 mol/l sodium citrate (pH 7.0) followed by fixation with ultraviolet irradiation. Filters were hybridized as described by Raines et al (1989) with cDNA probes (1.8-kb *Pst*I/*Hind*III fragment of human cyclin A cDNA or 1.2-kb *Pst*I/*Pst*I fragment of β-actin cDNA) radiolabelled to approximately 10^6 cpm/ml with [α-^{32}P]-deoxycytidine 5'-triphosphate (New England Nuclear) by random-primed DNA labelling. The filters were washed with a solution containing 15 mmol/l NaCl, 1.5 mmol/l sodium citrate and 0.1% (w/v) SDS at 65°C, and exposed to an X-ray film at -80°C with an intensifying screen for 12-48 h. RNA sizes were determined based upon the migration distances with 18S and 28S ribosomal RNA references stained with ethidium bromide.

NUCLEAR RUN-ON ASSAY

Isolated nuclei (1 x 10^8) suspended in 50 mmol/l Tris/HCl (pH 8.3), 5 mmol/l $MgCl_2$, 0.1 mmol/l EDTA and 40% (v/v) glycerol were mixed with an equal volume of buffer containing 80 mmol/l Tris/HCl (pH 8.3), 15 mmol/l $MgCl_2$, 300 mmol/l NH_4Cl, 400 units/ml RNase inhibitor (Toyobo), 1.25 mmol/l ATP, 0.625 mmol/l GTP, 0.625 mmol/l CTP and 14.8 MBq of [α-^{32}P]-UTP (New England Nuclear). The mixture was incubated at 30°C for 30 min to elongate the RNA chains. Labelled RNA (at least 10^7 cpm) extracted as described above was hybridized with cDNA fragments of human cyclin A (1.7-kb *Eco*RI/*Nco*I) and β-actin (1.2-kb *Pst*I/*Pst*I), which had been obtained from 5 μg cDNA-containing plasmids, electrophoresed on a 1% (w/v) agarose gel to separate from the vectors, and alkali-transferred to Hybond N+ (Amersham). Hybridization was performed in buffer (2 ml) containing 0.5 mol/l sodium phosphate (pH 7.2), 1 mmol/l EDTA, 7% (w/v) SDS and 1% (w/v) bovine serum albumin at 65°C for 40 h. The membrane was then incubated with 10 μg/ml RNase A (Sigma) in a solution containing 0.3 mol/l NaCl and 30 mmol/l sodium citrate (pH 7.0) at 37°C for 30 min to lower background radioactivity

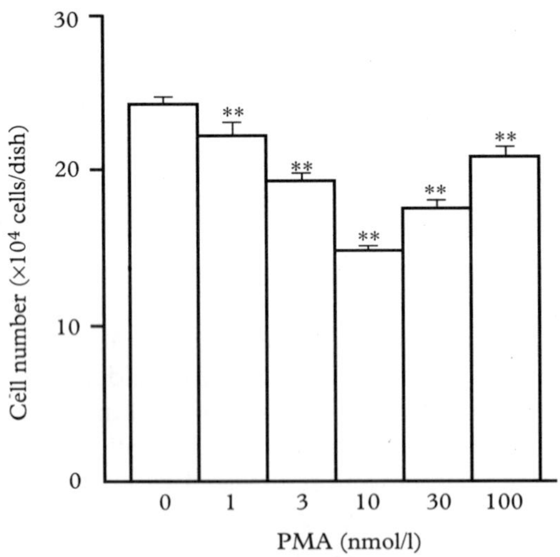

Fig. 17.1 Protein kinase C inhibition of endothelial cell proliferation. G_0-arrested cells were seeded at a density of 5 x 10^4 per dish (35-mm diameter), incubated in the presence of 20% FBS, 10 ng/ml bFGF and various concentrations of PMA for 5 days, and were counted with a Coulter counter. *Statistical significance:* ** p <0.01 versus control. *Abbreviations:* FBS = foetal bovine serum; bFGF = basic fibroblast growth factor; PMA = phorbol 12-myristate, 13-acetate. (Reproduced with permission from Kosaka et al 1993a)

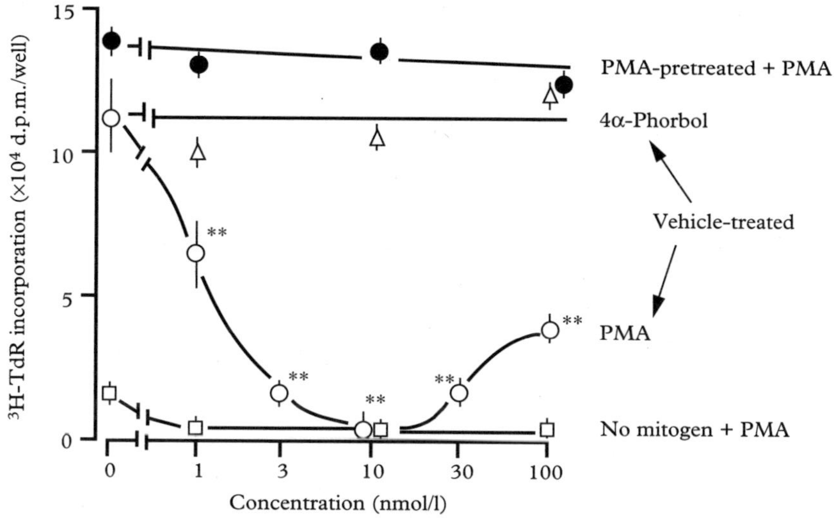

Fig. 17.2 PKC inhibition of DNA synthesis by endothelial cells. Effects of PMA on DNA synthesis. G_0-arrested cells were stimulated with 10 ng/ml bFGF and labelled with [^{3}H]-TdR from 12 until 24 h after stimulation. PMA (○,●) or 4α-phorbol (△) was added 8 h after bFGF. Cells pre-exposed to 1 μmol/l PMA for 24 h, after which PMA was washed out before stimulation with bFGF (●). Cells not stimulated with mitogen (□) [PMA was added at time 0]. Values are given as means ± SD of quadruplicate experiments. *Stastistical significance:* * $p < 0.05$, ** $p < 0.01$ versus control. *Abbreviations:* bFGF = basic fibroblast growth factor; PKC = protein kinase C; PMA = phorbol 12-myristate, 13-acetate; TdR = thymidine. (Reproduced in part and with permission from Kosaka et al 1993a)

followed by washing with solution containing 30 mmol/l NaCl, 3 mmol/l sodium citrate (pH 7.0) and 0.1% (w/v) SDS at 65°C for 30 min. Autoradiography was performed as described above.

Statistical analysis

The results were expressed as means ± SD of the number of observations. Statistical significance was assessed by the Student's t test for paired or unpaired values.

RESULTS

The increase in the endothelial cell population was inhibited by PMA in a concentration-dependent manner, with the maximal effect being obtained at 10 nmol/l. Above this concentration, the effect was partially reversed (Fig. 17.1). This effect seemed to be mediated through the PKC pathway, since the cells exhibited specific and saturable binding of PMA over a concentration range of 1.25-25 nmol/l, which is similar to that causing inhibition of their proliferation. Scatchard analysis of these data showed

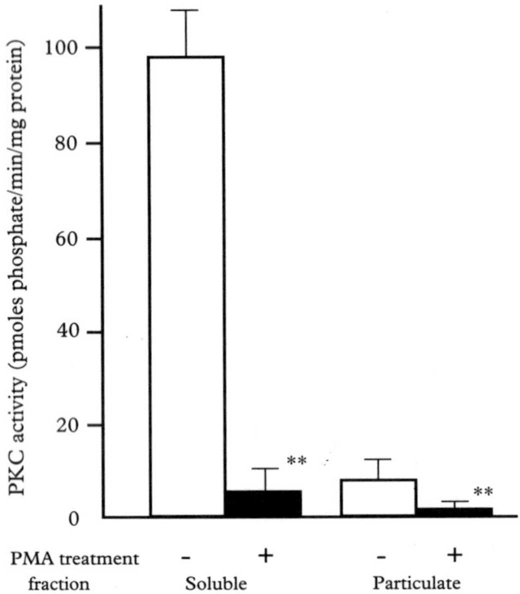

Fig. 17.3 PKC inhibition of DNA synthesis by endothelial cells. Down-regulation of PKC activity after 24-h exposure to 1 μmol/l PMA. Activity was measured at 8 h after bFGF addition. Values are given as means ± SD of quadruplicate experiments. *Statistical significance:* ** $p < 0.01$ versus control. *Abbreviations:* bFGF = basic fibroblast growth factor; PKC = protein kinase C; PMA = phorbol 12-myristate, 13-acetate. (Reproduced in part and with permission from Kosaka et al 1993a)

that PMA bound to a single class of sites, with an apparent K_D and B_{MAX} being 2.7 nmol/l and 29.8 fmol/10^5 cells, respectively, in agreement with the affinities of PMA for PKC reported in other systems.

To elucidate the mechanism underlying this effect, we analyzed their cell cycle. DNA synthesis stimulated with bFGF was strongly inhibited by PMA with a dose dependency similar to that obtained for the cell population (Fig. 17.2). 4α-Phorbol, which is unable to activate PKC, had no influence. The PMA effect was completely abolished by prolonged pre-exposure to 1 μmol/l PMA, which down-regulated PKC activities (Fig. 17.3). 1,2-Dioctanoylglycerol (DiC_8), a membrane-permeable DAG, also inhibited DNA synthesis (Fig. 17.4). DiC_8 was added repeatedly from late G_1, since this compound has been shown to be degraded rapidly by non-specific esterase or DAG lipase when added to live cells (Asaoka et al 1991b). The effect of DiC_8 was also inhibited in cells pre-exposed to PMA, although not completely. Therefore, PKC-independent mechanisms might partially contribute to this inhibition.

The effect of PMA was maximal when applied 8 h after bFGF (Kosaka et al 1993a). This implies that the check point for PKC is located in late G_1, since the entry into the S phase occurred about 12 h after stimulation.

This led us to the assumption that PKC influences an event that is essential for initiation of DNA synthesis and which occurs a few hours before entry into the S phase. The level of cyclin A mRNA was elevated from about 8 h (late G_1) and reached a maximal value at 16 h (early to middle S), followed by a decay (Kosaka et al 1993a). Concomitantly, the level of the protein increased from late G_1, reaching a maximal value at 20 h (middle to late S); it was reduced more slowly than mRNA (Kosaka et al 1993a). Therefore, the onset of cyclin A expression appeared to coincide with the moment of PKC action.

The level of cyclin A protein, determined by Western blotting, was markedly reduced by PMA added 8 h after bFGF, the most effective time for PMA to inhibit DNA synthesis (Fig. 17.5a). This effect was apparent 4 h after PMA addition and lasted for at least 16 h. The dose dependency was similar to that observed for proliferation (Fig. 17.5b). However, PMA did not inhibit protein expression in PKC-depleted cells, confirming that inhibition of cyclin A expression was caused by PKC, and suggesting that a down-regulable PKC isoform(s) was responsible for this effect (Fig. 17.5b).

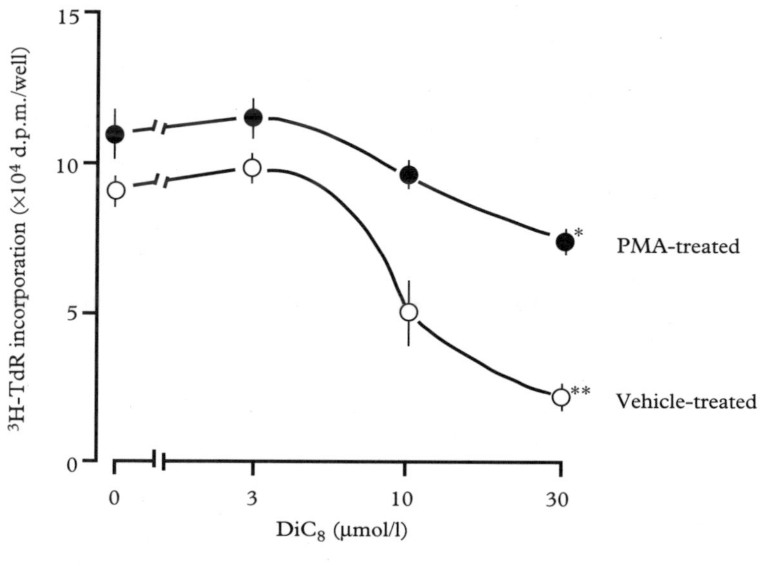

Fig. 17.4 PKC inhibition of DNA synthesis by endothelial cells. Effects of DiC_8 on DNA synthesis. DiC_8 was applied every hour from 8 until 16 h. Cells were labelled with [^{3}H]-TdR as described in figure 17.2. Filled symbols indicate cells pre-exposed to 1 μmol/l PMA for 24 h. The indicated concentrations of DiC_8 are those obtained by a single dose. Values are given as means ± SD of quadruplicate experiments. *Statistical significance:* *$p < 0.05$, **$p < 0.01$ versus control. *Abbreviations:* bFGF = basic fibroblast growth factor; DiC8 = 1,2-dioctanoylglycerol; PKC = protein kinase C; PMA = phorbol 12-myristate, 13-acetate; TdR = thymidine. (Reproduced in part and with permission from Kosaka et al 1993a)

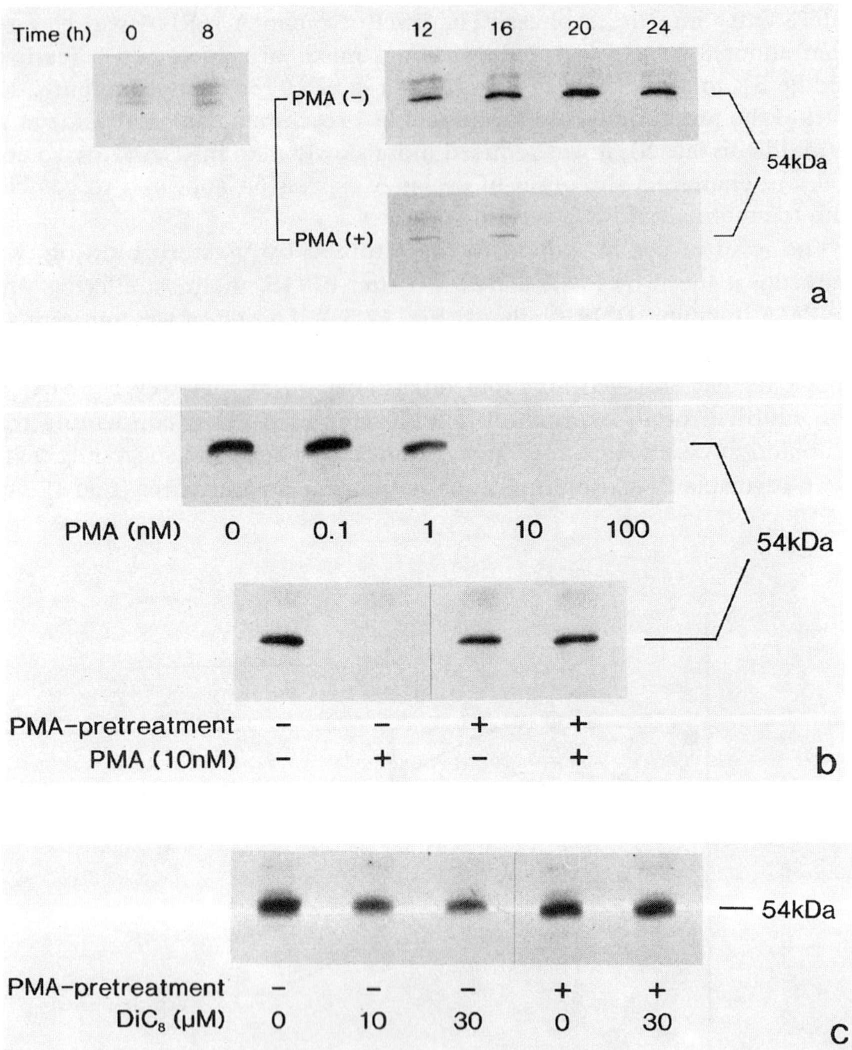

Fig. 17.5 PKC inhibition of cyclin A protein expression. (**a**) Time course of cyclin A protein expression. PMA (10 nmol/l) was added at 8 h after bFGF. Cells were harvested at the indicated times, and the extracted proteins were analyzed by Western blotting for human cyclin A using a monoclonal antibody C160. (**b**) Dependence of cyclin A protein expression on PMA concentration. PMA was added at 8 h, and cells were lysed at 20 h after bFGF addition. (**c**) Effects of DiC_8 on cyclin A protein expression. DiC_8 was added every hour from 8 until 19 h, and proteins were extracted at 20 h. *Abbreviations:* bFGF = basic fibroblast growth factor; DiC_8 = 1,2-dioctanoylglycerol; PKC = protein kinase C; PMA = phorbol 12-myristate, 13-acetate. (Reproduced with permission from Kosaka et al 1993a)

DiC_8 also inhibited the expression (Fig. 17.5). Although DiC_8 was not as potent as PMA, its potency appeared to parallel its effect on proliferation.

To determine whether the decrease in the amount of cyclin A protein was due to suppression of its gene expression, we performed Northern blotting. The level of cyclin A mRNA was potently reduced by PMA (Fig. 17.6). The dose dependency was, again, similar to that shown for the PMA effect on DNA synthesis. However, PMA failed to reduce mRNA levels in PKC-depleted cells (Fig. 17.6a). DiC_8 also reduced mRNA levels, with a dose dependency similar to that shown for the protein levels (Fig. 17.6b). To examine whether the decrease in cyclin A mRNA was caused by inhibition of transcription, we performed a nuclear run-on assay. PMA inhibited the nascent transcription of mRNA, indicating that cyclin A transcription was negatively regulated through the PKC pathway (Fig. 17.7).

With regard to pRB, hyperphosphorylated pRB moved more slowly in SDS-polyacrylamide gel than the underphosphorylated form. Underphosphorylated pRB was predominant in G_0-arrested cells, whereas the hyperphosphorylated form increased after the cells entered the S phase. PMA added in late G_1 markedly inhibited this phosphorylation (Kosaka et al 1993b).

We then examined whether the G_2/M transition is also regulated through the PKC pathway. Endothelial cells, the growth of which was arrested at the G_1/S boundary by aphidicolin (a DNA polymerase-α inhibitor), was released by washing out the inhibitor, and cultured in medium containing FBS and bFGF. DNA synthesis was completed by 12 h after the release, and the cell population began to increase at 24-27 h. PMA added by 21 h strongly inhibited the cell population increase. However, PMA did not interrupt the completion of the M phase in cells released from nocodazole-induced M-phase arrest.

Flow cytometry using propidium iodide demonstrated that cells in the G_2 or M phases accumulated in the presence of PMA, suggesting that the PKC pathway does not interrupt progression of the S phase. Furthermore, flow cytometry using acridine orange showed that cells did not enter the M phase in the presence of both PMA and colcemide, an M-phase inhibitor, whereas, in the presence of colcemide alone, cells in the M phase accumulated markedly. This suggests that the check point for PMA is located in G_2 and not in the M phase.

To elucidate the mechanism responsible for the G_2 inhibition, we examined the effect of PMA on Cdc2 (Cdk1) kinase activity. Cdc2 activity, determined using histone H1 as the substrate, was elevated around the traversal across the G_2/M border. PMA added in the G_2 phase strongly suppressed this activation.

To determine the PKC isoform(s) involved in the cell cycle inhibition, we performed Western blotting using antibodies specific to the isoforms. From the soluble proteins of the endothelial cells, PKC-α, -ε, and - ζ were detected (Kosaka et al 1993b).

DISCUSSION

We found that the cell cycle of cultured human vascular endothelial cells was negatively regulated by the PKC pathway at two independent points, i.e., the G_1 and the G_2 phases (Fig. 17.8). This inhibition paralleled the net effect of PKC activation on cell proliferation, since the increase in the cell population was also inhibited by PKC activators. Doctrow and Folkman (1987) reported that PKC inhibited proliferation in bovine capillary endothelial cells, but not in bovine aortic endothelial cells. They suggested that the inhibitory effect of PKC would be specific to capillary endothelial cells, and that this mechanism would play a role in angiogenesis. According to our findings, however, the proliferation of bovine aortic endothelial cells was also inhibited by PKC activators; the inhibition was maximal when PKC activators were added in the middle to

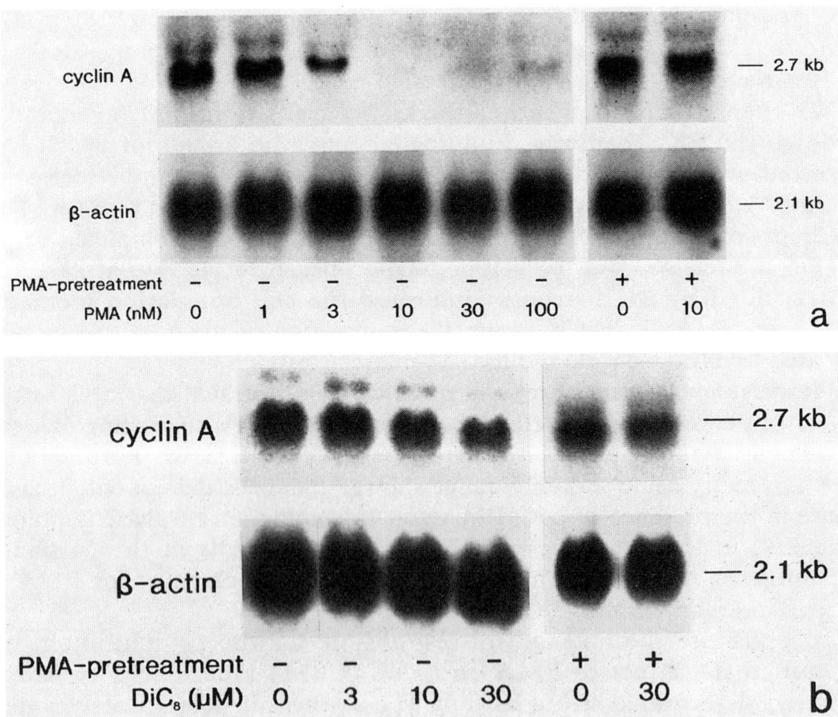

Fig. 17.6 PKC inhibition of cyclin A gene expression. (**a**) Effect of PMA on cyclin A mRNA amount. PMA was added 8 h after bFGF, and RNA was extracted at 16 h. Total cellular RNA (20 μg) was analyzed by Northern blotting for human cyclin A and β-actin. (**b**) Effects of DiC_8 on cyclin A mRNA. DiC_8 was added every hour from 8 until 15 h, and RNA was extracted at 16 h. *Abbreviations:* bFGF = basic fibroblast growth factor; DiC_8 = 1,2-dioctanoylglycerol; PKC = protein kinase C; PMA = phorbol 12-myristate, 13-acetate. (Reproduced with permission from Kosaka et al 1993a)

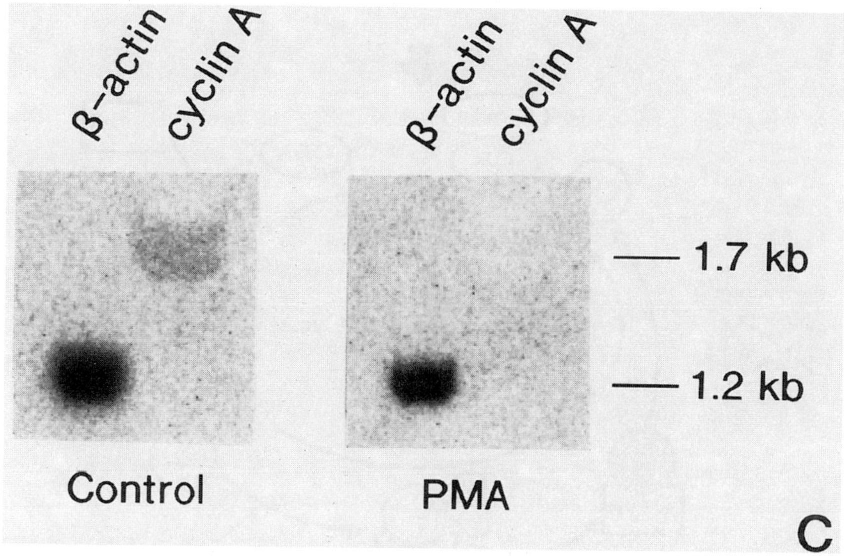

Fig. 17.7 PKC inhibition of cyclin A gene expression. Nuclear run-on analysis for cyclin A transcription. Nuclei isolated 12 h after bFGF addition were analyzed for nascent transcription. PMA (10 nmol/l) was added at 8 h. *Abbreviations:* bFGF = basic fibroblast growth factor; DiC_8 = 1,2-dioctanoylglycerol; PKC = protein kinase C; PMA = phorbol 12-myristate, 13-acetate. (Reproduced with permission from Kosaka et al 1993a)

late G_1 (data not shown). Together with the data presented in this article, G_1/S progression of vascular endothelial cells seems to be always inhibited regardless of their origin. Moreover, PKC-mediated growth inhibition is not a phenomenon limited to endothelial cells, but may be a more universal mechanism, as PKC has been reported to inhibit proliferation in several cell systems other than endothelial cells (Huang & Ives 1987; Kanakura et al 1991; Mackanos et al 1991; McKay et al 1983; Rovera et al 1979; Sasaguri et al 1993).

On the other hand, PKC can promote G_0/G_1 transition (early G_1 progression) in some cell systems (Rozengurt 1986). However, this effect may not be a fundamental mechanism in the regulation of the cell cycle, since according to our observations, the effects of PKC activators on early G_1 progression varied greatly with the cell system used in the experiment. Stimulation of an autocrine growth factor production has been suggested as a cause of PKC-mediated growth stimulation in human melanocytes (Arita et al 1992). Therefore, the effects of PKC on early G_1 progression could depend on the ability of cells to produce growth factors through the PKC pathway. By contrast, in our studies, G_1/S transition was inhibited by PKC activators without an exception, in experiments using rat, porcine, bovine and human arterial smooth muscle cells, bovine aortic and human umbilical vein endothelial cells, and a human fibroblast line, IMR-90. This

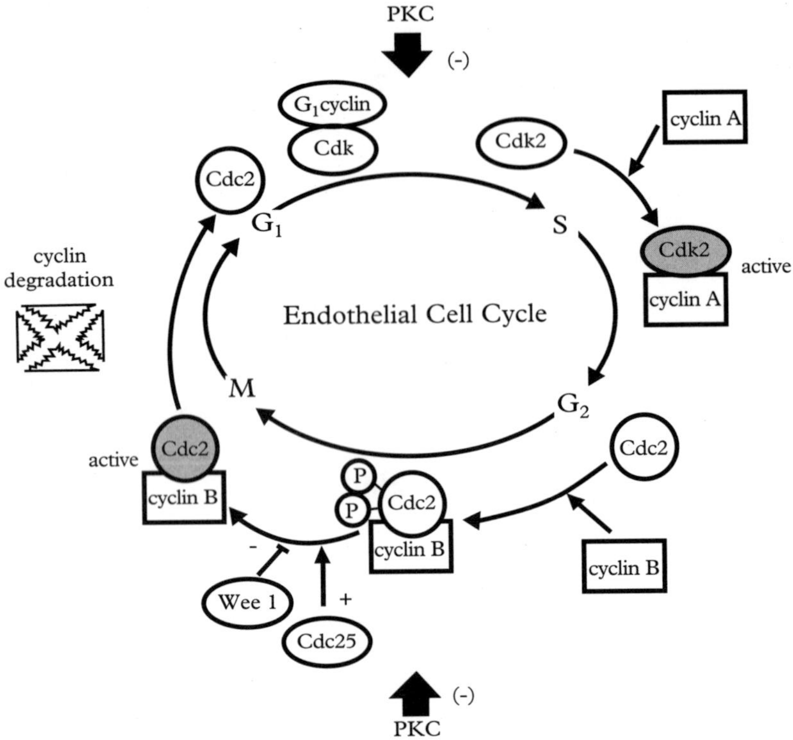

Fig. 17.8 Regulation of the endothelial cell cycle by the protein kinase C (PKC) pathway.

implies that PKC-mediated G_1/S inhibition is a fundamental mechanism in regulating the mammalian cell cycle. However, the way in which PKC inhibits cell proliferation has remained unknown.

Cyclin A has been shown to be essential for G_1/S progression of mammalian cells; plasmids encoding antisense cyclin A cDNA microinjected into G_1 cells inhibited their DNA synthesis, and re-injection of cyclin A protein relieved this inhibition (Girard et al 1991). Furthermore, anti-cyclin A antibodies injected into G_1 cells blocked their G_1/S transition (Girard et al 1991; Pagano et al 1992). Cyclin A/Cdk2 complex might phosphorylate a putative substrate essential to DNA replication, associating with a transcription factor, E_2F (Nevins 1992). We found that cyclin A expression is suppressed through the PKC pathway, and this effect seemed to be potent enough to be the cause of the G_1/S arrest. Therefore, our study may provide a crucial biochemical basis for PKC-mediated G_1/S inhibition. PKC also inhibited pRB phosphorylation. pRB has been shown to be phosphorylated by Cdk2 *in vitro* (Akiyama et al

1992). If pRB is the *in vivo* substrate for Cdk2, then the inhibition of pRB phosphorylation might be a result of the suppression of cyclin A expression. Recently, a pRB-related protein, p107, has also been suggested as playing an important role in G_1/S regulation (Schwarz et al 1993). Whether PKC modulates this protein should therefore be investigated.

The PKC target responsible for the G_1/S inhibition, which might be located upstream to cyclin A transcription, has not yet been determined. There are several candidates. PKC phosphorylates the epidermal growth factor receptor, thus inhibiting receptor binding (Lin et al 1986). PKC inhibits protein tyrosine phosphorylation caused by granulocyte-macrophage colony-stimulating factor, without affecting its receptor expression (Kanakura et al 1991). The autocrine production of transforming growth factor-β is involved in phorbol ester-induced growth inhibition of a human lymphoma cell line (Sing et al 1990). However, the fact that the most effective time for PKC activation coincided well with the onset of cyclin A expression implies that the PKC pathway interacts with a molecule closely related to cyclin A gene expression, such as transcription factors. Direct influence of PKC on nuclear function has been suggested in light of the findings that nuclear DAG levels in IIC9 cells were elevated by α-thrombin (Leach et al 1992), and that some isoforms of PKC, such as PKC-α, were localized in or translocated to nuclei (Buchner et al 1992; James & Olson 1992; Leach et al 1992). However, recent findings suggest that G_1 cyclins, such as cyclins D and E, play important roles in G_1 progression and in G_1/S transition, activating certain cyclin-dependent kinases (Sherr 1993). Their appearances may precede cyclin A expression, and therefore, it is possible that the effect of PKC on cyclin A transcription is secondary to its effect on these G_1 cyclins and their companion kinases. Investigation aimed at identifying the putative PKC substrate responsible for the G_1/S inhibition is now underway in our laboratory.

G_2/M progression is also interrupted by phorbol ester in endothelial cells, and this effect appeared to correlate with the suppression of Cdc2 (Cdk1) kinase activity. The cell cycle of CHO cells overexpressing PKC-δ is arrested by PMA in the M phase (Watanabe et al 1992). However, in endothelial cells, PMA seemed to interrupt the progression of the G_2 phase. If this interruption was mediated through the PKC pathway, such an effect of PKC has not previously been reported in other cell systems to our knowledge. Therefore, it remains to be determined whether the PKC-mediated G_2 inhibition is a fundamental mechanism for cell-cycle regulation common to various cell systems.

Endothelial cells possess three isoforms of PKC, i. e., PKC-α, -ε, and -ζ. We have previously reported that PKC-α and -ε are the most probable mediators of the G_1/S inhibition in vascular smooth muscle cells (Sasaguri et al 1993). The possible involvement of PKC-α in cell growth regulation is supported by the observation that overexpression of PKC-α diminished cell growth and promoted differentiation of melanoma cells (Gruber et al 1992).

Endothelial cells are exposed to several substances, such as Ca^{2+}-mobilizing hormones and growth factors, which stimulate phospholipase-linked receptors. One of the earliest events in their intracellular signalling is the activation of phospholipase C, which hydrolyzes membrane phospholipids, such as phosphoinositides and phosphatidylcholine, to produce DAG (Nishizuka 1992). Phospholipase D may also be activated following receptor stimulation to produce phosphatidic acid, which is further hydrolyzed by phosphatases to generate DAG (Nishizuka 1992). Therefore, our findings suggest that PKC could function as a negative feedback regulator against mitogenic signals. On the other hand, PKC could be involved in signalling pathways for antiproliferative agents, such as interferons (Pfeffer et al 1991; Tiefenbrun & Kimchi 1991). Interferon-α/β, transforming growth factor-β and interleukin-6 have recently been reported to reduce cyclin A protein levels in haematopoietic cells (Resnitzky et al 1992), and that tumour necrosis factor-α, interferon-γ, prostaglandin E_2, and 8-bromo-cAMP suppress cyclin D1 gene expression in macrophages (Cocks et al 1992). Therefore, it is possible that several antiproliferative agents, particularly those activating PKC or cAMP-dependent protein kinase, exert their effects through inhibiting the gene expression of cyclin A and/or G_1 cyclins.

However, PKC activation does not necessarily require receptor-mediated signalling. It would not be surprising if PKC activity were modulated by lipids deposited in the vessel wall, since PKC is a unique protein kinase, the activity of which depends on phospholipids. In fact, lysophosphatidylcholine, which accumulates in atherosclerotic lesions (Portman & Alexander 1969), has recently been reported to enhance PKC activity *in vitro* in the presence of DiC_8 and ionomycin, a calcium ionophore (Asaoka et al 1991a). As already mentioned, excess glucose-induced DAG accumulation is another means of PKC activation. Therefore, at least *in vitro*, the PKC pathway of endothelial cells can be activated by nonreceptor mechanisms, particularly under pathological conditions.

Lorenzi et al (1987) reported that an excess of ambient glucose prolonged the cell cycle of human umbilical vein endothelial cells, by disturbing the progression of the G_1 and G_2 phases. They stated that increased intracellular osmotic pressure due to activation of the polyol pathway was unlikely to cause the cell cycle delay, since intracellular sorbitol accumulation was lower by orders of magnitude than would be expected as causing the osmolar increase. They also excluded the possibility that depleted myo-inositol (Finegold et al 1983; Greene & Lattimer 1982) could cause the cell cycle delay, since a supplement of myo-inositol failed to prevent the delay (Lorenzi & Toledo 1986). Precise mechanisms for the prolongation of the G_1 and G_2 phases remain unknown, although they suggested that DNA damage caused by excess glucose could, at least in part, contribute to the cell cycle delay (Lorenzi et al 1986).

Our study shows that G_1/S and G_2/M transitions are both interrupted through the PKC pathway in endothelial cells of the same origin as those used by Lorenzi et al (1987) in their experiments. The check points for PKC appear to coincide with the phases in the cell cycle disturbed by excess glucose. This led us to speculation that excess glucose could inhibit endothelial cell growth through the PKC pathway. Therefore, a sustained elevation of endothelial PKC activity in the diabetic state could impair endothelial regeneration after vascular injury, resulting in retardation of intimal repair, and, therefore, in accelerated atherosclerotic lesion formation (Fig. 17.9). To evidence this hypothesis requires testing whether high concentrations of glucose lose the ability to inhibit the cell cycle after PKC is inactivated by certain means, such as specific inhibitors for PKC, phorbol ester-induced PKC down-regulation, and antisense oligonucleotide for the PKC isoform involved in cell cycle inhibition.

In addition, high concentrations of glucose impair the proliferation of cells other than endothelial cells, such as capillary pericytes (Li et al 1984) and renal mesangial cells (Togawa et al 1991). These effects could also, therefore, contribute to the pathogenesis of diabetic complications. Whether the activation of PKC is involved in these processes should be investigated to determine more precisely the role of the PKC pathway in the pathogenesis of diabetic complications.

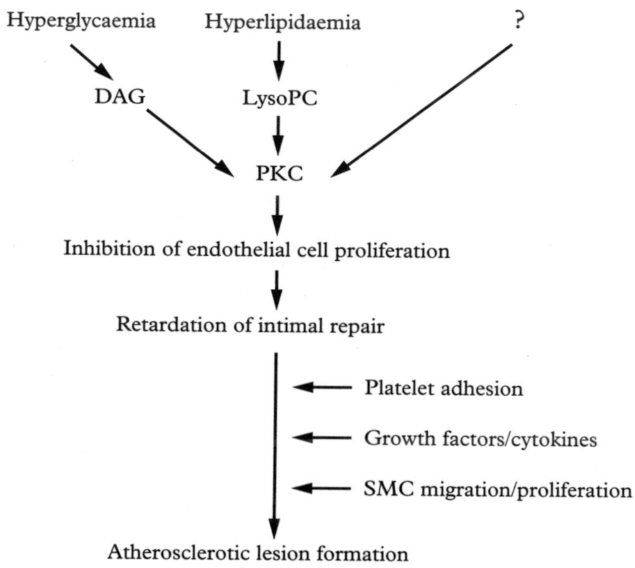

Fig. 17.9 The protein kinase C (PKC) pathway and atherogenesis (hypothesis). *Abbreviations:* DAG = diacylglycerol; LysoPC = lysophosphatidylcholine; SMC = smooth muscle cell.

ACKNOWLEDGMENTS

This study was supported by grants from the Japanese Science and Technology Agency, the Japanese Ministry of Health and Welfare, the Yamanouchi Foundation for Research on Metabolic Disorders, and the Uehara Memorial Foundation. We thank Drs. Jun Ogata, Kentaro Shimokado, Junichi Masuda, and Katsuhiro Zen for helpful discussions.

REFERENCES

Abe M, Ono J, Sato Y et al 1990 Effects of glucose and insulin on cultured human microvascular endothelial cells. Diabetes Res Clin Pract 9: 287-295

Akiyama T, Ohuchi T, Sumida S et al 1992 Phosphorylation of the retinoblastoma protein by cdk2. Proc Natl Acad Sci USA 89: 7900-7904

Arita Y, O'Driscoll K R, Weinstein I B 1992 Growth of human melanocyte cultures supported by 12-*O*-tetradecanoylphorbol-13-acetate is mediated through protein kinase C activation. Cancer Res 52: 4514-4521

Asaoka Y, Oka M, Yoshida K et al 1991a Lysophosphatidylcholine as a possible second messenger synergistic to diacylglycerol and calcium ion for T-lymphocyte activation. Biochem Biophys Res Commun 178: 1378-1385

Asaoka Y, Oka M, Yoshida K et al 1991b Metabolic rate of membrane-permeant diacylglycerol and its relation to human resting T-lymphocyte activation. Proc Natl Acad Sci USA 88: 8681-8685

Ayo S H, Radnik R, Garoni J A et al 1991 High glucose increases diacylglycerol mass and activates protein kinase C in mesangial cell cultures. Am J Physiol 261: F571-577

Brolin S E, Naeser P 1988 Sorbitol in aortic endothelium of diabetic rats. Diabetes Res 8: 59-61.

Buchner K, Otto H, Hilbert R et al 1992 Properties of protein kinase C associated with nuclear membranes. Biochem J 286: 369-375

Chomczynski P, Sacchi N 1987 Single-step method of RNA isolation by acid guanidinium thiocyanate-phenol-chloroform extraction. Anal Biochem 162: 156-159

Cocks B G, Vairo G, Bodrug S E et al 1992 Suppression of growth factor-induced CYL1 cyclin gene expression by antiproliferative agents. J Biol Chem 267: 12307-12310

Corkey R F, Corkey B E, Gimbrone Jr M A 1981 Hexose transport in normal and SV40-transformed human endothelial cells in culture. J Cell Physiol 106: 425-434

Craven P A, DeRubertis F R 1989 Protein kinase C is activated in glomeruli from streptozotocin diabetic rats: possible mediation by glucose. J Clin Invest 83: 1667-1675

Davies M J, Woolf N, Rowles P M et al 1988 Morphology of the endothelium over atherosclerotic plaques in human coronary arteries. Br Heart J 60: 459-464

Dolgov V V, Zaikina O E, Bondarenko M F et al 1982 Aortic endothelium of alloxan diabetic rabbits: a quantitative study using scanning electron microscopy. Diabetologia 22: 338-343

Doctrow S R, Folkman J 1987 Protein kinase C activators suppress stimulation of capillary endothelial cell growth by angiogenic endothelial mitogens. J Cell Biol 104: 679-687

Elledge S J, Richman R, Hall F L et al 1992 *CDK2* encodes a 33-kDa cyclin A-associated protein kinase and is expressed before *CDC2* in the cell cycle. Proc Natl Acad Sci USA 89: 2907-2911

Finegold D, Lattimer S A, Nolle S et al 1983 Polyol pathway activity and *myo*-inositol metabolism: a suggested relationship in the pathogenesis of diabetic neuropathy. Diabetes 32: 988-992

Girard F, Strausfeld U, Fernandez A et al 1991 Cyclin A is required for the onset of DNA replication in mammalian fibroblasts. Cell 67: 1169-1179

Greene D A, Lattimer S A 1982 Sodium- and energy-dependent uptake of *myo*-inositol by rabbit peripheral nerve: competitive inhibition by glucose and lack of an insulin effect. J Clin Invest 70: 1009-1018

Gruber J R, Ohno S, Niles R M 1992 Increased expression of protein kinase Ca plays a key role in retinoic acid-induced melanoma differentiation. J Biol Chem 267: 13356-13360

Harrison H E, Reece A H, Johnson M 1978 Decreased vascular prostacyclin in experimental diabetes. Life Sci 23: 351-356

Huang C-L, Ives H E 1987 Growth inhibition by protein kinase C late in mitogenesis. Nature 329: 849-850
Hunter T, Pines J 1991 Cyclins and cancer. Cell 66: 1071-1074
Inoguchi T, Battan R, Handler E et al 1992 Preferential elevation of protein kinase C isoform βII and diacylglycerol levels in the aorta and heart of diabetic rats: differential reversibility to glycemic control by islet cell transplantation. Proc Natl Acad Sci USA 89: 11059-11063
James G, Olson E 1992 Deletion of the regulatory domain of protein kinase C α exposes regions in the hinge and catalytic domains that mediate nuclear targeting. J Cell Biol 116: 863-874
Johnson M, Harrison H E, Raftery A T et al 1979 Vascular prostacyclin may be reduced in diabetes in man. Lancet 1: 325-326
Kanakura Y, Druker B, DiCarlo J et al 1991 Phorbol 12-myristate 13-acetate inhibits granulocyte-macrophage colony stimulating factor-induced protein tyrosine phosphorylation in a human factor-dependent hematopoietic cell line. J Biol Chem 266: 490-495
King G L, Buzney S M, Kahn C R et al 1983 Differential responsiveness to insulin of endothelial and support cells from micro- and macrovessels. J Clin Invest 71: 974-979
Kosaka C, Sasaguri T, Masuda J et al 1993a Protein kinase C-mediated inhibition of cyclin A expression in human vascular endothelial cells. Biochem Biophys Res Commun 193: 991-998
Kosaka C, Sasaguri T, Zen K et al 1993b Cell growth regulation through the protein kinase C pathway in cultured human vascular endothelial cells. Jpn Circ J 57 (suppl 4): 1207-1210
Leach K L, Ruff V A, Jarpe M B et al 1992 α-Thrombin stimulates nuclear diglyceride levels and differential nuclear localization of protein kinase C isozymes in IIC9 Cells. J Biol Chem 267: 21816-21822
Lee T-S, Saltsman K A, Ohashi H et al 1989 Activation of protein kinase C by elevation of glucose concentration: proposal for a mechanism in the development of diabetic vascular complications. Proc Natl Acad Sci USA 86: 5141-5145
Levine A J 1993 The tumor suppressor genes. Annu Rev Biochem 62: 623-651
Li W, Shen S, Khatami M et al 1984 Stimulation of retinal capillary pericyte protein and collagen synthesis in culture by high-glucose concentration. Diabetes 33: 785-789
Lin C R, Chen W S, Lazar C S et al 1986 Protein kinase C phosphorylation at Thr 654 of the unoccupied EGF receptor and EGF binding regulate functional receptor loss by independent mechanisms. Cell 44: 839-848
Lorenzi M, Cagliero E, Toledo S 1985 Glucose toxicity for human endothelial cells in culture: delayed replication, disturbed cell cycle, and accelerated death. Diabetes 34: 621-627
Lorenzi M, Montisano D F, Toledo S et al 1986 High glucose induces DNA damage in cultured human endothelial cells. J Clin Invest 77: 322-325
Lorenzi M, Nordberg J A, Toledo S 1987 High glucose prolongs cell-cycle traversal of cultured human endothelial cells. Diabetes 36: 1261-1267
Lorenzi M, Toledo S 1986 *Myo*-inositol enhances the proliferation of human endothelial cells in culture but fails to prevent the delay induced by high glucose. Metabolism 35: 824-829
Mackanos E A, Pettit G R, Ramsdell J S 1991 Bryostatins selectively regulate protein kinase C-mediated effects on GH_4 cell proliferation. J Biol Chem 266: 11205-11212
Masuda J, Ross R 1990 Atherogenesis during low level hypercholesterolemia in the nonhuman primate. I. Fatty streak formation. Arteriosclerosis 10: 164-177
McKay I, Collins M, Taylor-Papadimitriou J et al 1983 An inhibitory effect of tumour promoters on human epithelial cell growth can be dissociated from an effect on junctional communication. Exp Cell Res 145: 245-254
Meraji S, Jayakody L, Senaratne M P J et al 1987 Endothelium-dependent relaxation in aorta of BB rat. Diabetes 36: 978-981
Naeser P 1986 Cell replication in retinal vessels of streptozotocin diabetic mice. Acta Ophthalmol 64: 439-440
Nevins J R 1992 E2F: a link between the Rb tumor suppressor protein and viral oncoproteins. Science 258: 424-429
Nishizuka Y 1992 Intracellular signaling by hydrolysis of phospholipids and activation of protein kinase C. Science 258: 607-614
Norbury C, Nurse P 1992 Animal cell cycles and their control. Annu Rev Biochem 61: 441-470
Ono H, Umeda F, Inoguchi T et al 1988 Glucose inhibits prostacyclin production by cultured aortic endothelial cells. Thromb Haemost 60: 174-177

Pagano M, Pepperkok R, Lukas J et al 1993 Regulation of the cell cycle by the cdk2 protein kinase in cultured human fibroblasts. J Cell Biol 121: 101-111

Pagano M, Pepperkok R, Verde F et al 1992 Cyclin A is required at two points in the human cell cycle. EMBO J 11: 961-971

Pfeffer L M, Eisenkraft B L, Reich N C et al 1991 Transmembrane signaling by interferon a involves diacylglycerol production and activation of the ε isoform of protein kinase C in Daudi cells. Proc Natl Acad Sci USA 88: 7988-7992

Portman O W, Alexander M 1969 Lysophosphatidylcholine concentrations and metabolism in aortic intima plus inner media: effect of nutritionally induced atherosclerosis. J Lipid Res 10: 158-165

Raines E W, Dower S K, Ross R 1989 Interleukin-1 mitogenic activity for fibroblasts and smooth muscle cells is due to PDGF-AA. Science 243: 393-396

Reidy M A 1985 Biology of disease: a reassessment of endothelial injury and arterial lesion formation. Lab Invest 53: 513-520

Resnitzky D, Tiefenbrun N, Berissi H et al 1992 Interferons and interleukin 6 suppress phosphorylation of the retinoblastoma protein in growth-sensitive hematopoietic cells. Proc Natl Acad Sci USA 89: 402-406

Rosenblatt J, Gu Y, Morgan D O 1992 Human cyclin-dependent kinase 2 is activated during the S and G_2 phases of the cell cycle and associates with cyclin A. Proc Natl Acad Sci USA 89: 2824-2828

Ross R 1993 The pathogenesis of atherosclerosis: a perspective for the 1990s. Nature 362: 801-809

Rovera G, Santoli D, Damsky C 1979 Human promyelocytic leukemia cells in culture differentiate into macrophage-like cells when treated with a phorbol diester. Proc Natl Acad Sci USA 76: 2779-2783

Rozengurt E 1986 Early signals in the mitogenic response. Science 234: 161-166

Sasaguri T, Kosaka C, Hirata M et al 1993 Protein kinase C-mediated inhibition of vascular smooth muscle cell proliferation: the isoforms that may mediate G_1/S inhibition. Exp Cell Res 208: 311-320

Schwarz J K, Devoto S H, Smith E J et al 1993 Interactions of the p107 and Rb proteins with E2F during the cell proliferation response. EMBO J 12: 1013-1020

Sherr C J 1993 Mammalian G_1 cyclins. Cell 73: 1059-1065

Sing G K, Ruscetti F W, Beckwith M et al 1990 Growth inhibition of a human lymphoma cell line: induction of a transforming growth factor-β–mediated autocrine negative loop by phorbol myristate acetate. Cell Growth Differ 1: 549-557

Stout R W 1982 Glucose inhibits replication of cultured human endothelial cells. Diabetologia 23: 436-439

Tiefenbrun N, Kimchi A 1991 The involvement of protein kinase C in mediating growth suppressive signals of interferons in hematopoietic cells. Oncogene 6: 1001-1007

Togawa M, Kikkawa R, Haneda M et al 1991 Metabolic and mitogenic effects of insulin-like growth factor I on rat glomerular mesangial cells cultured under high concentration of glucose. Nippon Jinzo Gakkai Shi 33: 131-138

Tsai L-H, Harlow E, Meyerson M 1991 Isolation of the human cdk2 gene that encodes the cyclin A- and adenovirus E1A-associated p33 kinase. Nature 353: 174-177

Watanabe T, Ono Y, Taniyama Y et al 1992 Cell division arrest induced by phorbol ester in CHO cells overexpressing protein kinase C-δ subspecies. Proc Natl Acad Sci USA 89: 10159-10163

Yamauchi T, Ohnaka K, Takayanagi R et al 1990 Enhanced secretion of endothelin-1 by elevated glucose levels from cultured bovine aortic endothelial cells. FEBS Lett 267: 16-18

18

Role of insulin-like growth factor-I in proliferative diabetic retinopathy: a modulator of free radical-derived oxidant generation

M. B. Grant, E. A. Ellis, S. Caballero

INTRODUCTION

Diabetic retinopathy, the leading cause of blindness in individuals between the ages of 24 and 64 years, is a disease process for which the pathological (anatomical) stages are well described (Frank 1991). The underlying mechanisms, however, remain ill-defined or unknown. This is due to three factors: the extended time course of progression of the disease (10-30 years); the individual variability of expression; and the limited number of model systems available for study (Merimee 1990). An understanding of diabetic retinopathy is further complicated by the fact that different stages of retinopathy can exist within the same retina.

Much of our understanding of diabetic retinopathy has been gained by the study of the endothelium. Under normal circumstances, endothelial cells function as an antithrombogenic, fibrinolytic surface with selective barrier characteristics. Upon specific perturbation, such as occurs in diabetics, the endothelium may become prothrombotic and permeable to cellular elements. This enhanced thrombosis may be due in part to decreased levels of plasminogen activators, increased levels of plasminogen activator inhibitor-1 (PAI-1), or both. In addition, diabetic individuals have hyperfibrinogenaemia (Ganda & Arkin 1992), increased blood viscosity (McMillan 1983), increased tissue factor (a procoagulant on the endothelial surface) [Boeri et al 1971] and increased von Willebrand factor (required for platelet-plug formation) [Lufkin et al 1979].

Diabetic individuals with vascular complications also have abnormal platelet function, including increased release of thromboxane A_2, a potent vasoconstrictor and inducer of platelet aggregation (Butkus et al 1982), and increased release of platelet factor 4 (PF-4) [Chmielewski & Farbiszewski 1970]. PF-4 can interact with heparin-like glycosaminoglycans on endothelial cells to exert a procoagulant effect (Chmielewski & Farbiszewski 1970). Upon platelet activation, growth factors which are inducers of PAI-1 secretion in endothelial cells (Grant & Guay 1991; Loskutoff 1991) are released from platelets (Assoian & Sporn 1986; Slivka & Loskutoff 1991).

Platelets, by synthesizing PAI-1 and acquiring PAI-1 from the blood, contain 300- to 3000-fold higher concentrations of PAI-1 than plasma (Konkle et al 1993; Slivka & Loskutoff 1991) and can significantly inhibit fibrinolysis in a platelet-rich thrombus.

The production of an antifibrinolytic state (e.g. increased PAI-1) would cooperate with the induction of procoagulant activity (e.g. increased tissue factor and increased von Willebrand factor) to stabilize a fibrin clot. This localized suppression of the fibrinolytic system, with stabilization of fibrin and increased platelet aggregation, would contribute to the formation of microthrombi and the propagation of an occlusive thrombus. This microthrombus formation could lead to retinal nonperfusion and retinal ischaemia.

It has been postulated for longer than 40 years that the ischaemic retina of the diabetic is a source of proliferative factors, which induce the aberrant new vessel growth on the retinal surface so typical of proliferative retinopathy (Michaelson 1948). Growth factors that have been implicated in this process include basic and acidic fibroblast growth factor (Sivalingam et al 1990), vascular endothelial growth factor (Taylor et al 1989) and insulin-like growth factor-I (Grant et al 1986; Merimee et al 1983). Our laboratory has focused on the role of insulin-like growth factor-I (IGF-I) in the pathogenesis of diabetic retinal neovascularization (Grant & Guay 1991; Grant et al 1986, 1987, 1993b, c; Merimee et al 1983).

IGF-I and IGF-II are single-chain polypeptides with structural homology to proinsulin. The IGFs regulate proliferation and differentiation of numerous cell types and can exert insulin-like metabolic effects. *In vivo*, IGF-I acts in a paracrine manner to meditate the activity of growth hormone (Zaph et al 1984). Both IGF-I and IGF-II are produced under specific conditions by most tissues in the body, are abundant in the circulation, and thus have the potential to act via endocrine, paracrine and autocrine mechanisms (Zaph et al 1984). IGF-I, together with platelet-derived growth factor (PDGF), is considered to account for most of the growth-promoting activity of serum *in vitro*. According to the dual control concept of cell proliferation, IGF-I is one of the progression factors which prompt 'competence factor'-primed cells to proceed through G_1 phase (Zaph et al 1984).

Even though IGFs are present in high concentrations in plasma, only 1-5% exist in free form, with the rest tightly complexed to specific IGF-binding proteins, which prolong the half-life of the IGFs in the circulation and represent a reservoir of IGFs (Clemmons 1992).

A role for IGF-I in the pathogenesis of diabetic retinopathy found its origin from the well-established involvement of growth hormone in the development of proliferative diabetic retinopathy (Kohner et al 1976; Lundbaeck 1976; Poulsen 1953). Merimee and coworkers demonstrated markedly elevated serum IGF-I levels in patients with rapidly accelerating proliferative retinopathy (Merimee et al 1983). Hyer et al (1989) demonstrated elevated serum IGF-I levels in diabetic individuals at the time of development of retinal neovascularization compared with 3 months earlier. After controlling for glycosylated haemoglobin, blood pressure, proteinuria, duration of disease and age at diagnosis, a large population-based study of 928 diabetic patients revealed higher levels of IGF-I associated with an increased frequency of proliferative diabetic retinopathy (Dills et al 1991). We have shown elevated vitreous levels of IGF-I in diabetics undergoing therapeutic vitrectomy and documented the presence of IGF binding proteins in human vitreous (Grant et al 1986). These studies support the importance of an endocrine mode of IGF-I action in the pathogenesis of diabetic proliferative retinopathy.

Danias and Stylianopoulou (1990) demonstrated that the rat retina has high levels of mRNA for IGF-I, levels exceeding those detected in the liver. The autocrine/paracrine actions of IGF-I in proliferative retinopathy are corroborated by our studies, demonstrating that retinal endothelial cells constitutively express IGF-I and that IGF-I acts on all the steps relevant to angiogenesis, including endothelial cell proliferation (Grant et al 1993c), migration (Grant et al 1987) and production of the proteases, plasminogen activators (Grant & Guay 1991) and MMP-2 (type IV collagenase or gelatinase) [Grant et al 1993a], and basement membrane degradation (Docherty et al 1992). IGF-I is thus validated as an angiogenic agent independent of any induction of inflammation.

We developed animal models of retinal angiogenesis using IGF-I (Grant el al 1993b, c). Employing these systems, we identified IGF-I as a factor which may be altered in diabetic retinopathy. Our data suggested that, in addition to the direct angiogenic effect on endothelial cells, IGF-I may activate leucocytes resulting in an enhancement of the traditional (noninflammatory) angiogenic response. The aim of this study was to determine whether IGF-I activated leucocytes *in vivo* to express increased amounts of free radical-derived oxidants and then to determine whether the degree of activation correlated with the occurrence of angiogenesis. We characterized the effects of IGF-I, insulin, high glucose concentration and H_2O_2 on cultures of human retinal endothelial cells. These *in vitro* studies are complemented by cytochemical and immunocytochemical studies using a previously described rabbit model of angiogenesis (Grant el al 1993b, c).

MATERIALS AND METHODS

Recombinant human IGF-I was kindly provided by Dr. J. Merryweather, Chiron Corporation (Emeryville, California, USA). Monoclonal antibody specific for IGF-I was obtained from Upstate Biotechnology Inc. (Waltham, Massachusetts, USA). Monoclonal antibody specific to human IGF-I receptor, αIR-3, was provided by Dr. S. Jacobs, The Wellcome Research Laboratories (Research Triangle Park, North Carolina, USA).

CELL CULTURES

Primary isolation of human retinal endothelial cells was performed as previously described (Grant & Guay 1991) and culture purity was verified by incorporation of fluorescent-labelled acetylated low-density lipoprotein and factor VIII staining.

Endothelial cell proliferation was measured by incorporation of ^{3}H-thymidine following exposure to either IGF-I, insulin, high glucose concentration or H_2O_2. Early-passage (up to passage 3) human retinal endothelial cells isolated from the retinal microvasculature were seeded in 6-well tissue culture-grade plates at a density of 5 x 10^4 cells per well and allowed to adhere for 24 h at 37 °C. The medium was washed from the wells with isotonic saline, and either serum-free medium or the test agent diluted in serum-free medium was then added. The cells were exposed to IGF-I or insulin (1, 10, 100, 1000 nmol/l), glucose (10 µg or 20 mmol/l) for 24 h or H_2O_2 (1, 10, 100 or 1000 nmol/l) for either 1 or 4 h at 37 °C.

The test agent was removed by several washes with isotonic saline and ^{3}H-thymidine (specific activity 13.2 Ci/mmol) was then added at a concentration of 12.5 µCi/well in serum-free medium. The cells were then incubated for 24 h at 37 °C. Free label was removed with several washes in isotonic saline. The well contents were then solubilized with alkaline detergent solution and precipitated with cold trichloroacetic acid (TCA). TCA-precipitable counts were then recovered on Whatman GF/D filter discs and counted in scintillant for 10 min.

INTRAVITREAL INJECTION STUDIES

For the intravitreal studies, pigmented rabbits were anaesthetized with ketamine hydrochloride (30 mg/kg) and xylazine (5 mg/kg) and their pupils were dilated with topical tropicamide 0.25% and phenylephrine 0.5%. Each animal was placed beneath an operating microscope, a 30-gauge needle was inserted into the anterior chamber, and 0.08 ml of fluid was withdrawn. Another 30-gauge needle was then inserted through the sclera and retina, 4 mm posterior to the corneoscleral junction, in the superotemporal quadrant. Under stereomicroscopic control, with the bevel of the needle directed up, 0.1 ml of balanced salt solution containing IGF-I 600 µg was injected directly over the optic nerve head. The injection was made close to the retinal surface to disperse the growth factor and promote the settling of the growth factor solution onto the vascularized medullary ray and disc. Control animals received either heat-inactivated IGF-I 600 µg (n = 12) or balanced salt solution (n = 6) [Grant et al 1993b].

CYTOCHEMICAL LOCALIZATION OF HYDROGEN PEROXIDE

Animals were killed by intracardiac injection with sodium pentobarbital and eyes were enucleated. The globe and attached optic nerve were dissected out and fixed for 1 h in cold 5.0% acrolein in 0.1 mol/l sodium cacodylate-HCl buffer (pH 7.4). Specimens were washed overnight in cold 0.15 mol/l sodium cacodylate-HCl buffer (pH 7.4) plus 5% sucrose and 1% dimethylsulphoxide.

Specimens were brought to room temperature in the final two buffer washes, which contained 0.1 mol/l glycine, and reacted in the NADH oxidase reaction mixture of Briggs et al (1975) as follows. Specimens were preincubated for 30 min at 37 °C with agitation in the following medium: 2.0 mmol/l cerium chloride, 10 mmol/l 3-amino-1,2,4,-triazole, 0.1 mol/l Tris-maleate buffer (pH 7.5), 7% sucrose and 0.0002% Triton X-100. They were than incubated for 1 h at 37 °C with agitation in the following complete reaction medium: 2 mmol/l cerium chloride, 10 mmol/l 3-amino-1,2,4-triazole, 0.8 mmol/l NADH, 0.1 mol/l Tris-maleate buffer (pH 7.5), 7% sucrose and 0.0002% Triton-X 100. The reaction was terminated by a washing in cold 0.1 mol/l Tris-maleate buffer (pH 7.5) and 7% sucrose followed by a wash in cold 0.15 mol/l sodium cacodylate-HCl buffer (pH 7.4), and 7% sucrose.

Specimens were postfixed overnight in 1% osmium tetroxide, 0.1 mol/l sodium cacodylate-HCl buffer (pH 7.4) and 7% sucrose in the cold, dehydrated through an ethanol series (20%, 40%, 60%, 80%, 95% ×2, 100% ×2) to propylene oxide, and then infiltrated and embedded in epoxy resin (Quetol 651® 1.15 g, Eponate 12® 1.83 g, dodecenyl succinic anhydride 7.02 g, benzyl dimethylamine 0.14 ml). Grids were examined and photographed at 75 kV in a transmission electron microscope without poststaining.

IMMUNOCYTOCHEMICAL LOCALIZATION OF PROLIFERATING CELL NUCLEAR ANTIGEN

Gold sections on nickel grids were oxidized for 30 min with 1% periodic acid, washed 5 times for 5 min each time with deionized water, followed by a phosphate buffered saline (PBS) wash. Grids were treated for 15 min with blocker [PBS containing 0.1 mol/l NaCl, 1% bovine serum albumin (BSA), 1% cold water fish gelatin (CWFG), 1% nonfat dry milk (NDM)] followed by an overnight incubation at 4°C in affinity-purified monoclonal mouse anti-rat proliferating cell nuclear antigen (clone PC 10 antibody) [Boehringer Mannheim Corp., Indianapolis, USA] diluted 1:200 in PBS plus the same additives as contained in the blocker. After two 5-min washes in PBS containing the same additives as used above, grids received two 5-min washes in Tris-buffered saline (TBS) [0.1 mol/l NaCl, 1% BSA, 1% CWFG, 1% NDM] followed by incubation for 1 h at room temperature in polyclonal goat anti-mouse polyvalent (IgG, IgA, IgM) secondary antibodies labelled with 10-nm colloidal gold (Sigma Chemical Co., St. Louis, Missouri, USA). Grids received three 5-min washes in TBS followed by three 5-min washes in deionized water. Grids were examined and photographed in an electron microscope at 75 kV without

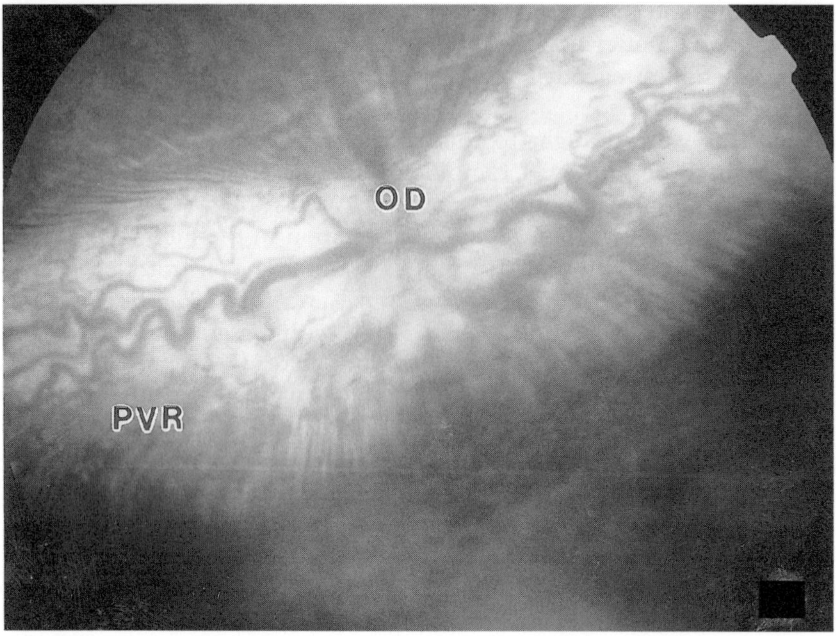

Fig. 18.1 Rabbit fundus 7 days after intravitreal injection of balanced salts solution with 600 μg of insulin-like growth factor-I. The vasculature is engorged with marked tortuosity of the vessels, hyperaemia surrounding the optic disc (OD) and areas of distended preretinal vessels (PRV).

poststaining. Controls for nonspecific labelling consisted of reaction with preimmune mouse serum in place of the primary antibody and reaction with secondary antibody without exposure to primary antibody.

RESULTS

Exposure of human retinal endothelial cells to recombinant IGF-I resulted in increased ^{3}H-thymidine incorporation in a dose-dependent manner (over the range 1-100 nmol/l). The stimulatory effect of IGF-I was abolished by addition of monoclonal IGF-I antibody, which recognized both IGF-I and IGF-II (but not insulin), and by the addition of αIR-3, a monoclonal antibody which is a specific antagonist of the type-I receptor. The stimulatory effect of 10 μg/ml of insulin was similar to that of 10 ng/ml of IGF-I. This stimulatory effect of insulin, confirmed by thymidine incorporation and growth curves, was inhibited by αIR-3, suggesting to us that the mitogenic effect of insulin on human retinal endothelial cells is mediated through the IGF-I receptor.

Exposure of human retinal endothelial cells to media containing glucose 20 mmol/l inhibited endothelial cell proliferation and thymidine incorporation in a dose-dependent manner. Cells of nondiabetic origin were inhibited to a greater extent than cells of diabetic origin ($p < 0.05$) [data not shown].

Following achievement of confluence, human retinal endothelial cells formed capillary tubes and invaded their extracellular matrix (ECM) when the cells were cultured in the presence of IGF-I. We developed an *in vivo* mode of retinal angiogenesis, with which we were able to validate that IGF-I induced capillary morphogenesis. This animal model system used intravitreal injections of IGF-I. A time-course study of this system showed that at days 2-4 there was microscopic evidence of microthrombi, as well as areas of capillary nonperfusion on fluorescein angiograms. Funduscopic examination revealed hyperaemia and vascular engorgement in all rabbits ($n = 30$) by day 4, and vascular tortuosity, intraretinal haemorrhage and vascular proliferation by day 8 (Fig. 18.1). Fluorescein angiograms at day 8 demonstrated late-phase fluorescein leakage, indicative of altered permeability of the blood-retinal barrier in the IGF-I-treated eyes. The fundus of control animals remained normal in appearance (Fig. 18.2) throughout the 3-week study period. At day 6, correlative light and

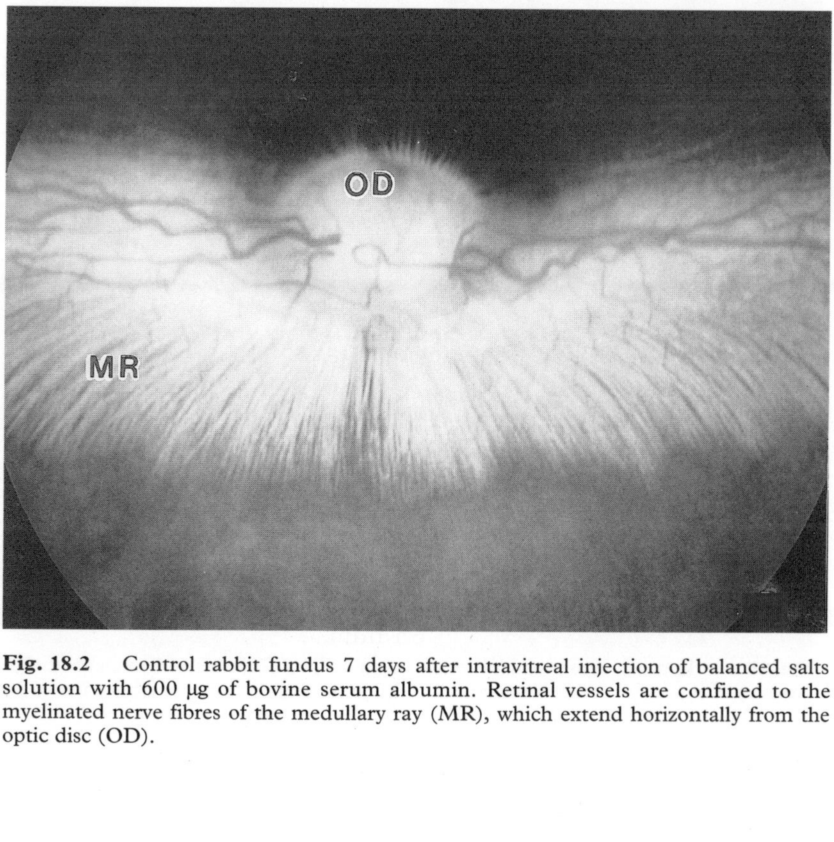

Fig. 18.2 Control rabbit fundus 7 days after intravitreal injection of balanced salts solution with 600 μg of bovine serum albumin. Retinal vessels are confined to the myelinated nerve fibres of the medullary ray (MR), which extend horizontally from the optic disc (OD).

transmission electron microscopy studies showed large abnormal vessels with oedematous endothelial cells, extravasation of leucocytes, activated macrophages and proliferation of the ECM. Immunocytochemical localization of proliferating cell nuclear antigen (Figs 18.3 and 18.4) validated proliferation of the endothelial cells in IGF-I injected eyes. These changes were maintained for 3 weeks following a single injection of IGF-I.

We postulated that reperfusion injury could be contributing to the late retinal changes (days 8-14) and that the generation of H_2O_2 by IGF-I-activated leucocytes could contribute to the observed angiogenic response. To validate this hypothesis we localized H_2O_2 cytochemically by the NADH oxidase method of Briggs et al (1975) in eyes injected intravitreally with IGF-I. The respiratory burst of activated leucocytes appeared to be the source of H_2O_2 and was readily apparent throughout the 3-week time-course (Fig. 18.5). In areas of angiogenesis, there was a dramatic increase

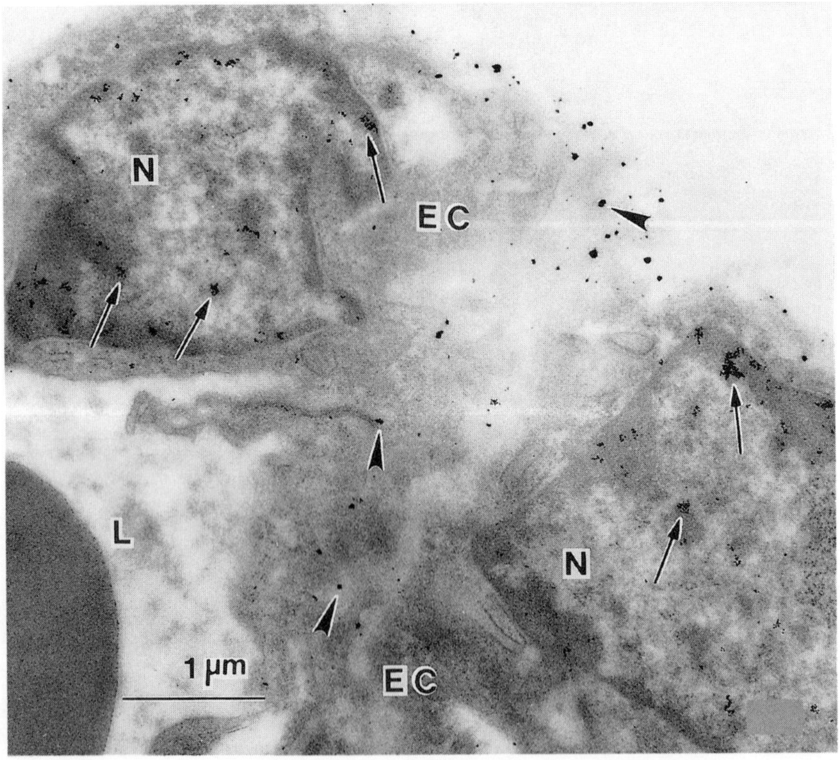

Fig. 18.3 Immunocytochemical localization of proliferating cell nuclear antigen (arrows) in nuclei (N) of endothelial cells (EC) 6 days after intravitreal injection of 600 μg insulin-like growth factor-I. H_2O_2 (arrowheads) localizes in the endothelial cells and basement membranes. Lumen (L). ×19,000.

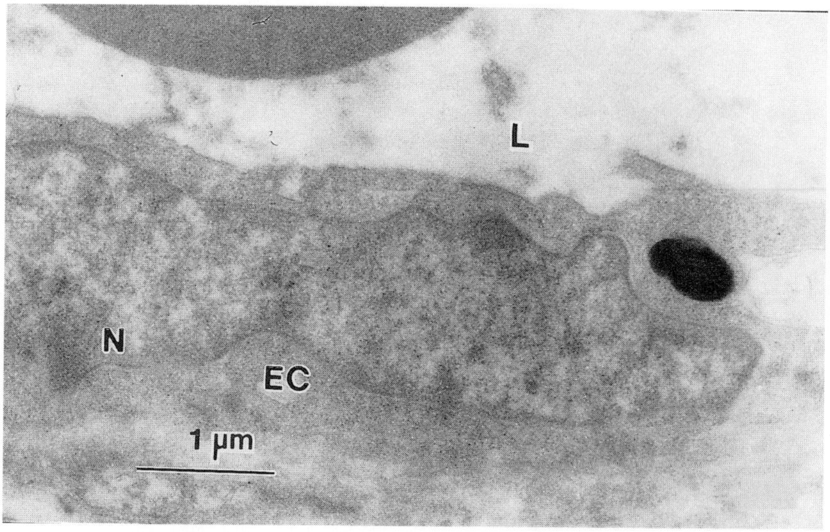

Fig. 18.4 Lack of proliferating cell nuclear antigen localization in the nucleus (N) of an endothelial cell (EC) 6 days after intravitreal injection of balanced salts solution with 600 µg of bovine serum albumin. Lumen (L). ×19,000.

in the amount of H_2O_2 the detected. The cytochemical localization suggested that H_2O_2 may facilitate the development of angiogenesis by directly stimulating endothelial cell proliferation.

To test this hypothesis, we examined the effect of nanomolar concentrations of H_2O_2 on human retinal endothelial cells *in vitro*. When H_2O_2 was added to cultures of human retinal endothelial cells, we observed increased levels of thymidine incorporation at concentrations of 1 to 100 nmol/l, while we observed decreased thymidine incorporation at higher concentrations (1000 nmol/l) [Fig. 18.6].

DISCUSSION

Fluorescein angiographic evidence for functional (clinical) nonperfused areas of retinal vessels exists in diabetic individuals early in their retinopathy (Schroder et al 1991). Diabetic animal models also support these findings. Both red and white blood cells of diabetics are poorly deformable and could contribute to capillary occlusion (Schmid-Schonbein et al 1981). Diabetic individuals have increased numbers of activated granulocytes and monocytes (Schroder et al 1991). Systemic activation of leucocytes in diabetics may be mediated in part by exposure to elevated serum levels of growth hormone and IGF-I (Merimee et al 1983, Poulsen 1953) since IGF-I has been shown to activate leucocytes (Edwards et al 1988). These activated leucocytes exhibit increased

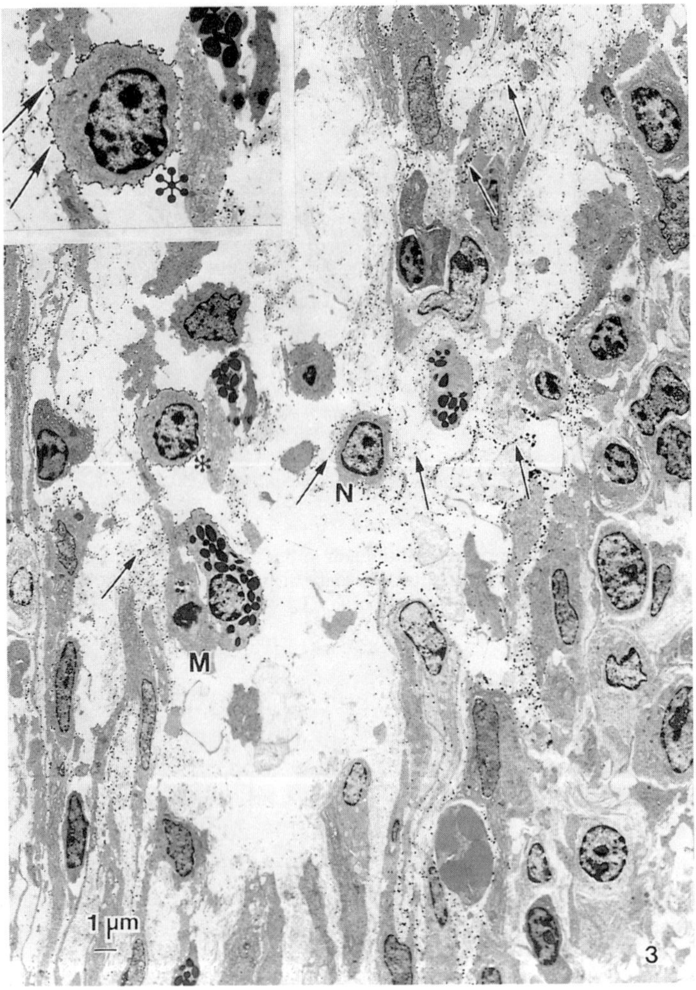

Fig. 18.5 Infiltration of inflammatory cells, macrophages (M) and neutrophils (N), with profuse secretion of H_2O_2 (arrowheads) in the optic disc 18 days after intravitreal injection of 600 μg of insulin-like growth factor-I. ×2100. Inset shows dense cerium perhydroxide precipitate (arrows) on the plasma membrane of a neutrophil. ×3900.

adhesiveness to endothelial cells, have large cell volumes, and high cytoplasmic rigidity (Schmid-Schonbein et al 1981). Single leucocytes often completely fill the capillary lumen, causing capillary occlusion, endothelial swelling and further narrowing of the capillary lumen by perivascular oedema (Schroder et al 1991).

Leucocyte-endothelial adhesion is followed by diapedesis of mononuclear cells and their proliferation to macrophages. Cell contact between monocytes and endothelial cells strongly enhances the prothrombotic nature of the endothelium (Hakkert et al 1990). Activated macrophages in the retina, probably derived both from a circulating pool of cells and from the resident microglia population, provide a rich source of cytokines (such as interleukin [IL-1] and tumour necrosis factor-alpha [TNF-α]) and growth factors (such as transforming growth factor-β and platelet-derived growth factor [PDGF]), which can attract more leucocytes (Mantovani & Dejana 1989; van Hinsbergh et al 1990). Specifically, IL-1 alters the functional properties of endothelial cells by: suppressing cell surface anticoagulant activity; stimulating PAI-1 while decreasing t-PA

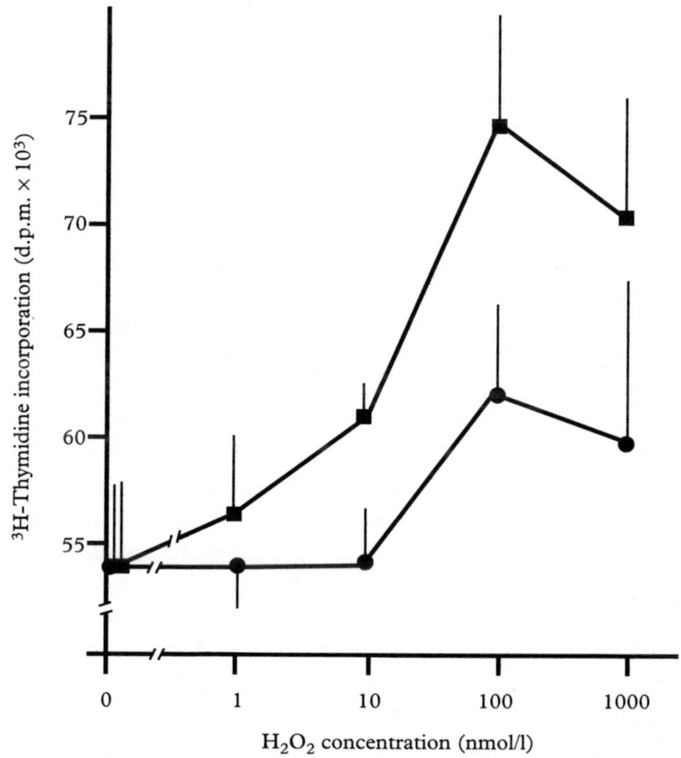

Fig. 18.6 Induction of retinal vascular endothelial cell (REC) proliferation in response to H_2O_2 exposure as measured by ^{3}H-thymidine incorporation. Early-passage human RECs were seeded in 6-well tissue culture-grade plates and allowed to adhere for 24 h at 37°C. The medium was removed by washing, then either medium or H_2O_2 at the concentrations indicated was added for either 1 h (●) or 4 h (■) at 37°C. The H_2O_2 was removed by several washes, then ^{3}H-thymidine was added for 24 h at 37°C. Free label was removed with several washes in normal saline. The well contents were then solubilized with alkaline detergent solution and precipitated with cold trichloroacetic acid (TCA). TCA-precipitable counts were then recovered on filter disks and counted in scintillant for 10 min. Values are given as means ± SEM from triplicate wells of 2 separate experiments.

production; increasing the production of platelet-activating factor (a potent vasoconstrictor and activator of platelets and leucocytes); inducing leucocyte adhesion molecules; and even inducing the production of other cytokines (Mantovani & Dejana 1989). Interleukin-β (IL-1β) increases tissue factor, and high levels of glucose intensify the expression of tissue factor by endothelial cells in response to IL-1β (Mantovani & Dejana 1989).

The red blood cell and leucocyte abnormalities of diabetics contribute to capillary nonperfusion and the development of ischaemic damage to the retina. We believe that the areas of acellular capillaries present in the retina of diabetics actually represent areas where oxygen deprivation, due to microthrombus formation, leucocyte adhesion and subsequent non-perfusion, was so severe that the cellular injury became irreversible. However, if the period of ischaemia does not cause irreversible damage, the restoration of blood flow and O_2 (albeit beneficial overall) causes increased free radical-derived oxidant formation in the damaged tissue and temporarily worsens the injury.

Free radical-derived oxidants are highly reactive chemical species which damage cells by direct oxidation, specifically causing DNA damage, membrane disruption, release of calcium ions within cells and activation of calcium-dependent enzymes (Oberley 1988). Free radical-derived oxidants and their lipid hydroperoxides are cytotoxic to endothelial cells, stimulate cyclooxygenase and prostaglandin (PG) synthesis, including PGE_2 which is angiogenic (Ginsburg et al 1989; Halliwell 1987), and at the same time inhibit prostacyclin production. The generation of free radical-derived oxidants may result from release of iron ions (catalytic for free radical reactions) from their normal storage site within the cell and/or disruption of mitochondrial respiratory chains so that more electrons 'escape' to oxygen to form superoxide anion ($O_2^{\bullet-}$) [Halliwell 1987]. There is increased free radical activity in diabetes, e.g., there are elevated $O_2^{\bullet-}$ levels in diabetic serum (Shah et al 1983; Wierusz-Wysocka et al 1987) and monocytes of diabetic patients and animals made diabetic release increased amounts of $O_2^{\bullet-}$ *in vitro*. Animal models of diabetic retinopathy and diabetics with microangiopathy (Armstrong & Al-Awadi 1991; Ginsburg et al 1989; Halliwell 1987; Murata et al 1981; Nishigaki et al 1981; Shah et al 1983; Wierusz-Wysocka et al 1987) demonstrated increased levels of lipid peroxides.

Advanced glycosylation end-products (AGEs) accumulating in basement membranes of diabetic individuals are resistant to degradation and are more susceptible to free radical-induced modification (Baynes 1991; Vlassara et al 1988). Receptor-mediated uptake of AGEs by macrophages and monocytes initiates the release of cytokines, particularly IL-1β and TNF-α (Kirstein et al 1990). It has more recently been demonstrated that exposure of monocytes to AGEs, derived from hyaluronic acid, results in the cells' ability to express IGF-I and appears to be dependent on IL-1 and PDGF secretion (Kirstein et al 1992; Noble et al 1993). These data support the notion that the natural formation of AGE-proteins in diabetic tissues can contribute to the induction first of inflammatory cytokines, then of competence factors, and finally of progression factors such as IGF-I.

Exposure of endothelial cells to low levels of H_2O_2 induces prolonged expression of the adhesion molecule p-selectin and facilitates enhanced leucocyte adherence (Patel et al 1991). Free radical-derived oxidants are implicated in TNF-α-mediated injury, as a synergistic effect between superoxide anion and TNF-α has been observed. TNF-α also mediates vascular permeability and neutrophil accumulation via up-regulation of adhesion molecules on both endothelial cells (ICAM-1, adhesion complex CD11/CD18, and E-selectin) [Nathan et al 1989] and neutrophils (β_2-integrins) [Luscinaskas et al 1991]. TNF-α induces IL-1β, which then induces IL-6. All three cytokines enhance neutrophil-endothelial cell adhesion (Luscinskas et al 1991). Free radical-derived oxidants could initiate increased leucocyte adhesion, which is perpetuated by the cytokines released by the leucocytes directly. Neutrophils and lymphocytes, responding to inflammatory stimuli, undergo an oxidative burst to produce free radical-derived oxidants such as $O_2^{\bullet-}$ and H_2O_2, which, in conjunction with hydrolytic enzymes, could injure neighbouring endothelial cells (Rao 1990). Interestingly, IGF-I activates neutrophils for $O_2^{\bullet-}$ secretion *in vitro* (Fu et al 1991) and the endothelium itself produces small amounts of $O_2^{\bullet-}$ (Oberley 1988).

An essential cytoprotective mechanism against oxidant-induced injury is the glutathioneredox cycle, which depends on the availability of NADPH/NADH (Williamson et al 1993). Hyperglycaemia in diabetic individuals leads to the intracellular generation of sorbitol by aldose reductase, a process that consumes NADPH and may therefore weaken the defense mechanisms against free-radical injury (Williamson et al 1993). Diabetics also have lower concentrations of the antioxidants, ascorbate and vitamin E, and decreased glutathione peroxidase (Oberley 1988).

CONCLUSION

Our previous *in vitro* studies have demonstrated that IGF-I can stimulate endothelial cell proliferation (Grant et al 1993c), chemotaxis (Grant et al 1987) and protease production (Grant and Guay 1991), and support the concept that IGF-I can induce all the steps required for retinal neovascularization, and thus by itself is an angiogenic agent. Our current studies demonstrate that the mitogenic effects of insulin are mediated by the IGF-I receptor and that high glucose concentration inhibits endothelial cell proliferation in human retinal endothelial cells derived from the retina of nondiabetics, whereas cells of diabetic origin do not appear to be inhibited to the same degree. As shown by the studies of Rao and Berk (1992), H_2O_2 can act as a smooth muscle cell mitogen. Our studies demonstrate that H_2O_2 acts as an endothelial cell mitogen at low concentrations, whereas it acts to inhibit cell proliferation at higher concentrations.

In vivo studies demonstrate that IGF-I can induce retinal neovascularization in the rabbit. However, our animal studies emphasized to us that the 'IGF-I angiogenic response' was truly multifactorial. It appeared that IGF-I could be activating leucocytes to express free radical-derived oxidants and secrete inflammatory cytokines and, in this manner, IGF-I may be unique as a retinal growth factor. Intravitreal IGF-I induced microthrombus formation and the capillary thrombosis resulted in localized areas of ischaemia. This localized ischaemia could result in 'local' expression of other growth factors by the ischaemic retina. Reperfusion of these ischaemic areas then resulted in additional retinal injury by the generation of free radical-derived oxidants. The role of free radical-derived oxidants cannot be minimized, since in our experience, the temporal association of H_2O_2 localization with the onset of angiogenesis is striking.

ACKNOWLEDGMENTS

This work was supported in part by funds from the National Institutes of Health Grant EY07739, grants from the American Heart Association and Diabetes Research and Education Foundation, and by a contract with the Department of Health and Rehabilitative Services of the State of Florida for the University of Florida Diabetes Research, Education and Treatment Center.

REFERENCES

Armstrong D, Al-Awadi F 1991 Lipid peroxidation and retinopathy in streptozotocin-induced diabetes. Free Radic Biol Med 11: 433-436

Assoian R K, Sporn M B 1986 Type beta transforming growth factor in human platelets: release during platelet degranulation and action on vascular smooth muscle cells. J Cell Biol 102: 1217-1223

Baynes J W 1991 Role of oxidative stress in development of complications in diabetes. Diabetes 40:405-412

Boeri D, Almos F, Maiello M et al 1971 High glucose induces increased tissue factor activity in human endothelial cells. Diabetes 20 (suppl) 2: 104a

Briggs R T, Drath D B, Karnovsky M L et al 1975 Localization of NADH oxidase on the surface of human polymorphonuclear leukocytes by a new cytochemical method. J Cell Biol 67: 566-586

Butkus A, Shiney E K, Schumacher O P 1982 Thromboxane biosynthesis in platelets of diabetic and coronary artery diseased patients. Artery 11: 238-251

Chmielewski J, Farbiszewski R 1970 Platelet factor 4 (PF4) release during human platelet aggregation in diabetic patients. Thromb Heamost 24: 203-205

Clemmons D R 1992 IGF binding proteins: regulation of cellular actions. Growth Regul 2: 80-87

Danias J, Stylianopoulou F 1990 Expression of IGF-I and IGF-II genes in the adult rat eye. Curr Eye Res 9: 379-386

Dills D G, Moss S E Klein R et al 1991 Association of elevated IGF-I levels with increased retinopathy in late-onset diabetes. Diabetes 40: 1725-1730

Docherty A J P, O'Connell J, Crabbe T et al 1992 The matrix metalloproteinases and their natural inhibitors. Trends in Biotechnology 10: 200-207

Edwards E K, Ghiasuddin S, Schepper A N et al 1988 Newly defined property of somatotropin: priming macrophages for production of superoxide anion. Science 239: 769-771

Frank R N 1991 On the pathogenesis of diabetic retinopathy. Ophthalmology 98: 586-593

Fu Y, Arkins S, Wang B S et al 1991 A novel role of growth hormone and insulin-like growth factor-1. Priming neutrophils for superoxide anion secretion. J Immunol 146: 1602-1608

Ganda O P, Arkin C F 1992 Hyperfibrinogenemia. An important risk factor for vascular complications in diabetes. Diabetes Care 15: 1245-1250

Ginsburg I, Gibbs D F, Schuger L et al 1989 Vascular endothelial cell killing by combinations of membrane-active agents and hydrogen peroxide. Free Radic Biol Med 7: 369-376

Grant M, Guay C 1991 Plasminogen activator production by human retinal endothelial cells of non-diabetic and diabetic origin. Invest Ophthalmol Vis Sci 32: 53-64

Grant M, Jerdan J, Merimee T J 1987 Insulin-like growth factor I modulates endothelial cell chemotaxis. J Clin Endocrinol and Metab 65: 370-371

Grant M B, Caballero S, Millard W J 1993a Inhibition of IGF-I and b-FGF stimulated growth of human retinal endothelial cells by the somatostatin analogue, octreotide: a potential treatment of neovascularization. Regul Pept 48: 267-278

Grant M B, Mames R N, Fitzgerald C et al 1993b Insulin-like growth factor I acts as an angiogenic agent in rabbit cornea and retina: comparative studies with basic fibroblast growth factor. Diabetologia 35: 282-291

Grant M B, Mames R N, Fitzgerald C et al 1993c Insulin-like growth factor I as an angiogenic agent. Ann NY Acad Sci 692: 230-242

Grant M B, Russell B, Fitzgerald C et al 1986 Insulin-like growth factors in vitreous: studies in controls and diabetics with neovascularization. Diabetes 35: 416-420

Hakkert B C, Rentennar J M, VanMourik J A 1990 Monocytes enhance the bidirectional release of type I plasminogen activator inhibitor by endothelial cells. Blood 76: 2272-2278

Halliwell B 1987 Oxidants and human disease: some new concepts. FASEB J 1: 358-364

Hyer S L, Sharp P S, Brooks R A et al 1989 A two year follow-up study of serum insulin-like growth factor I in diabetics with retinopathy. Metabolism 38: 586-589

Kirstein M, Aston C, Hintz R et al 1992 Receptor-specific induction of insulin-like growth factor I in human monocytes by advanced glycosylation end product-modified proteins. J Clin Invest 90: 439-446

Kirstein M, Brett J, Radoff S et al 1990 Advanced protein glycosylation induces transendothelial human monocyte chemotaxis and secretion of platelet-derived growth factor: role in vascular disease of diabetes and aging. Proc Natl Acad Sci USA 87: 9010-9014

Kohner E M, Hamilton A M, Joplin G F 1976 Florid diabetic retinopathy and its response to treatment by photocoagulation or pituitary ablation. Diabetes 25: 104-110

Konkle B A, Schick P K, He X et al 1993 Plasminogen activator inhibitor-1 mRNA is expressed in platelets and megakaryocytes and the megakaryoblastic cell line CHRF-288. Arterioscler Thromb 13: 669-674

Loskutoff D J 1991 Regulation of PAI-1 gene expression. Fibrinolysis 5: 197-206

Lufkin E G, Fass D N, O'Fallon W M et al 1979 Increased von Willebrand factor in diabetes mellitus. Metabolism 28: 63-66

Lundbaeck K 1976 Growth hormone's role in diabetic microangiopathy. Diabetes 25 (suppl 2): 845-849

Luscinskas F W, Cybulsky M I, Kiely J et al 1991 Cytokine-activated human endothelial monolayers support enhanced neutrophil transmigration via a mechanism involving both endothelial-leukocyte adhesion molecule-1 and intercellular adhesion molecule-1. J Immunol 146:1617-1625

Mantovani A, Dejana E 1989 Cytokines as communications signals between leukocytes and endothelial cells. Immunol Today 10: 370-375

McMillan D E 1983 The effect of diabetes on blood flow properties. Diabetes 32 (suppl 2): 56-63

Merimee T J, Zapf J, Froesch E R 1983 Insulin-like growth factors: studies in diabetics with and without retinopathy. N Engl J Med 309: 527-530

Merimee, T J 1990 Diabetic retinopathy: a synthesis of perspectives. N Engl J Med 322: 978-983

Michaelson I C 1948 The mode of development of retinal vessels. Transactions of the Ophthalmology Society UK 68: 137-138

Murata T, Nishida T, Eto S et al 1981 Lipid peroxidation in diabetic rat retina. Metab

Pediatr Syst Ophthalmiol 5: 83-87
Nathan C, Srimal S, Farber C et al 1989 Cytokine-induced respiratory burst of human neutrophils: dependence on extracellular matrix proteins and CD11/CD18 integrins. J Cell Biol 109: 1341-1349
Nishigaki I, Hagihara M, Tsunekawa H et al 1981 Lipid peroxide levels of serum lipoprotein fractions of diabetic patients. Biochem Med Metab Biol 25: 373-378
Noble P W, Lake F R, Henson P M et al 1993 Hyaluronate activation of CD44 induces insulin-like growth factor-1 expression by a tumor necrosis factor-dependent mechanism in murine macrophages. J Clin Invest 91: 2368-2377
Oberley L W. Free radicals and diabetes. Free Radic Biol Med 1988 5:113-124
Patel K D, Zimmerman G A, Prescott S M et al 1991 Oxygen radicals induce human endothelial cells to express GMP-140 and bind neutrophils. J Cell Biol 112: 749-759
Poulsen J E 1953 The Houssay phenomenon in man: recovery from retinopathy in a case of diabetes with Simmond's disease. Diabetes 2: 7-12
Rao G N, Berk B C 1992 Active oxygen species stimulate vascular smooth muscle cell growth and proto-oncogene expression. Circ Res 70: 593-598
Rao N A 1990 Role of oxygen free radicals in retinal damage associated with experimental uveitis. Trans Am Ophthalmol Soc 88: 797-850
Schmid-Schonbein G W, Sung K P, Tozeren H et al 1981 Passive mechanical properties of human leukocytes. Biophys J 36: 243-256
Schroder S, Palinski W, Schmid-Schonbein G W 1991 Activated monocytes and granulocytes, capillary nonperfusion, and neovascularization in diabetic retinopathy. Am J Pathol 139: 81-100
Shah S V, Wallin J D, Eilen S D 1983 Chemiluminescence and superoxide anion production by leukocytes from diabetic patients. J Clin Endocrinol Metab 57: 402-409
Sivalingam A, Kenney J, Brown G C et al 1990 Basic fibroblast growth factor levels in the vitreous of patients with proliferative diabetic retinopathy. Arch Ophthalmol 108: 869-872
Slivka S R, Luskotoff D J 1991 Platelets stimulate endothelial cells to synthesize type 1 plasminogen activator inhibitor. Evaluation of the role of transforming growth factor beta. Blood 77: 1013-1019
Taylor C M, Kissun R D, Schor A M et al 1989 Endothelial cell-stimulating angiogenesis factor in vitreous from extraretinal neovascularizations. Invest Ophthalmol Vis Sci 30: 2174-2178
van Hinsbergh V W, Bauer K A, Kooistra T et al 1990 Progress of fibrinolysis during tumor necrosis factor infusions humans. Concomitant increase in tissue-type plasminogen activator, plasminogen activator inhibitor type 1, and fibrin(ogen) degradation products. Blood 76: 2284-2289
Vlassara H, Brownlee M, Manogue K R et al 1988 Cachectin/TNF and IL-1 induced by glucose-modified proteins: role in normal tissue remodeling. Science 240: 1546-1548
Wierusz-Wysocka B, Wysocky H, Siekirka H et al 1987 Evidence of polymorphonuclear neutrophlis activation in patients with insulin-dependent diabetes mellitus. J Leukoc Biol 42: 519-523
Williamson J R, Chang K, Frangos M et al 1993 Hyperglycemic pseudohypoxia and diabetic complications. Diabetes 42: 801-813
Zaph J, Schmidt C H, Froesch E R 1984 Biological and immunological properties of insulin-like growth factors (IGF) I and II. Clin Endocrinol 13: 3-30

Index

A23187, 24, 35, 118, 120, 133
Acetylcholine, 22, 35, 112-114, 117-119, 123, 125, 128, 133, 134, 138
β-Actin, 81
Actomyosin ATPase, 80
Acyl-coenzyme A, 66, 67
Adhesion molecule, 145-155, 277
AGE (*see* glycosylation end-product, advanced)
Alanine, 184
Albumin, 41
Aldose reductase, 82, 219, 277
  inhibitor, 7, 22, 24, 68, 81, 82, 139
Allopurinol, 150-152, 155
Amadori product, 189, 190
Aminoguanidine, 137, 139, 191, 192, 194
Angiogenesis, 215-226, 231-241, 267, 273
Angiogenin, 216, 217
Angiogram, 270, 271
Angiopathy, 25, 40, 74, 194
Angiotensin converting enzyme, 89
Angiotensin II, 34, 64, 109, 160
Antioxidant, 277
α_2-Antiplasmin, 37, 39
Antithrombin III, 26, 33, 34, 39-42, 174-186
Aphidocolin, 247, 255
Apolipoprotein
  A-1, 19
  B-100, 41, 45
Apolipoprotein(a), 45-48
Apoprotein B, 124
Aprotinin, 234, 238
Arachidonic acid, 17, 23, 24, 66, 129, 135, 139, 151, 153, 189, 190, 207
Arginine, 123, 124, 127-130, 134
Ascorbic acid, 11, 277
Asparagine, 174
Atherogenic index, 205
Atherosclerosis, 23-25, 36, 58, 105, 117-122, 127-130, 145, 159-169, 173-186, 201-213, 245, 246
Basement membrane thickening, 40, 74, 78, 80
Blood viscosity, 265
Blood-brain barrier, 5
Blood-retinal barrier, 219
Body mass index, 36-38
Bradykinin, 124, 126
Ca^{2+}, 57, 58, 60, 64, 105-115, 121, 126-129, 134, 138, 155, 260, 276
Caldesmon, 79, 80, 84, 247
Calmodulin, 121, 126, 129, 134
Catalase, 8, 136, 146-155, 183, 185
Catecholamine, 115
CD11, 145-155, 277
CD11a, 146-149, 152-155
CD11b, 146-149, 154, 155
CD11c, 145, 148, 149, 152-155
CD18, 145-155, 277
Cdc1, 247
Cdc2, 247, 249, 255, 258, 259
Cdc25, 258
Cdk1, 255, 259
Cdk2, 246, 258, 259
Cell cycle, 246-262
Cholesterol, 122, 129
  transport, 127
Cholesteryl ester, 24
Chondroitin, 174, 181, 186
Citrulline, 127, 129, 134
Coagulation, 33-49, 173-186
Coenzyme A, 67
Colecemide, 247, 255
Colesteryl ester, 192, 193
Collagen, 40, 74, 84, 136
  disease, 43
  type I, 79, 81, 161, 234
  type III, 81, 161
  type IV, 74, 78, 79, 81, 83
  type VI, 79
Collagenase, 40, 224, 231, 247, 267
Cu^{2+}, 122, 183, 184, 191, 192
Cyclic AMP, 160
Cyclic GMP, 117, 118, 135
Cyclin, 246-262
  A, 246, 250, 253-259
  B, 258

(Cyclin contd)
D, 259, 260
E, 259
Cyclohexamide, 26
Cyclooxygenase, 18, 19, 35, 276
inhibitor, 163
Cystathione β-synthase deficiency, 180
Cysteine, 184
Deferoxamine mesylate, 146, 151
Dermatan, 174
Diabetes
endothelial dysfunction, 133-139
vascular complication, 73-84
Diacylglycerol, 7, 57-69, 81, 82-84, 126, 127, 137, 138, 246, 259, 260
lipase, 17
Dihydroxyacetone phosphate, 57, 64, 67, 68
Dioctanoylglycerol, 252-260
1,3-Diphosphoglycerate, 67, 68
Disseminated intravascular coagulation, 44
DNA damage, 276
Eicosanoid, 135, 136
Elastin, 40, 164
Elongation factor-2, 79
Endothelial cell
gene transfection, 89-100
giant, 201-213
injury, 145-155
migration, 215-226
multinucleate, 201-213
permeability, 89, 118, 201-213
proliferation, 215, 226, 245-262
variant, 201-213
Endothelial cell-derived growth factor, 160-163
Endothelial cell-stimulating angiogenesis factor, 221, 224
Endothelial-derived relaxing factor, 10, 11, 133-139
Endothelin, 34, 117, 89-100, 160, 207, 209
prepro, 89-100
Endothelin-1, 83, 91-100, 201, 209-211
big, 92, 96, 98, 100
converting enzyme, 92
prepro, 92-100
Endothelin-2, 92, 209
Endothelin-3, 209
Endothelium-dependent relaxing factor, 194
Endothelium-derived growth factor, 33-36
Endothelium-derived relaxing factor, 117-121, 124-126, 129
Endotoxin, 43, 161
Epidermal growth factor, 26, 90, 160, 163, 216, 217, 233, 234, 238
receptor, 58, 259
Euglobulin fibrinolytic activity, 36, 37
Extracellular matrix, 271, 272
protein (*see* protein)
Extrinsic pathway inhibitor (*see* tissue factor pathway inhibitor)
Factor
V, 180
Va, 34, 42
VII, 34, 39, 45
VIIa, 45
VIII, 268
VIIIa, 42
IX, 45
IXa, 34
Xa, 34, 45, 161, 163, 174
XIa, 41
XII, 34
Fatty acid, 66
oxidized, 122
Fe^{2+}, 151, 276
Fe^{3+}, 153
Fibrin, 36, 40, 42, 46, 160, 266
cap, 206
Fibrinogen, 36, 39-42, 265
Fibrinolysis, 33-49, 266
Fibroblast growth factor
acidic, 90, 216, 217, 221, 233, 266
basic 160, 162-164, 168, 216, 217, 221, 225, 226, 233-235, 247, 250-257, 266
Fibronectin, 40, 69, 74, 78-80, 83, 84, 89, 98, 164
specific integrin receptor, 78
Foam cell, 166
Focal adhesion kinase, 80
Free radical, 265-278
Fructosamine, 189
Fructose, 67, 68, 82
1,6-diphosphate, 10, 67
6-phosphate, 9, 10, 67
transporter, 5
Fura-2, 107
Galactose, 68
Gelatinase, 267
Gene
expression, 73-84
extracellular matrix, 81
glucose-induced, 73-84
NO synthetase, 130
transfection, 89-100
Glucocorticoid, 18
Glucosamine, 174-185
Glucose
metabolism, 3-13
3-phosphate, 68
6-phosphate dehydrogenase, 77
6-phosphate, 9, 10, 67, 68, 77, 83
transporter, 3-13
Glucuronic acid, 174, 185
GLUT-1, 3-6
GLUT-2, 3, 4, 6
GLUT-3, 4, 6

GLUT-4, 4,6
GLUT-5, 4
Glutathione, 8, 9
peroxidase, 9, 277
redox cycle, 8, 9-11, 205, 277
reductase, 9
Glycation (*see* glycosylation)
Glyceraldehyde-3-phosphate dehydrogenase, 10
Glyceraldehyde, 67, 68
3-phosphate, 67, 68
Glycerol, 67
3-phosphate acyltransferase, 66
3-phosphate, 57, 64, 67, 68, 246
Glyceryl trinitrate (*see* nitroglycerine)
Glycolysis, 67, 68
Glycosamine, 174, 175
Glycosaminoglycan, 34, 173-186, 265
Glycosylation, 40, 90 139, 189-195
lipid, 24
lipoprotein, 189, 190
nonenzymatic, 7, 11, 39-43, 57, 77, 78, 83, 84
protein, 91, 136, 189-195
Glycosylation end-product
advanced, 83, 136, 137, 139, 189-195, 217, 276, 277
advanced, receptor, 194, 195
early, 189-195
Granulocyte-macrophage colony-stimulating factor, 259
Growth hormone, 221, 222, 273
Guanylate cyclase, 117, 118, 133
H-7, 138
Haemoglobin, 134, 136
glycosylated, 36-38, 41, 136, 139, 189, 267
Haemoprotein, 134
Harber-Weiss reaction, 152
Heparan sulphate, 90, 173-186
proteoglycan, 83, 173-186
Heparin-binding epidermal growth factor-like growth factor, 160
Heparin, 25, 26, 41, 46, 160-164, 176, 177, 180, 233, 265
Heparinase, 164
Hexokinase, 68
High-density lipoprotein, 19, 23, 24, 127, 128, 189-195
Hills and valley pattern, 165, 166
Histamine, 24, 35, 43, 133
Histone, 247, 249, 255
Homocysteinaemia, 184
Homocysteine, 176-186
Hyaline, 207
Hyaluronic acid, 90, 174, 276
Hydrogen peroxide, 6, 8-11, 145-155, 183, 277, 267, 268, 272-277
15-Hydroeicosatetraenoate, 35
Hydroperxyeicotetraenoic acid, 153
Hydroxyl radical, 145, 149-153
Hypercholesterolaemia, 118-121, 129
Hyperinsulinism, 38, 105, 115
Hyperlipidaemia, 117
Hypertension, 105, 115
Hypoxia, 6
ICAM-1, 145-155, 277
Iduronic acid, 174, 185
Indomethacin, 18, 22, 26, 112, 113, 136, 180
Inositol, 66
phosphate, 7, 65, 82, 126
phospholipid, 65
1,3,4,5-tetrakisphosphate, 127
1,4,5-triphosphate, 126, 127, 138
Insulin
receptor, 35
resistance, 38, 39, 105, 115
vasodilator action, 105-115
Insulin-like growth factor, 28, 43, 44
Insulin-like growth factor I, 216, 217, 221-223, 234, 265-278
receptor, 267, 270
Insulin-like growth factor II, 221, 238, 266, 270
receptor, 238
Integrin, 80
Interferon, 26, 260
α, 260
β, 260
γ, 160, 161, 260
Interleukin-1, 26, 43, 160-164, 176, 177, 276
Interleukin-1β, 137, 163, 168, 177-180, 276, 277
Interleukin-2, 26
Interleukin-6, 160, 260, 277
Ionomycin, 260
Ischaemia, 276
Keratan, 174
6-Keto-prostaglandin $F_{1\alpha}$, 18, 20, 21, 25, 189, 190, 208
L-N^{G}-monomethylarginine monoacetate, 112, 113
Lactate dehydrogenase, 190, 191
Lactic acid, 10, 67, 68
Lactoferrin-like polypeptide, 194
Laminin, 40, 78, 79, 81, 83, 160, 164, 247
Latency-associated peptide, 236-239
Latent transforming growth factor-β, 235, 236
Left ventricular ejection fraction, 225
Leucine, 41
Leucocyte, 117, 145-155, 272-276
activated, 145-155, 266, 267, 272-274
adhesion, 118, 145-155, 276, 277
adhesion molecule, 276
phorbol-stimulated, 145-155

Leukotriene, 153
Leukotriene C_4, 217
Lipid
  amphiphilic, 123-129
  hydroperoxide, 191, 192, 276
  peroxide, 23, 24, 35, 191, 192, 276
  peroxidation, 153
Lipocortin, 18
Lipopolysaccharide, 134, 163
Lipoprotein(a), 45-48
Lipoprotein-associated coagulation factor (*see* tissue factor pathway inhibitor)
Lipoxygenase, 18, 153
  pathway, 35
Low-density lipoprotein, 23, 24, 45, 46, 121, 122, 125, 126, 160, 166, 189-195
  acetylated, 161, 166, 268
  endothelial cell-modified, 189-195
  oxidized, 117, 121-128, 161, 166, 191-195
  receptor, 125
Lysolipid, 117, 122
Lysophosphatidate, 67
Lysophosphatidylcholine, 122, 127, 260
Lysophosphatidylethanolamine, 122
Lysophosphatidylinositol, 129
Lysophospholipase, 123
α_2-Macroglobulin, 160
Macrophage colony-stimulating factor, 166
  receptor, 166
Mannitol, 21
Mannose-6-phosphate, 238, 240
MARCKS protein, 63, 64, 65
Meclofenamic acid, 136
Mellitin, 22
2-Mercaptoethanol, 184
Metalloproteinase, 40, 231-233
  inhibitor, 224, 232
Metformin, 38, 39
Methionine, 184
MMP-2, 267
Monoacylglycerol-3-phosphate acyltransferase, 66
Monoclonal antibody, 146-149, 154, 155, 239, 254, 267-270
Monocyte adhesion, 145
mp41, 92-100
Mutation, 77, 78
Myo-inositol, 7, 62, 82, 260
Myosin, 117
Na^+, resorption, 115
Na^+,K^+-ATPase, 137-139
NADPH oxidase, 152, 272
Nephropathy, 44, 46-48, 61, 62, 83, 206, 207
N^G-Monomethyl L-arginine, 134, 137
Nicotinamide, 217
Nitrosothiol, 121
Nitrite, 137
Nitroglycerine, 118, 122, 124
Nitroprusside, sodium, 118, 135
Nitrosovasodilator, 118
NO (nitric oxide) [*also see* endothelium-derived relaxing factor]: 113, 114, 117-121, 125-129, 134-138, 194
  synthetase, 117, 119, 121, 126-130, 134, 194
  synthetase inhibitor, 112
Nododazole, 247, 255
Noradrenaline (*see* norepinephrine)
Norepinephrine, 106, 109-114, 125
Oleic acid, 66, 129
Oxidative stress, 7, 11
Oxygen radical, 7, 8, 35, 36, 120, 135, 136, 139, 145, 151, 154, 192-206, 265-278
Oxyhaemoglobin, 136
Palmitic acid, 66, 129
1-Palmitoyl-2-oleoyl-sn-glycerol, 67
Partial thromboplastin time, 39
Pentose phosphate pathway, 9-11
Pentose shunt, 67
Pericyte, 215-226, 231-241
Peroxide, 146-155
Pertussis toxin, 121
Phenotypic modulation, 159-13
Phenylephrine, 115, 119, 125
Phorbol, 83, 145-155
  ester, 69, 137, 138, 161, 163, 169, 248, 251-257
Phosphatidic acid, 67, 129, 160, 260
Phosphatidylcholine, 122, 129, 260
Phosphatidylethanolamine, 122, 129
Phosphatidylinositol-4,5-diphosphate, 65, 126, 127
Phosphatidylinositol, 66, 129, 138
Phosphatidylserine, 58, 129
Phosphoglucose isomerase, 77
Phosphoinositide, 57
Phosphoinositol, 260
Phospholipase, 260
  A_2, 17-19, 122
  A_2-activating protein, 18
  B (*see* lysophospholipase), 123
  C, 65, 126, 127, 138, 217, 260
  D, 260
Phospholipid, 17, 24, 57, 60, 62, 64, 122, 194, 260
Placental growth factor, 233
Plasma-derived serum, 25-27, 35
Plasmin, 36, 37, 39, 40, 231-233, 237-240
Plasmin-α_2-antiplasmin, 36, 37
α_2-Plasmin, 238
Plasminogen, 36, 39, 40, 46, 47, 232, 233, 238-241
Plasminogen activator, 33, 37, 231-241, 265, 267, 276
  inhibitor, 34, 36-39, 177, 232, 235, 240, 241, 265, 266, 275

(Plasminogen activator contd)
receptor
urokinase-type, 234
tissue-type, 34, 36-40, 173, 177, 232, 234, 275
urokinase-type, 36, 37, 40, 232, 234
Platelet, 17, 18, 33-49, 266, 276
aggregation, 19, 20, 23, 24, 26, 33, 118, 128, 129, 134, 164, 265, 266
Platelet-activating factor, 34, 153, 177, 276
Platelet-derived growth factor, 26, 83, 129, 159-169, 216, 217, 221, 246, 266, 275, 277
receptor, 162, 169
Platelet factor 4, 265
Poly G, 125
Polyol pathway, 6, 7, 11, 57, 62, 68, 81, 82, 220
pRB (*see* retinoblastoma gene product)
Pro-urokinase, 36
Probucol, 121
Procollagen, 79
Proinsulin, 39, 266
Proliferating cell nuclear antigen, 269, 272, 273
Prometalloproteinase, 224
Prostacyclin, 17-28, 33, 34, 35, 89, 90, 113, 117, 160, 163-166, 173, 189, 190, 201, 207-210, 217, 245, 276
stimulatory activity, 24-27
stimulatory factor, 27, 28
synthetase, 18, 23
Prostaglandin, 69, 113, 135, 138, 139, 180, 276
D_2, 18
E_1, 160, 217
E_2, 18, 22, 35, 113, 217, 260, 276
$F_{2\alpha}$, 18, 19
G_2, 18
H_2, 18, 22
I_2 (*see* prostacyclin)
endoperoxide, 18
metabolism, 17-28
Protease, 151, 153, 154, 223, 267
inhibitor, 174, 176, 178, 238
serine, 33
Protein
C, 33, 34, 39, 42, 43, 173, 176, 180, 183
contractile, 111
extracellular matrix, 40, 78, 83
Gi, 120, 121
S, 34, 42, 176
Protein kinase C, 7, 57-69, 80-84, 121, 126, 127, 137-139, 161, 221, 245-262
activator, 256, 257
inhibitor, 138
isoforms, 58-60, 255, 259
Proteinase, 231, 232
Proteinuria, 42
Proteoglycan, 173-186
heparin-containing, 33, 41
regulation, 173-186
Prothrombin, 39
time, 39
Pyruvic acid, 67
RAGE (*see* glycosylation end-product receptor, advanced)
Raji, 92-100
Respiratory burst, 272
Retinoblastoma gene product, 247, 255, 259
Retinoic acid (*see* tretinoin)
Retinopathy, 19, 20, 23, 42, 44, 61, 62, 206, 218-224, 233, 265-278
Rieske FeS reductase, 79
Scavanger
mechanism, 205
pathway, 166, 169
receptor, 125
Schiff base, 189
Selectin, 277
Serotonin, 83, 123, 125, 129
Smooth muscle cell
growth, 159-169
proliferation, 118
phenotype, 164-169
Smooth muscle cell-derived growth factor, 160, 165-168
Smooth muscle cell-derived migration factor, 166
Somatomedin C, 160
Sorbinil, 7, 68
Sorbitol, 6, 7, 68, 82, 277, 246
dehydrogenase, 82
pathway, 67
Sphingomyelin, 122
Sphingosine, 138
SQ 29548, 22
1-Steroyl-2-arachidonyl-sn-glycerol, 66, 67
Stromelysin, 231
Superoxide, 120, 276
anion, 145, 153
dismutase, 8, 11, 120, 136, 139, 146, 148-152, 183, 185
Sympathetic nervous system, 115
Syndrome X, 105
Thrombin, 21, 33, 41, 42, 160, 161, 173, 174
α-Thrombin, 259
Thrombin-antithrombin complex, 39
Thrombogenesis, 33-49, 173-186
Thrombomodulin, 33, 34, 42-44, 46, 83, 173, 176, 180, 184, 186
Thromboplastin, 39
Thrombospondin, 34
Thromboxane A_2, 17-20, 22, 28, 33, 35, 138, 246, 265

Thromboxane B_2, 20
Thrombus, 266
TIMP (*see* metalloproteinase inhibitor), 232
Tissue factor, 34, 44, 83, 176, 265, 266, 276
  pathway inhibitor, 34, 44, 45
D-α-Tocopherol, 24
Transducin, 79
Transferrin, 90
Transforming growth factor-α, 26, 216, 217, 233, 234
Transforming growth factor-β, 160-164, 168, 216, 217, 220-223, 231-241, 260, 275
  binding protein, latent, 236-239
  large latent, 236, 239
  latent, 235-241
  prepro, 236
  pro, 236
  receptor, 235
  small latent, 236
Transforming growth factor-β1, 81, 163, 235
Transforming growth factor-β2, 235
Tretinoin, 43
Tricarboxylic acid cycle, 10
Triose phosphate, 82
Tube formation, 161, 215, 15,2, 231, 234
Tumour necrosis factor-α, 6, 18, 26, 43, 44, 161-180, 216, 217, 221, 260, 275-277
Tyrosine kinase, 39, 79, 80
Uronic acid, 174, 185
Vascular endothelial growth factor, 216, 217, 221, 233, 235, 266
Vascular permeability factor, 6
Vascular relaxation
  endothelium-dependent, 105-115, 117-130, 133-139
  endothelium-independent, 105-115
Vasoactive intestinal vasocontractor, 92
  prepro, 92
Vasopressin, 64
Vimectin, 247
Vitamin E, 11, 24, 35, 277
Vitronectin, 40
von Willebrand factor, 34, 202, 203, 265, 266
Weibel-Palade body, 202
Xanthine
  dehydrogenase, 152, 155
  oxidase, 150-155
Xanthine-xanthine oxidase system, 150, 154